PRAISE HEALING THE VEGAN WAY

"*Healing the Vegan Way* is more than just an amazing cookbook. It's an invaluable guide for anyone in search of the way to optimum health through a plant-based diet. A must-read!!"

—Marco Borges, plant-based advocate and *New York Times* best-selling author, founder of 22 Days Nutrition program

"If you're interested in how eating plants can heal your body and nourish your spirit, look no further. Mark Reinfeld is a superb guide on the journey. His recipes are fabulous and his wisdom reliable."

—John Robbins, author of *Diet for a New America*, cofounder and president of the Food Revolution Network

"*Healing the Vegan Way* is a rich document that goes clearly beyond a cookbook. It is a thorough scientific resource with excellent documentations surrounding great recipes."

—Hans A. Diehl, DrHSc, MPH, CNS, FACN, clinical professor of preventive medicine, School of Medicine, Loma Linda University, founder, CHIP and Lifestyle Medicine Institute

"This guy can seriously cook. Went to a conference where Mark made all the meals, and incredible does not begin to describe the culinary experience. If the whole world had Mark as their chef, I would be out of business. His new recipe book is beautiful and practical."

—Dr. Garth Davis, author of *Proteinaholic*

"No one I know can make [culinary] magic happen better than Mark Reinfeld. In *Healing the Vegan Way*, Mark presents principles for creating a delicious menu that will help heal all the tissues and organs of the body—while also bringing delight to the tongue and palate. Bon appétit!"

—Michael Klaper, MD

"*Healing the Vegan Way* is a wonderfully written resource for anyone interested in the countless health benefits of a plant-based diet. Mark Reinfeld combines comprehensive expert testimonies with an extensive array of delicious, easy-to-prepare recipes that will impress everyone at the table."

 —Neal Barnard, MD

"When plant foods are incorporated into healthy recipes and diets, they can play a critical role in treating and even reversing the common diseases we face today. *Healing the Vegan Way* is a valuable, practical guide that shows us the way to enjoy optimal health."

 —John Westerdahl, PhD, MPH, RD, chair, Vegetarian Nutrition Dietetic Practice
  Group of the Academy of Nutrition and Dietetics

"*Healing the Vegan Way* underlies the recipes with a message, and in this case, the title says it all. The selling point for [Mark Reinfeld's] whole-food, plant-based dietary agenda is the recipes themselves."

 —*Milwaukee Shepherd-Express*

The ULTIMATE AGE-DEFYING PLAN

ALSO BY MARK REINFELD

Healing the Vegan Way: Plant-Based Eating for Optimal Health and Wellness

The 30-Minute Vegan: Soup's On!: More Than 100
Quick and Easy Recipes for Every Season

The 30-Minute Vegan's Taste of Europe: 150 Plant-Based Makeovers
of Classics from France, Italy, Spain . . . and Beyond

The 30-Minute Vegan's Taste of the East: Asian-Inspired
Recipes—from Soba Noodles to Summer Rolls

The 30-Minute Vegan: Over 175 Quick, Delicious,
and Healthy Recipes for Everyday Cooking

The Complete Idiot's Guide to Eating Raw

Vegan Fusion World Cuisine: Extraordinary Recipes & Timeless
Wisdom from the Celebrated Blossoming Lotus Restaurants

ALSO BY MICHAEL KLAPER, MD

Vegan Nutrition: Pure and Simple

Pregnancy, Children and the Vegan Diet

The ULTIMATE AGE-DEFYING PLAN

The Plant-Based Way to Stay Mentally Sharp and Physically Fit

MARK REINFELD & ASHLEY BOUDET, ND
WITH MICHAEL KLAPER, MD

Da Capo
LIFE LONG

Copyright © 2019 by Mark Reinfeld and Ashley Boudet, ND

Cover design by Kathleen Lynch
Cover photograph © Okea/Dreamstime.com
Cover copyright © 2019 Hachette Book Group, Inc.

Salt-Free Seasoning, Balsamic Reduction, Vegan Mayonnaise, Vegan Sour Cream, and Raw Cashew Sour Cream were originally printed in *Healing the Vegan Way* © 2016 by Mark Reinfeld.

Da Capo Press
Hachette Book Group
1290 Avenue of the Americas, New York, NY 10104
dacapopress.com
@DaCapoPress

Printed in the United States of America

First Edition: February 2019

Published by Da Capo Lifelong Books, an imprint of Perseus Books, LLC, a subsidiary of Hachette Book Group, Inc.

The Hachette Speakers Bureau provides a wide range of authors for speaking events. To find out more, go to www.hachettespeakersbureau.com or call (866) 376-6591.

The publisher is not responsible for websites (or their content) that are not owned by the publisher.

Photographs by Elizabeth Arraj, Olivia Wallace, and Mark Reinfeld

Print book interior design by Amy Quinn

Library of Congress Cataloging-in-Publication Data

Names: Reinfeld, Mark, author. | Boudet, Ashley, author. | Klaper, Michael, author.
Title: The ultimate age-defying plan: the plant-based way to stay mentally sharp and physically fit / Mark Reinfeld and Ashley Boudet, ND, with Michael Klaper, MD.
Description: First edition. | New York, NY: Da Capo Press/Hachette Book Group, 2019. | Includes index.
Identifiers: LCCN 2018028374| ISBN 9780738234731 (pbk.) | ISBN 9780738234748 (ebook)
Subjects: LCSH: Nutrition. | Vegetarian cooking. | Health. | Rejuvenation. | LCGFT: Cookbooks.
Classification: LCC TX837 .R449 2019 | DDC 641.5/636—dc23
LC record available at https://lccn.loc.gov/2018028374

ISBNs: 978-0-7382-3473-1 (paperback), 978-0-7382-3474-8 (ebook)

LSC-C

10 9 8 7 6 5 4 3 2 1

To all those who inspire us to live in the truth that every day and every age is an exciting adventure in being human

CONTENTS

INTRODUCTION

With age usually comes some form of health "reality check." Suddenly you notice your joints are increasingly creaky, new wrinkles are popping up, it's getting harder to read that label, you've misplaced your keys once again. You might feel that you're slowing down physically, with nagging fatigue or a need for more recovery time after strenuous activities; perhaps you have new aches and pains or chronic ones; or possibly brain changes, such as slower recall, forgetfulness, difficulty concentrating, or a lowered ability to multitask. You might ask yourself, *How did I get here?*

It all seems to happen out of nowhere, and there seems to always be someone nearby assuring you not to worry—that this is all normal and you need to accept the fact that you are getting older.

And yet, chalking up these symptoms to the normal effects of aging just doesn't feel right, when you know deep down you have a lot more life to experience.

If you have a sneaking suspicion that you do not need to believe that feeling "old" is normal, and you just know that you are capable of more, we are here to support your emergence from the "trap" of aging. Let's start by considering the suggestion that the human body is dynamic and ever-changing, and that healing and growth are always possibilities when given a proper healing environment. People are much like a garden that needs healthy soil, basic nutrients, water, sunshine, diversity, and an ability to recover easily from environmental stresses.

What if we told you there is a simple solution that will allow you to feel more in control of your health and vitality? If you want to defy your age, step one is as easy as this: eat more plants instead of animal products, every day.

No matter how old you are, a plant-based vegan diet can help you live longer, look younger, feel younger, and stay active for life—steering clear of cognitive decline, heart disease, diminished senses, and other common age-related health challenges. Stronger bones and muscles and smoother skin are ours for the taking.

Before we dive further into the book, when we say *plant-based*, we are referring to a diet that eschews all animal products. It's essentially a vegetarian diet (no meat, fish, or fowl) that also eliminates animal by-products, such as dairy and eggs. A vegan diet is synonymous with a plant-based diet, though vegan tends to extend to eliminating the use of animals in any way from your lifestyle as well as your diet. By emphasizing whole foods, as opposed to processed and junk foods (yes, there are even vegan junk foods!), you can enjoy the vast array of delicious plant nutrition choices that nature provides. These include the colorful and exciting world of vegetables, fruits, grains, nuts, seeds, legumes, and vegan dark chocolate!

That said, please know that the vegan police are not part of the plan! Even if you want to get started and dip your feet into the water by having just one meatless meal a week, the rewards are sure to follow.

There is a difference between your chronological age—how long you have been alive—and your "physiological age" or "biological age," which takes into account not only your genetic makeup, but also lifestyle factors, such as your diet, activity level, and sleep habits. Physician Swapnil Jaiswal tells us, "Biological age is a truer measure of your age than your date of birth." While we cannot halt the aging process entirely, we can help slow it down.

Believe it or not, you really can change the rate at which your body ages! It all comes down to your basic dietary choices and habits—making simple changes to your daily routine. By understanding how to best prevent damage over time and to boost the body's natural rejuvenation abilities, you can continue to enjoy vitality well into maturity.

Healthy aging is not only about the number of years lived, but the quality of your life, too. Most important is how old you feel. And most would agree that you want to feel young! Here's the good news: Everyone gets to choose. Feeling in control, empowered, and energized is always within reach. You can experience the joy and satisfaction of knowing that you are doing everything possible to maintain mental sharpness and physical fitness throughout your life.

Who We Are

We are Mark Reinfeld, a vegan chef, and Ashley Boudet, a naturopathic doctor, who have teamed up to share our experience and knowledge with those seeking a more elevated state of health through our business, The Doctor and the Chef. We have over thirty years' combined experience in the world of plant-based cuisine and natural healing modalities. For us, this represents the future both of food and of medicine: a return to a sustainable way of feeding ourselves, and of preventing many illnesses before they have a chance to develop, as well as reversing those that have already advanced. It is putting Hippocrates's edict to "let food be thy medicine" into practice in our everyday lives.

Our passion is to show others just how easy it is to succeed on a plant-based lifestyle.

Through our seasonal wellness retreats, as well as in our online membership community, we have had the privilege of witnessing countless people who chose to take their health back into their own hands

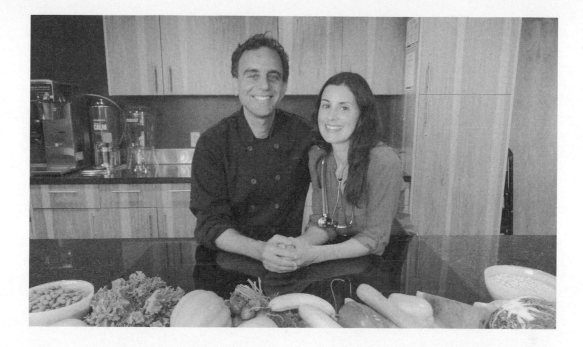

through positive diet and lifestyle choices. Oftentimes they even surprised themselves in how extreme the results have been: swift drops in cholesterol levels, reversing diseases, getting off medications, sudden pain relief, and pushing themselves even further than they thought they could go. We are inspired by seeing more stories about people defying age everywhere: The ninety-year-olds taking up yoga, the seventy-plus-year-olds competing in and winning marathons, the sixty-plus-year-old body builders. The list goes on! Twenty years ago, you rarely, if ever, heard of such stories. Now they are becoming more commonplace.

In our own personal lives, too, we have experienced what you might consider a health renaissance, looking and feeling much younger than our chronological age. We have more energy now as truly nourished vegans than we did in our twenties and thirties.

Joining us is an expert on the matter of living well, the renowned Michael Klaper, MD, a physician with decades of experience treating people and helping them to live a healthy and active lifestyle on a plant-based diet. His famous three words explain so many of our modern diseases and how to treat them: "It's the Food!" Dr. Klaper reviewed the manuscript and contributed feedback based on his vast scientific knowledge and clinical expertise.

Turning Back the Clock

We want to show you how a plant-based diet can help you reclaim your health, extend your life, and thrive at any age. A vast number of scientific research studies clearly show a wide gap in the health effects of a whole food, plant-based diet versus one heavily laden with animal products and highly processed foods. To sum it up, scientific evidence supports that animal-based/processed-food diets contribute to premature aging, and that eating more plant foods is the solution we seek to defy the aging process.

The basics of maintaining a young physiologic age are to avoid the toxins and foods that lead to potential cell and organ damage, and to eat the foods and nutrients that fuel your cells, help you naturally eliminate potential toxins, and directly strengthen and balance your body. We also aspire to show you how easy it is to include these life-giving foods and practices in your life through the delectable vegan recipes and simple wellness tips we have to share. This will help you on your way to continued health and longevity.

The first half of this book will introduce you to the astounding evidence that supports increasing the plant foods in your diet as a way of optimizing your health as you age. Then, we'll show you how and what to eat for an aging intervention! Enter the second part of this book, "Age-Defying Vegan Recipes." This section features over 175 simple recipes—using just seven main ingredients or less—so you can ace vegan meal preparation and never miss the meat. This section also introduces you to some simple kitchen hacks that will allow you to quickly become your own plant-based chef, no matter your level of cooking experience. Recommended kitchen gear, pantry items, techniques, and more will have you chiffonading like a pro in no time.

Be sure to rotate through as many of the recipes in the book as possible. This will provide you with a wide array of important nutrients that stave off age-related decline and other illnesses, and keep you looking and feeling great.

Use these recipes as a starting point for creating your own versions and specialties based on your preferences and whatever ingredients are on hand and available locally. Once you learn the simple concept of a Template Recipe (see page 98), you will discover how easy it is to create dozens of variations to please any palate.

We chose recipes that feature easy-to-prepare, everyday ingredients that can help you stay energized for a lifetime. You'll be enjoying a wide selection of colorful, plant-based whole foods. And while these recipes are oh-so-flavorful, what you won't find here are excesses of sodium, processed oil, and sugar. Excessive daily use of these three flavor enhancers are well known to significantly increase the risk for the very degenerative changes we are looking to prevent. As Dr. Klaper says, "You are as old as your arteries." It is important to take good care of them by avoiding damage from high blood pressure (excess sodium), protein-damaging molecules (excess sugar), and inflammatory lesions (oxidized vegetable oils).

Food for Our Future

We recommend using organic ingredients. Organic food is grown without the use of chemical fertilizers and pesticides, most of which have not been fully tested for their long-term effects on humans. Pesticides are known to be direct neurotoxins, so it is always a good idea to protect your brain from them when possible. Also, these are chemicals that can actively contribute to the oxidation processes we are working to repair. Our grandparents never had to question whether their food was organic. It was just food. Now with all of these toxic chemicals infiltrating our food system, it is more important than ever to choose organic when possible to protect ourselves from the ravages of aging.

We also recommend cooking with whole foods whenever possible, and minimizing the use of processed and packaged ingredients. This is much better not only for your life, but the life of the planet as well. Also, eating locally grown foods ensures they'll be at their best flavor. Grow foods in your own garden if you have the opportunity. Community supported agriculture (CSAs) and farmers' markets, where you can meet the people growing your food, are the next best choice. Ask the vendors how the food was grown, if not labeled "certified organic."

Sidebars and Symbols

Throughout these pages you will see the following sidebars:

Age-Defying Advice: A quick-reference checklist and wellness tips on the nutrients and lifestyle practices that will help you incorporate the information in the chapter into your own life.

Fountain of Youther: These stories highlight real people who exemplify what it means to thrive on a plant-based lifestyle at any age.

Timeless Tips: Here we feature quick and easy kitchen tips and techniques you can easily learn that will help you prepare your meals like a boss.

NOURISH Your Way to a Younger You

When it comes to healthy aging, there's no question nutrition plays a crucial role. But several other important factors also have been shown to contribute to creating a long, healthy, and happy life. We have created a simple acronym that can help you remember all these factors so you can easily include them in your day-to-day. Our philosophy, in a word, is **NOURISH**.

N is for **Nutrition**. What you eat is the foundation for a healthy body, and nutrition is the central focus of this book. Plant foods provide the raw materials needed for your cells' proper function, structure, balance, repair, and energy maintenance. Nutrition is all about optimizing how your body takes in, digests, absorbs, stores, and releases nutrients. You can protect and strengthen your body by learning how to prioritize great nutrition. That's where all of the amazing recipes in this book come into play!

O is for **Oxytocin**, the "happiness hormone." There are many simple ways to help stimulate this hormone in your brain. Things you can do every day include exercise, getting outside and connecting with nature, physical touch, laughing, creating gratitude lists, meditating, giving to others, volunteering your time, exploring your creative interests, or spending time with animals. The possibilities are endless—the point is to find out what brings you pleasure, and make sure you prioritize getting plenty of that! This is the best way to manage unavoidable stress.

U is for "**Use It or Lose It.**" It is never too late to strengthen your body or stretch your brain. Your body is meant to move regularly, and the benefits of regular exercise, no matter how gentle or strenuous, are phenomenal in keeping your body functioning optimally. Likewise, keeping your mind active, alert, calm, and stimulated is amazingly important to brain health. Stay curious and your mind can remain sharp. Create daily routines around both physical and mental exercise. Choose activities you enjoy and that will keep you motivated. Besides, life is much more interesting and manageable that way!

R is for **Relationships**. Having meaningful social interactions is more important than ever. The fast-paced digital culture we live in can make it more challenging to maintain close relationships, but the time and effort is well worth it to connect to people who are important to you. Reach out to those friends who share your interests and values. Offer support to others. Find and participate in group activities that you resonate with. Sharing your story and being willing to open yourself to others in service can be true medicine for the soul.

I is for **Intention**. Intentional living means being mindful and present in your actions and proactive in your life choices. It includes taking time to reflect and really dig deep to be aware of what is most important to you personally. Know your values and your vision for your life well, and act from that place. Do not compromise on what is important to you just to maintain the status quo. Remember that waiting for something to change rarely results in success. You create the life you desire by taking necessary actions. It is never too late to choose to up your level of vitality, and personal growth work is always worth it.

S is for **Sleep**. Sleep serves a very important function: a daily reset of your body and mind. Regular circadian rhythms, or sleep-wake cycles, are essential for regulating all hormonal and metabolic processes in the body. Your tissues can repair and recover only when you reach a deep state of rest. This is why sleep is usually the first thing your body needs when you get sick. Be sure to make sleep a high priority, and listen to your body's needs, which can change day to day. It is possible to make up for lost sleep after a period of insomnia. Do this for your body!

H is for **Hydration**. Water is life! Your body is made mostly of water, and needs an adequate intake daily to function properly. The common recommendation to drink half your weight in ounces daily is the bare minimum, and most people will need even more than that. (For example, if you weigh 140 pounds, you'll want to drink at least 70 ounces of water a day.) Having a large, toxin-free water bottle that you like can help you to get enough by sipping and refilling it throughout the day. Remember that water is the number one medicine for fatigue, sinus congestion and allergies, dry skin, headaches, heart palpitations, constipation, spasms, indigestion, and many more common ailments.

There are so many ways your body can become depleted of water, and it is up to you to replenish regularly. (If you find it challenging to drink a lot of water, in Chapter 10 you'll find options for more flavorful hydrating beverages.) In addition, the act of immersing yourself in water can help bring balance to your body and your mind. The use of hot and cold temperatures either through compresses, steam, or immersion baths can have a truly powerful effect on the body's circulation and detoxification pathways, helping to direct the blood and lymphatic fluids to where they are needed, and to flush out areas where these fluids can become congested. This powerful naturopathic practice is called hydrotherapy.

For optimal results, bring love into each of these areas on a daily basis. For a NOURISH worksheet that you can print out and use daily to stay on top of your game, please visit www.doctorchefresources.com.

There's Never Been a Better Time to Start

With current knowledge about how food and lifestyle choices can impact aging becoming more mainstream, there's a growing shift in attitude toward what it means to grow older and wiser. For us and many others, 50 is the new 30, 70 is the new 50, and 90 is the new 70! It is an exciting time to join the movement of those who look toward aging as an opportunity for expansion, rather than an acceptance of degeneration as a normal part of growing old.

The most important thing to remember is that you *can* do this. You can defy the conventional assumptions and instead learn how to live longer, stronger, and happier with age. We want to make it easy for you to embark on a plant-based lifestyle— whether or not you choose to fully go vegan from the start—and cut down your learning curve dramatically by sharing what we have discovered over many years immersed in the wellness field. Many people, including those featured in the Fountain of Youther sidebars, have discovered the secret to maintaining a physically active and mentally sharp lifestyle as they gracefully age the vegan way. You, too, can experience your own health revolution, and we are here to help get you started. Now is the time to give yourself the gift of lasting health and longevity.

We also want to stay connected with you on this journey. Please visit our Facebook page where you can interact with others on a similar path to receive inspiration and support. Learn more at www.doctorchef resources.com. Remember, there may be many twists and turns in the road; the path to optimal health typically does not proceed in a straight line. Always be gentle with yourself along the way!

part one

HEALTHY AGING THE PLANT-BASED WAY

ONE

LIVE LONGER, LIVE BETTER

A recent study reported that the average life expectancy in the United States has now begun to decrease, after two decades of rising steadily. While these are small decreases, they are concerning enough to bring about a real sense of urgency around Americans' personal lifestyle choices. Heart disease and cancer persist as the top causes of death in both men and women. And Alzheimer's has been gaining ground. So, now is the time to take the steps needed to be an outlier rather than a statistic! The choices you make could make a real difference in your longevity—and how you experience all the next decades of your life.

A six-year study by the Centers for Disease Control and Prevention found that three behaviors have an enormous impact on mortality: consuming a healthier diet, not currently smoking, and moderately exercising for at least twenty-one minutes a day. People who practiced just one of the three behaviors had a 40 percent lower risk of dying within that six-year period. Those with two out of three more than halved their

chances of dying, and those with all three reduced their chances of dying in that time by 82 percent!

Interestingly, meal preparation may be a significant factor: a large ten-year observational study published in *Public Health Nutrition*, a Cambridge University journal, showed that those who cooked at home up to five times a week were 47 percent more likely to still be alive after ten years than those who did not. This was found to be the most significant lifestyle factor connected to longevity. The group who cooked most often also tended to eat more vegetables and less meat.

This book will help make it easy for you to cook your own meals and consume the healthiest diet there is—a plant-based one!

How Can You Grow Old Better?

Of course, healthy aging isn't only about living longer—it's also about living better. We want you to enjoy doing the things you love decade after decade, not be dragged down by chronic illness. Unfortunately, these days most Americans over age sixty-five endure the opposite. The National Council on Aging recently outlined the top 10 most common chronic diseases. How common? The council reported that *80 percent* of adults aged sixty-five and older have at least one of these conditions, while 68 percent have two or more from the list. If you are fortunate enough to be living outside of the typical pattern here, you very likely have a friend or family member dealing with at least one of these. The list, along with some commonly known risk factors for each, is as follows:

1. **Hypertension**, a.k.a. high blood pressure, is currently defined as a blood pressure reading of greater than 130/80, and can be diagnosed after three consecutive high readings. These readings can fluctuate throughout the day, and high blood pressure that continues over time can put great stress on the heart's ability to function.

    Risk factors: lack of exercise, low nutrient/inflammatory diet, poor sleep quality, excess weight, chronic unmanaged emotional/mental stress, anxiety

2. **High cholesterol:** High levels of cholesterol (see page 53) circulating in your blood, as revealed by a blood test. Total cholesterol levels above 240 mg/dL are considered high, with an ideal number being below 200 mg/dL. LDL should be less than 100, while HDL should ideally be above 60 mg/dL. You

may have high cholesterol or an unhealthy balance of LDL to HDL and not have any noticeable symptoms.

    Risk factors: lack of exercise, highly processed diet, animal fats, low fiber intake, alcohol intake, smoking, inflammation, chronic emotional/mental stress

3. **Arthritis:** Inflammation of the joints between small and large bones can be caused by wear and tear over time, or an overall inflammatory process in the body. Joint swelling, redness, stiffness, creaking, and warmth can be signs before notable pain occurs.

    Risk factors: sedentary lifestyle, excess weight, joint strain, chronic inflammation, smoking, highly processed foods, food additives, environmental toxin exposure, microbial infection

4. **Coronary heart disease:** A buildup of inflammatory plaque that narrows the arteries leading to the heart, decreasing the amount of oxygen-rich blood delivered to the heart. This can cause other complications, such as blood clots, angina, or a heart attack.

    Risk factors: high-salt diet, saturated and trans fat consumption, sugar in diet, alcohol use, smoking, lack of exercise, poor sleep quality, high emotional/mental stress

5. **Diabetes:** An impairment of the body's ability to produce adequate insulin in response to a meal, or an impaired ability for the body to respond adequately to insulin signaling,

resulting in high amounts of glucose remaining in the blood rather than being used by the tissues. This can eventually lead to serious consequences of loss of circulation to eyes, limbs, and major organs.

Risk factors: lack of exercise, excess weight, high alcohol intake, low nutrient and highly processed food diet, chronic excess saturated fats, low fiber, environmental toxin exposure

6. **Chronic kidney disease:** A gradual loss of kidney function over months or years, leading to serious problems with fluid retention and, eventually, heart disease.

    Risk factors: Diabetes, high blood pressure, smoking, excess weight, chronic dehydration, a low-fiber and high-sodium diet

7. **Heart failure:** Congestive heart failure occurs when the heart cannot adequately supply blood and oxygen to all of the organs in the body, due to either structural or functional changes.

    Risk factors: high blood pressure, smoking, inflammatory diet, excess weight, prior heart damage, circulation issues

8. **Depression:** Defined by several symptoms, notably a depressed mood with difficulty concentrating and a gradual loss of interest in activities that does not improve over time and interferes with normal routines.

    Risk factors: lack of exercise, low-nutrient diet, emotional stress, lack of connection, loss of self-expression or creative outlets, lowered exposure to fresh air and natural environments

9. **Alzheimer's disease and dementia:** Both are characterized by progressive losses in both memory and cognitive functions.

    Risk factors: sedentary lifestyle, insomnia, emotional stress, dehydration, highly processed foods, artificial sweeteners, environmental toxins and heavy metal accumulation

10. **Chronic obstructive pulmonary disease:** Any type of lung disease that results in a blockage of airflow and difficulty breathing, requiring supplemental oxygen or pharmaceutical intervention.

    Risk factors: smoking, environmental toxin exposure, inflammatory diet

Often, one of these conditions leads to another. Here's the thing: these conditions are largely preventable! What's the common denominator? As you can see, certain lifestyle factors are implicated in every single one of these chronic diseases, and a major one is a diet high in animal products, processed foods, saturated fats, sugar, and sodium, and low in fiber, vitamins, and minerals. This fact has been shown over and over again in observational research studies, and is borne out by research, that vegetarians live on average almost eight years longer than the general population. Luigi Fontana, director of the longevity research program at Washington University in St. Louis, has said that only about 25 percent of your risk of premature death is due to genetics. Of the remaining 75 percent, diet is likely the *most* important factor.

Why Do You Age, Anyway?

Why do you develop wrinkles, begin to lose some of your memory, and experience declines in organ system function as you get older? The answers may be found inside your cells.

Oxidative stress is thought to be one reason. Oxidative stress occurs when oxygen in the body splits into what are called free radicals—highly reactive and unstable molecules. They can build up in the body as waste products from metabolizing the foods and medicines you consume, or from contaminants in the air you breathe and water you drink. While some free radical action is normal, too much can cause a chain of events leading to cell disruption. Unchecked damage over time overwhelms your cells' repair mechanisms, causing constant stress to those cells. In each one of your trillions of cells, there is an engine called the mitochondria. You can think of mitochondria as a cell's power source. Free radicals damage the mitochondria, leading to a loss of cellular energy and function over time. Scientists believe this resulting cellular damage is what essentially causes aging. Early signs of free radical oxidative stress can show up as fatigue, headaches, memory loss, graying and loss of hair, wrinkles, vision changes, sensitivity to noise, and lowered immune responses.

Here's another finding: A particular enzyme called the target of rapamycin (TOR) is a nutrient-sensitive central controller of cell growth and aging. Its action is involved in the development of cancer, heart disease, diabetes, Alzheimer's, and other diseases.

Eating less animal protein has been shown to hamper TOR activity. A 2012 paper found that the amino acid leucine, found mostly in animal foods, has the greatest effect on TOR signaling compared to other proteins. On the other hand, fruits and vegetables have phytochemicals that function as natural TOR inhibitors. Plant-based diets may have a cancer-protective effect, which is thought to be in part due to this natural TOR inhibition.

One more recent cellular discovery has been shown to have a major impact on how people age: the telomere, a structure at the end of chromosomes that essentially protects the chromosome from damage. (Chromosomes, which house your DNA, are found in the nucleus of each cell). The average cell divides between fifty and seventy times before cell death. Each time the cell divides, the telomeres on the end of the chromosome get shorter, until the cell can no longer divide, reaching what is called senescence. Telomeres can start shortening as soon as you're born, and when they're gone, you're gone.

Studies have now shown that people with longer telomeres live longer and healthier lives than do those with shorter telomeres. Even more exciting, scientists have begun to understand the factors that can influence telomere length. In 2009, scientist Dr. Elizabeth Blackburn was awarded the Nobel Prize for her discovery of the telomerase enzyme. She was curious about how the oldest living organism on Earth, a five-thousand-year-old bristlecone pine tree in the White Mountains of California, could live so long and also age so well. Bristlecone pines have telomerase in their roots, an enzyme that rebuilds telomeres and keeps DNA from fraying. And it turns out that humans also have telomerase in certain highly active cells.

In 2008, Dr. Dean Ornish teamed up with Blackburn and found that just three months of eating a diet rich in plant-based protein, fruits, vegetables, unrefined grains, and legumes significantly boosted telomerase activity. In a 2013 follow-up study published in *Lancet Oncology*, Ornish again noted that telomere length had increased in the plant-based diet group. Although the group eating plant foods also exercised and lost weight, other studies have shown that even more vigorous exercise and similar amounts of weight loss have not affected telomere length. And in a 2013 review, fiber (found exclusively in plant foods) was associated with longer telomeres. Along with fiber, plant foods are filled with antioxidants that

---

AGE-DEFYING ADVICE:
WHAT ARE THE MOST ANTIOXIDANT-RICH FOODS?

Phytochemicals is the name for any of the active compounds obtained from plant-based foods (*phyto* is Greek for "plant"), and the most common action of phytochemicals is to oppose the action of dangerous free radicals, which are known to cause cellular damage and disease. The superheroes of the phytochemical world are antioxidants.

The Antioxidant Food Table is a comprehensive database that was developed to help with research on the antioxidant benefits of plant foods. It demonstrates that there are several thousand–fold differences in the antioxidant content of foods! Spices, herbs, and supplements are among the most antioxidant-rich products in this study, with some exceptionally high. Berries, fruits, nuts, chocolate, and vegetables constitute common foods with very high antioxidant values.

This information validates eating a wide variety of plant foods, and consuming them in their most whole form. Eating antioxidant-filled plant foods equals less free radical damage! Besides promoting better absorption and a wider range of benefits to the body, eating a rainbow of plant foods is much more enjoyable than taking in nutrients in supplement form.

The database is available online at the University of Oslo's website. Top antioxidant-rich foods include:

Blackberries
Prunes
Kale
Beets
Broccoli
Cacao
Garlic
Artichokes
Pumpkin
Kidney beans
Walnuts
Cloves, parsley, rosemary, cilantro

---

can directly oppose the oxidative stress responsible for telomere shrinking, preventing and even reversing cellular aging.

Dr. Ornish stated, "Shortened telomeres have been shown to play a role in heart disease, colon cancer, stroke, dementia, and premature death. But our study is the first to show that any intervention could lengthen telomeres."

Although the study was conducted on a small scale, Dr. David Katz, a prevention medicine specialist at Yale University's Prevention Research Center, believes the finding to be very valuable. He said, "The message we're getting from this and other studies is consistent: We don't have the medical capacity to tweak genes and make chronic diseases go away, but we can refashion our fate at the level of our DNA by the behavior choices we make."

What You Eat Can Add Years to Your Life

Simply put, the power of plants is your strongest defense against cellular degeneration. A whole foods, plant-based diet comprised primarily of vegetables, fruits, legumes (beans, peas, and lentils), whole grains, nuts, and seeds is the absolute best diet for health. A plant-based diet reduces inflammation, helps with ideal body weight maintenance, promotes glowing skin, optimizes sexual function, sends energy levels soaring, increases mental capabilities, and lengthens life span. It has been proven to reduce the risk for, and help reverse, cardiovascular disease, obesity, hypertension,

digestive disorders, cancer, and dementia. Studies have found that within just ten days of sticking to a whole foods, plant-based diet, you can reduce your triglyceride and cholesterol levels (two major heart disease risk factors) by a whopping 10 percent.

A conventional animal- and processed food–based diet, laden with sugar and fat, does the opposite. Sugars and fats cause blood cells to clump together, resulting in thicker blood and a type of inflammatory response in the endothelium (the inner lining of blood vessels), which in turn reduces the blood flow to your heart, kidneys, liver, sexual organs, and all your other organs. One study showed that just ten minutes after consuming a conventional fast-food meal (a hamburger, French fries, and a soft drink), participants' blood flow was vastly restricted and their triglyceride levels were notably increased. The study was repeated using whole, plant-based foods and there was no postmeal effect at all on the participants' blood vessels or triglyceride levels.

Load up on veggies and fruits, on the other hand, and you can't go wrong. Eating a variety of fruits, vegetables, herbs, and spices at each meal continuously floods your body with antioxidants that help ward off age-related diseases. How much healthier is a vegan diet than a meat-based one? On average, plant foods may contain up to sixty-four times more antioxidants than animal foods!

In a 2003 eight-week dietary intervention study, 102 healthy male smokers were randomized to either a diet largely consisting of various antioxidant-rich foods, a kiwi diet (three kiwis/day added to the regular diet), or a control group. Positive blood cell gene expression changes, such as regulation of cellular stress defense, DNA repair, and removal of toxic compounds from cells, were all significantly increased in both the antioxidant foods and kiwi diet groups. These observed changes in the blood suggest that a plant-based diet can directly promote cell defense from disease.

A follow-up study used a variety of fruits, juice, green tea, veggies, dark chocolate, spices, and nuts. Measuring the effects of a plant-based diet on the expression of hundreds of different genes at a time, a research group found that an antioxidant-rich diet of plant foods, such as berries, pomegranates, purple grapes, red cabbage, oregano, and walnuts, was able to normalize healthy gene expression.

Finally, calorie restriction is linked to anti-aging. Calorie restriction is marked by a limited calorie intake (as few as 1,000 to 1,200 calories per day). This often is accompanied by a low intake of protein (10 to 18 percent of daily calories), and high-density nutrition from seeds, berries, and greens. Calorie restriction has been shown to decrease levels of a hormone called IGF-1, correlating to a younger cellular age and increased life span. A vegan diet based upon whole plant foods with their naturally high content of fiber and water is inherently lower in calories compared to an animal-based diet, and most important, is more nutrient dense, meaning the calories come from bioactive nutrients that are used up in the body rather than taken in excess of need.

Longevity Superfoods

Superfoods to the rescue! Also known as nutrient-dense foods, superfoods are the true champions of the plant kingdom, especially when it comes to antiaging. They help counter the effects of a not-so-healthy diet and are loaded with antioxidants, fiber, minerals, vitamins, healthy fats, and all the other nutrients you need to thrive. If you want to age gracefully, superfoods need to be a part of your diet!

Eat dark chocolate and berries. These contain resveratrol, known as the red wine antioxidant, but also found in even higher quality and quantities in berries, grapes, and dark chocolate. Researchers believe that resveratrol may mimic the effects of calorie restriction.

Especially blueberries. Pterostilbene is a brain-boosting antioxidant found in blueberries. Studies have shown that pterostilbene may be even more effective than its cousin, resveratrol, at both preventing and reversing degenerative and sugar-related conditions of the brain. In another study, blood markers of cellular stress, inflammation, and Alzheimer's disease pathology were all positively lowered by pterostilbene. All in all, research findings indicate that pterostilbene in the diet can be a potent modulator of cognition, memory, and cellular stress. This information is especially promising for the prevention of Alzheimer's.

Eat less meat, and more walnuts, soy, and flaxseeds. In a clinical trial with 106 healthy, sedentary, overweight middle-aged and elderly individuals who were supplemented with 2.5 g of omega-3 fatty acids, researchers assessed whether omega-3 poly-unsaturated fatty acid (PUFA) supplementation could affect telomere length, telomerase, and oxidative stress. The study concluded that telomere length increased with decreasing omega-6 to omega-3 ratios, suggesting the possibility for nutritional prevention and longevity.

Replace animal protein with plant protein. In a Harvard study published in *JAMA*, the study authors found that substituting 3 percent of daily calories from animal protein with plant protein was associated with a lower risk for death from all causes—a 34 percent drop when participants swapped out processed red meat for plant protein, and a 19 percent decrease when they replaced eggs with plant protein. By contrast, participants who increased their animal-source protein by 10 percent had an 8 percent higher risk of death from heart disease, and a 2 percent higher risk of death from all causes.

Eat more whole grains. A report published in the journal *Circulation* reviewed the data in fourteen studies that combined had more than 786,000 participants. That analysis made the finding that people who ate the most whole grains had a 16 percent reduction in all-cause mortality compared to those who ate the least whole grains. This supports what we have learned from the planet's longest-living people in the "Blue Zones"—areas where about 65 percent of the diet is whole grains, beans, and starchy tubers. Grains, including oats, barley, brown rice, and ground corn, play a key role in the world's Blue Zone diets.

Eat greens. While greens are well known for being chock-full of health-preserving and energy-boosting nutrients, a recent study has gotten the attention of many people looking to increase their brainpower. The study, published in *Neurology*, was conducted at Rush Medical College in Chicago, and quite simply looked at the difference in memory, sharpness of mind, and overall cognition in seniors based on the amount of greens they ate over a five-year observational period. The results were extremely positive, with a huge difference in the rates of cognitive decline between groups that had at least an average of 1.3 servings a day versus no greens at all. Daily ½-cup serving sizes of spinach, kale, collards, lettuce, and other greens all seemed to be protective. The rate of cognitive decline among those who consumed the most to those who consumed the least was equivalent to being eleven years younger cognitively, based on average global cognitive scores over time.

These studies are a small sample of the continually mounting evidence that demonstrate the power of plants to extend your life and truly heal, taking you to a higher state of health and vitality. They show that your food and lifestyle choices can be a major influence, especially regarding those body systems that are commonly affected by aging, which we will explore in the upcoming chapters.

TWO

BRAIN HEALTH—STAY MENTALLY SHARP: COMBAT COGNITIVE DECLINE

Aging often leads to glitches with brain function, and moments of forgetfulness and "foggy thinking" become more frequent. If you're constantly forgetting where you put things, have a hard time staying on task, or find yourself searching for the right word that's on "the tip of your tongue," you're definitely not alone! But what if we told you that clarity of thought, memory, and concentration can be recovered with proper self-care? The brain is an organ and needs to be nourished with food, hydration, and healthy circulation just like all the others.

According to the Alzheimer's Association, currently Alzheimer's disease affects approximately 5.4 million Americans and 30 million people globally. Researchers predict that by 2050, without effective treatment, the disease could impact an estimated 160 million people globally.

Alzheimer's progresses over time, often many years, through several stages starting with what is called mild cognitive impairment or mild cognitive decline. Although symptoms of mild decline don't necessarily lead to Alzheimer's, the early stages are characterized by slight impairments in memory and thinking that may progress further toward dementia as the impairments begin to interfere more and more with daily living activities. These earlier stages are where we can most effectively see results and even reversal of progression with healthy dietary and lifestyle changes.

As people get older, cognitive decline may seem inevitable—but it doesn't have to be. It was once widely thought that brain cells continually die off and the brain can never recover what was lost. Now we know that this is just not true!

"The dogma for the longest time was that adult brains couldn't generate any new brain cells. You just use what you were born with," says Dr. Amar Sahay, a neuroscientist with Harvard-affiliated Massachusetts General Hospital. "But the reality is that everyone has the capacity to develop new cells that can help enhance cognitive functions." In this process, called neurogenesis, new neurons, which are cells that transmit signals along nerves to and from the brain, develop in the hippocampus, the brain region responsible for learning information, storing long-term memories, and regulating emotions.

New discoveries indicate that the brain is able to reorganize its connections and form new neural connections throughout life. This phenomenon, called neuroplasticity, allows the neurons in the brain to compensate for injury and adjust their activity in response to new situations. Existing neural pathways that are inactive or used for other purposes show the ability to take over and carry out functions lost to degeneration. Understanding the brain's ability to reorganize itself helps scientists understand how patients can recover brain functions damaged by injury or disease.

New connections can form at amazing speed, but to be able to reconnect, the neurons need to be stimulated through regular activity. Simple brain exercises, such as presenting oneself with intellectual challenges, interacting in social situations, or getting involved in physical activities will boost the general growth of connections. Remember that these nerve cells also require optimal nutrition to perform well, so adequate nutrients, such as B vitamins, magnesium, omega-3 essential fats, and antioxidants, such as vitamin E from whole plant foods, are absolutely essential to this process.

A New Perspective on Alzheimer's

Until now, the gradual loss of normal brain functioning in dementia and Alzheimer's disease has been seen as irreversible, and most treatment has been focused on educating family members on how to best support their loved ones and learn to cope with unavoidable behavior changes. The cause of the tangles and plaques found in and around brain cells of Alzheimer's patients has long been a mystery. Since the disease was discovered one hundred years ago, there has not been a pharmaceutical drug that has succeeded in stopping or slowing its progression more than moderately or temporarily, and none without potentially worsening side effects. Over a billion dollars have been spent on hundreds of clinical trials conducted just in the past decade, none of which has been successful in finding a cure.

But a National Institutes of Health (NIH) study known as the MEND study, conducted by researchers at UCLA's Easton Center for Alzheimer's Disease Research and the Buck Institute for Research on Aging, has been the first of its kind to show a significant reversal in memory loss associated with Alzheimer's. Even more amazing, the remarkable results did not come from a new and exciting drug. The researchers instead have been exploring an idea that has been the foundation of naturopathic medicine for many years: that disease is actually a process, the body's attempt to rebalance itself; and that the body can and will heal when its needs are met.

Based on broader, more holistic approaches to chronic diseases, such as heart disease and diabetes, researcher and professor of neurology Dale Bredesen, MD, decided to explore this idea by using a combination of therapies, instead of a drug, to address the root cause of Alzheimer's disease. His UCLA laboratory found evidence that an *imbalance* in nerve cell signaling is the true cause of Alzheimer's, rather than a brain "broken down" from an accumulation of toxicity. The idea of imbalance makes more sense if you look at the brain as one part of the complex neurological system, connected to the entire body through interconnected biochemical pathways.

Excess amyloid protein makes up the sticky plaques found in the brain of Alzheimer's patients. These plaques cause signals to become scrambled, causing loss of necessary memory. Bredesen suggests that amyloid protein may actually have a normal function in helping the brain to forget unnecessary memories and hold on to important ones. His researchers are not interested in "curing" the amyloid protein, but in understanding how to *rebalance* this functional process, which they think has likely gone awry due to a combination of factors. If the underlying cause is in fact multifactorial, then it is understandable that a targeted approach, such as a medication, will not be successful.

Bredesen uses the analogy of a leaky roof with several holes in it. If you use a drug to patch one hole, the drug may have done its job well, but with all the other holes left open, the problem remains. Without seeking to understand why the roof has been damaged, you may not get very far in fixing it.

Similarly, in naturopathic medicine, there is never a one-size-fits-all protocol. A personal treatment plan is created after a comprehensive assessment of a person's current state and health history. That way, no hole will be left uncovered, and the "roof" can be properly mended.

This is the approach the researchers took, proposing that brain plasticity, just like that of other tissues in the body, can be affected by basic lifestyle factors, such as quality of diet, sleep, exercise, and stress levels.

Because "each roof may have a different pattern of leaks," the treatment protocols had to be personalized for each participant. The therapies used included simple improvements in lifestyle, such as:

Diet: increasing fruits and vegetables; eliminating processed foods, sugars, and farmed fish; keeping blood sugar steady by eating regularly and only at mealtimes; not eating 3 hours before sleep or for 12 hours after dinner

Exercising: 30 minutes of exercise 4 to 6 days per week

Sleep: increasing both quality and number of hours by creating routines and supplementing melatonin as needed

Stress: making needed changes to daily schedule; introducing yoga and/or meditation

Assessing and optimizing hormonal activity, to make sure thyroid, insulin, and other hormones are working properly and not adding to brain dysfunction

Supplementing: Participants were given vitamins B_{12}, D_3, coenzyme Q (CoQ10), and DHA as needed.

Assessing and optimizing oral hygiene, taking into account the potential that periodontal disease can be connected to brain health as well

All participants had been diagnosed with memory loss associated with Alzheimer's disease (AD), amnestic mild cognitive impairment (aMCI), or subjective cognitive impairment (SCI).

Incredibly, reversal of memory loss was reported in 9 out of 10 participants when following their personalized therapeutic program for three to six weeks. Sustained improvements have been reported up to two and a half years so far.

The "side effects" most commonly reported in the MEND study participants? Overall *improved* health, energy, and body weight. Never has a drug done this! These results are far more positive than any previous clinical trials, and further study is now being pursued.

We can think of several other simple things that can be done daily to improve brain health by helping the body process unnecessary toxins and function properly through nutrition rather than waiting for disease to begin. We are very excited to see the results of this small study in such a short period of time, and hope that this is only the beginning of a new understanding of Alzheimer's and other chronic diseases.

The Vegan Solution

The MEND study isn't the only one to indicate that a plant-based diet can boost your brain.

According to Dr. Michael Greger, looking at rates of dementia all around the world, data showed two to three times less dementia in those cultures that eat vegetarian than in others with a meat-heavy diet. It seems the longer one goes meat-free, the lower the associated risk of dementia, regardless of other lifestyle factors. Globally, the lowest validated rates of Alzheimer's in the world are in rural India, where the typical diet is low in meat and high in carbohydrates, especially whole grains and beans.

And, in a new book on brain health, *The Alzheimer's Solution*, doctors at Loma Linda University also recommend eating a plant-based diet for optimal brain health. They describe their study of two different population groups. One group was composed of their patients from Loma Linda—these were mainly Seventh-Day Adventists who followed a vegetarian diet, exercised regularly, and had good social ties. They were known to be some of the healthiest people in the world. In contrast, the second group included patients in San Bernardino, in a medically underserved area plagued by chronic disease.

After years of working and studying both groups, the doctors found that "people living a healthy lifestyle had a much lower prevalence of dementia." The Adventist population, on average, lived ten years longer than the other group; their lifestyle promoted a healthy heart and kidneys and "appeared to be beneficial for the brain."

The doctors formed these conclusions:

- Eating meat is bad for your brain.
- Physical exercise increases both the number of brain cells and the connections between them.
- Chronic stress puts the brain in a state of high inflammation, causing structural damage.
- Restorative sleep is essential for cognitive and overall health.
- Higher education and other complex cognitive activities protect your brain against decline.
- Social support has an undeniable influence on the way your brain ages.

Meat and dairy are detrimental to brain health mostly because of the overall inflammatory processes associated with consuming them. Plant proteins are much better digested and absorbed, and come in a package along with plenty of fiber and beneficial micronutrients that help keep blood sugar stable and inflammation under control. There is an addictive potential associated with animal fats, particularly dairy, which can make it very challenging to address mood

stability and focus when there is an underlying emotional connection to such foods. The essential vitamins, minerals, and antioxidants provided by plants are helpful in keeping energy metabolism steady, which in turn prevents the sudden mood changes and foggy thinking associated with inflammatory foods.

The Most Important Nutrients for the Brain and Nervous System

Certain nutrients are essential for the brain to function properly, and others serve as bonus fuel to allow the brain and nervous system to truly heal and thrive continuously. As you will see from the following list, all these brain-loving nutrients can be found in abundance in plant foods. A whole food, varied vegan diet is easily the way to go to ensure you will maintain a brain that is high functioning, alert, clear, and adaptable!

Magnesium is an important nutrient in the health of the brain and nervous system. Deficiencies of magnesium have been implicated in both depression and dementia. Because it is necessary for so many biochemical processes, magnesium can become easily depleted with both high mental work and emotional stress.

Magnesium stimulates the neurotransmitter serotonin, which regulates sleep and mood patterns and relieves pain. It is important for healthy sleep by helping to relax muscles and regulating the cortisol/melatonin cycle, which governs a person's sleep/wake rhythms. Magnesium also helps alleviate anxiety by modulating receptors as needed: it will stimulate those needed to promote calming neurotransmitters and inhibit those promoting the stimulating neurotransmitters in the brain. Magnesium is also important in activating ATP, the energy that fuels your cells.

How to consume more magnesium: dark leafy greens, dark chocolate, figs, nuts, seeds, beans, avocados, quinoa

Omega-3 fatty acids are essential fatty acids that build and protect the brain, so named because they have a double bond at the third carbon atom in their chain. The short-chain version, found in such plant foods as flaxseeds and walnuts, can be converted in the body to DHA and EPA forms. DHA is concentrated in the membranes of brain cells, where it provides structure to the membrane and is involved in signaling, connectivity between cells, and neurotransmitter production, whereas EPA seems more influential on behavior and mood, showing promise in clinical studies to significantly lower depression and other mood disorders.

In adulthood, getting enough omega-3s helps maintain optimal brain function, prevents depression, and lays the groundwork for a healthy brain later in life. For example, a six-month study of young adults (18–45 years of age) showed that supplementing with DHA and EPA omega-3s resulted in improvements in memory. Additionally, twelve weeks of DHA supplementation was found to improve blood flow to the brain of healthy young adults during a cognitive task.

Another study found that higher omega-3 levels in the blood are associated with larger brain volume in older people, implying that abundant DHA and EPA could help prevent brain shrinkage with age.

Alzheimer's and Parkinson's are the two most common neurodegenerative diseases. Whereas Alzheimer's is known to affect mental functions, Parkinson's usually has more physical symptoms, such as tremors and challenges with muscle control. Consuming omega-3 fatty acids appears to be useful for preventing these diseases. Low omega-3 intake and low levels of DHA in the blood are associated with age-related cognitive decline and Alzheimer's disease. Also, DHA depletion in certain areas of the brain occurs in Alzheimer's disease. In some studies, low plasma EPA is also associated with the risk of dementia or cognitive decline.

DHA not only turns on the growth of new brain cells, but offers protection for existing brain cells while it enhances neuroplasticity. In addition, DHA is known to reduce the action of a particular inflammatory enzyme, COX-2. Ultimately, this translates into DHA's acting as a natural anti-inflammatory. This becomes quite significant when you recognize that inflammation is in fact a key player in both Alzheimer's and Parkinson's disease, and in virtually every other neurodegenerative condition, for that matter.

Diets heavy in processed foods, cholesterol, and meat (a higher omega-6 to omega-3 fat ratio) can lead to excess inflammation, which has been implicated in Alzheimer's disease. Evidence shows DHA acts to oppose this, exerting multiple protective activities.

One great way to get more omega-3s is to consume chia seeds. Chia seeds are tiny packages of pure goodness, known for their ability to boost energy, stabilize blood sugar, and nourish the brain. These seeds are native to Mexico and Guatemala, where the Mayan word *chia* means "strength." They are easy to add to your diet and add a hefty amount of omega-3 fats, sustaining minerals, and protein. They help keep the arteries of the brain clear of plaque and promote communication between brain cells, improving memory.

How to consume more omega-3s: flaxseeds (freshly ground), chia seeds, walnuts, leafy greens (purslane is a good source), cabbage, squash

The B vitamins: The eight vitamins—thiamine (B_1), riboflavin (B_2), niacin (B_3), pantothenic acid (B_5), pyridoxine (B_6), biotin (B_7), folate (B_9), and cobalamin (B_{12})—that make up the B vitamins play key roles in the majority of your cellular functions. One or more B vitamins are involved in every aspect of the absolutely essential process of generating energy within cells. B vitamins are also critical for brain function; they are so important that they actually have dedicated vehicles to transport them across the blood-brain barrier for use in brain cells. Deficiency in any one B vitamin will have negative consequences, including neurological and psychiatric symptoms. For example, the primary symptoms of vitamin B_6 deficiency are neurological, including depression, cognitive decline, and dementia, and vitamin B_{12} deficiency manifests in the form of neurological symptoms even at early stages. More than a third of psychiatric admissions were found to be suffering deficiencies in folate (B_9) or cobalamin (B_{12}), according to a 2006 *Lancet Neurology* article.

As B vitamins are water-soluble, any excess is generally excreted in urine. On the one hand, this means they are typically safe in high amounts, so it's hard to consume too many. On the other hand, you need to eat them more often than the fat-soluble vitamins, such as A, E, or K. So, eat those Bs! Fortunately, B vitamins are found in so many plant foods. To ensure you get enough of all eight, be sure to eat fruits, veggies, grains, beans, seeds, and mushrooms. Note that vitamin B_{12} is made by bacteria that live in the soil and is not naturally found in the plants we eat. Animals have B_{12} in their muscles from eating grass with these B_{12}-producing microbes clinging to the roots. When humans were living Earth-connected lives, foraging for roots and tubers and drinking from streams, B_{12} was naturally ingested into our GI tracts and supplements were not necessary. Today, however, modern sanitation dictates washing vegetables in chlorinated water and no more drinking from streams—so the "natural" sources of B_{12} have disappeared from our diets. If you are avoiding all animal products, you will need to assure a supplemental source of B_{12} that furnishes approximately 200 mcg of B_{12} daily, or 1,000 mcg once weekly. Ask your doctor to test your levels once or twice a year until you are sure of your intake and the levels that amount produces in your body.

B_{12}, in the form of cyanocobalamin or methylcobalamin, is often added to fortified foods, like plant-based milks and certain nutritional yeast products. Liquid or sublingual "microdots" of B_{12} are inexpensive, widely available, and easy to take.

How to consume more B vitamins: vitamin B_6: pistachios, pinto beans, avocados, sesame seeds, sunflower seeds, blackstrap molasses; vitamin B_9 (folate): avocados, legumes, peas, broccoli, citrus, okra; vitamin B_{12}: fortified foods, such as nutritional yeast

Choline is a water-soluble nutrient that is related to other vitamins in the B vitamin complex family. Just like B vitamins, choline plays a role in supporting energy and brain function as well as in keeping the metabolism active. It's important for the functioning of the key neurotransmitter acetylcholine, which is responsible for memory, mental clarity, and the healthy formation of synaptic connections between neurons.

Low acetylcholine levels are associated with Alzheimer's, and research has found that optimizing choline intake, through supplementation or regular dietary sources, tends to improve memory. Men may require more choline than postmenopausal women, who in turn need more than premenopausal women.

How to consume more choline: fermented foods, kidney beans and chickpeas, cauliflower, Brussels sprouts

Low-GI carbs: Population studies have continually found that dietary grains appear strongly protective in relation to Alzheimer's disease. Of course we are talking about whole, low-processed, high-fiber grains from the earth, not from a box.

Brown rice, sweet potatoes, and whole grains, such as oats, give you energy in the form of glucose. These brain-friendly complex carbs are low on the glycemic index (GI), which ranks foods on a 0–100 scale according to the rate at which sugar from food enters the brain and body cells. Eating low-GI foods will keep your energy steady throughout the day. Other low-GI carbs include legumes (chickpeas, lentils, and kidney beans). If you do eat a high-GI food, it is better to consume it *right after* a meal or with some protein, to slow the entry of sugar into your bloodstream and brain, preventing a crash later on. Also, consuming spices, such as cinnamon and cardamom, can help better balance energy by slowing the sugar release.

How to consume more low-GI carbs: whole grains, starchy veggies, legumes, carrots, most fruits

Chlorophyll is the green "blood" of plants. Nearly identical in chemical structure to your blood, chlorophyll delivers an energy transfusion, providing your cells with long-lasting vitality. This, of course, optimizes your brain function. The darker the leafy green, the more chlorophyll within. So, green up your life with a fresh salad or juice on a daily basis. At the next level, we suggest eating the nutrient-dense algae, such as chlorella, which is conveniently available in powdered form to spruce up your power smoothie. Wheatgrass is also one of the best sources of chlorophyll available.

How to consume more chlorophyll: greens, such as kale, Swiss chard, and arugula; herbs, such as parsley and cilantro; sprouts; algae; wheatgrass

Anthocyanins: Berries to the rescue! A protein called brain-derived neurotrophic factor (BDNF) is essentially the fountain of youth for brain health and plasticity, helping to promote new nerve connections associated with healthy cognitive function. BDNF has been found to play a significant role in the growth of nerve cells. A new study proves that the anthocyanins of blueberries very powerfully boost BDNF levels.

Anthocyanins seem to help reduce brain-cell damage from Parkinson's disease. They work by firing up mitochondria, the tiny biological power plants that provide energy to cells, allowing them to resist the neurotoxins linked to the disease.

Blueberry supplementation also improves memory in older adults, suggesting that "consistent supplementation with blueberries may offer an approach to forestall or mitigate" brain degeneration with age, according to a study at the University of Cincinnati that looked at cognitive performance in adults diagnosed with mild cognitive decline after twelve weeks of supplementation with pure pressed wild blueberry juice.

In addition, consuming blueberries and strawberries is associated with delayed cognitive aging by as much as two and a half years—thought to be because these anthocyanins tend to have an affinity for specific learning areas in the brain as shown on functional MRI scans.

How to consume more anthocyanins: blueberries, cranberries, black currants, raspberries, cherries, elderberries, black "forbidden" rice, red and purple grapes, red cabbage, eggplant peel, blue corn, red onion

Avoid Heavy Metals

Is the food you're eating contaminated with heavy metals? It could be wreaking havoc on your mind. When such metals as iron, copper, aluminum, or mercury over-accumulate in the body, they produce free radicals, which are like little sparks that damage brain cells, according to Neal Barnard, MD, an adjunct associate professor of medicine at the George Washington University School of Medicine. These metals have been linked to dementia and everyday mental fuzziness. Conversely, a study of roughly 1,450 adults in the *Journal of Nutrition, Health & Aging* found that women who performed highest on cognition tests had the lowest levels of copper and iron in their blood.

Although some **iron** is necessary for blood cell production and function, it turns out that your body cannot regulate heme iron (from animal products) as well as it can nonheme iron (from plants). Eating dark leafy greens can help you safely meet the recommended daily allowance (RDA) for iron (18 mg for women aged 19 to 50; 8 mg for women 50+). Greens are rich in antioxidants that seem to bind to any excess iron to prevent risk of damage.

Copper is needed in trace amounts for functions, such as tissue repair and melanin production. But again, too much is not a good thing. Inorganic copper—the type in multivitamins and tap water and different from that in plant foods—largely bypasses the liver's filtration system and heads directly to the blood and brain. It is especially dangerous when combined with saturated and trans fats, such as on a meat-heavy diet: Research has found that individuals whose high-fat diet included 1.6 mg or more of copper a day experienced a loss of mental function equivalent to an *extra nineteen years of aging*, compared with those who took in an average of 0.9 mg a day.

According to Dr. Barnard, "We need traces of iron to make the hemoglobin our blood cells use to carry oxygen. And you need traces of copper to make several key enzymes. But iron rusts. Copper corrodes, too, which is why a penny does not stay shiny forever. This is oxidation. And it doesn't just happen in a frying pan you accidentally left on your backyard picnic table for a few days. It also happens to the iron and copper within your body." This is another example of balance being the key, and plants, when consumed often and in a great variety, provide the balance the body needs to utilize essential nutrients without becoming overburdened by them.

Your body does not need **aluminum** to function. It seeps into your diet through antacids, soda cans, and even tap water. In one British study, people with high levels of aluminum in their tap water had a 50 percent increased risk for Alzheimer's compared to those with the least exposure. The Environmental Working Group has a tap water database where you can search any American zip code and find out about the quality of your tap water, as well as recommendations on avoiding or how to properly filter it. (Visit www.ewg.org/tapwater.)

And **mercury** is one heavy metal your body doesn't need under any circumstances. It's a known neurotoxin found commonly in fish and shellfish, where it accumulates in their bodies from water pollution. Whether fish come from the ocean, lakes, rivers, or streams, nearly all sources are contaminated with mercury. It is important to remember that fish are carnivores, which sets them apart from many other animals people eat. That means they are part of a long food chain, and they accumulate whatever toxins their prey have swallowed.

Be aware of other known dietary "brain toxins," too, such as those found in processed foods, sugar, artificial sweeteners, and pesticides. While many pesticides are directly neurotoxic, the brain is also particularly sensitive to the array of chemicals used as preservatives, colorings, flavorings, additives, and so on, in processed foods. Excess sugar and sweeteners can lead to insulin resistance, which affects brain functions as well. Your best defense? Organic vegetables! Continue to load up on protective antioxidants.

More Ways to Protect Your Brain Function

While food is the foundation, providing the brain with essential nutrients and supporting its constant activity, keep in mind that there are other simple ways to boost your brainpower throughout your day.

Move Your Body

Your body is made to move! Not only does it feel good and give your mood an immediate boost, but movement also stimulates your blood circulation, bringing more fresh oxygen to all your organs, including your brain. Exercise reminds your body that you are alive, stimulating your metabolism to prepare for the next burst of energy you will need! (For more on energy and metabolism, see Chapter 8.)

A recent study of exercise and improvements in brain function and cognitive changes looked at individuals with mild cognitive impairment who showed significant improvements after twelve weeks of moderate-intensity walking exercise training.

It seems the best overall health results—mental and physical—for people over age fifty appear to come from a combination of aerobic workouts and resistance training. This could include anything from high-intensity interval training, like the seven-minute workout, to dynamic flow yoga, which intersperses strength-building poses with heart-pumping dancelike moves.

Why does movement work so well to boost the brain? In *Healthy Brain, Happy Life*, Wendy Suzuki describes that during physical exercise, attention is increasing, memory is increasing, and mood is increasing. A bigger part of your brain is being activated, therefore you're building more motor circuits.

Not a fan of the gym? There are plenty of other easy ways to get moving:

Dance the night away: Dancing increases neural connectivity because it forces you to integrate several brain functions at once—kinesthetic, rational, musical, and emotional. If you're dancing with a partner, learning both "lead" and "follow" roles will increase your cognitive stimulation.

Older people who routinely partake in physical exercise can reverse the signs of aging in the brain—and dancing has the most profound effect, says a new study published in the journal *Frontiers in Human Neuroscience*. "In this study, we show that two different types of physical exercise (dancing and endurance training) both increase the area of the brain that declines with age. In comparison, it was only dancing that lead to noticeable behavioral changes in terms of improved balance." The traditional fitness program conducted was mainly repetitive exercises, such as cycling or Nordic walking, but the dance group were challenged with something new each week.

Play Ping-Pong: A 1992 Japanese study published in the *International Journal of Table Tennis Sciences* suggested the sport can delay the onset of dementia. Table tennis requires quick thinking, good hand-eye coordination, and fine motor skills control, all of which can stimulate expansion in certain areas of the brain through frequent practice.

Try the "cross-crawl": Walking with swinging arms, crawling, marching in place, alternately touching each hand to the opposite knee. The motion of "cross-crawling" coordinates opposite sides of the body, activating the nerve cells in the brain and stimulating them to create synapses between the left and right sides of the brain. This improves focus, short-term memory, and overall brain function. It is wonderful exercise for improving reading, listening, writing, learning, and memory. It coordinates the whole brain and nervous system.

Neurobics: Stimulate Your Mind

Think of it as aerobics for your mind! This can be any nonstressful, familiar activity that is changed slightly to focus and stimulate your brain in a new way. More simple ways to support growth of new neurons:

Learn to play music. Brain scans of musicians show heightened connectivity between brain regions. If you've always wanted to learn an instrument, consider brain health as a motivator to get started.

Switch hands. Using your nondominant hand to do simple tasks, such as brushing your teeth, texting, or stirring your coffee/tea can help you form new neural pathways.

Read fiction. Reading a novel "can transport you into the body of the protagonist," according to an Emory study published in the journal *Brain Connectivity*, which found that positive brain changes can linger in the brain for days after reading an influential novel. This ability to shift into another mental state is a crucial skill because it allows you to practice empathy, which keeps your brain flexible and allows for more creative problem solving.

Expand your vocabulary. Learning new words activates the brain's visual and auditory processes and memory processing. Learn one new word each day to expand your vocabulary and give your brain a workout. Practice speaking in other languages as well whenever you have the opportunity. Use apps or online courses to make it fun.

Create a work of art. Participants in a ten-week art course (a two-hour session, one day per week) showed enhanced connectivity of the brain at a resting state known as the default mode network (DMN). The DMN influences such mental processes as introspection, memory, and empathy. Engaging in art also strengthens the neural pathway that controls attention and focus. Whether it's creating mosaics, jewelry, pottery, painting, or drawing, the combination of motor and cognitive processing will promote better brain connectivity. Pull out the crafts or join a local art class; just once a week will help your brain grow.

Venture out. Travel promotes neurogenesis by exposing your brain to new, novel, and complex environments. Simply taking a weekend road trip to a different city gives your brain the same stimulation. Even simpler—take a different route than usual to your daily activities.

Get Better Sleep

Did you know that your brain cells shrink while you sleep? A recent study in the *Journal of Science* found that this opens up the gaps between neurons and allows fluid to "wash" the brain clean, showing that one purpose of sleep is to be a waste removal system. This builds on another recent discovery of the brain's own network of plumbing pipes—known as the glymphatic system—which carries waste material out of the brain.

The brain only has limited energy at its disposal, and interestingly, it appears that it must choose between two different functional states—"awake and aware" or "asleep and cleaning up," said researcher Dr. Maiken Nedergaard. Aim for seven to eight hours of sleep each night to ensure that the brain has had adequate "cleanup" time. If you're struggling to get a consistently good sleep, try creating a nightly ritual; for example, going to bed at the same time; drinking some sleep-inducing tea; and making your room as dark as possible. Remember that you can make up for lost sleep. Listen to your body's needs and respond accordingly.

Silence Is Brain Medicine

How much time a day do you spend in complete silence? Florence Nightingale, the nineteenth-century British nurse and social activist, once wrote, "Unnecessary noise is the most cruel absence of care that can be inflicted on sick or well." Nightingale argued that needless sounds could cause distress, sleep loss, and alarm for recovering patients. Today, her concern is borne out by research. There is overwhelming evidence that exposure to environmental noise has adverse effects on health, according to a 2011 World Health Organization report that called noise pollution a "modern plague."

Loud noises raise stress levels by activating the brain's amygdala and causing the release of the stress hormone cortisol. When those attention resources are depleted, you become distracted and mentally fatigued, and may struggle to focus, solve problems, and come up with new ideas.

In your everyday life, sensory input is being thrown at you from every angle. When you can finally get away from these sonic disruptions, your brain's attention centers have the opportunity to restore themselves.

The brain can restore its finite cognitive resources in environments with lower levels of sensory input. In silence—for instance, the quiet stillness you find when walking alone in nature—the brain can let down its sensory guard. A 2006 study published in the journal *Heart* found two minutes of silence to be more relaxing than listening to "relaxing" music, based on changes in blood pressure and blood circulation in the brain.

When the brain is idle and disengaged from external stimuli, you can finally tap into your inner stream of thoughts, emotions, memories, and ideas. In a 2013 study, two hours of silence daily led to the development of new cells in the hippocampus, a key brain region associated with learning, memory, and emotion. While preliminary, the findings suggested that silence could be therapeutic for such conditions as depression and Alzheimer's, which are associated with decreased rates of neuron regeneration in the hippocampus.

AGE-DEFYING ADVICE:
PROTECTING YOUR SENSES

Diminished eyesight and hearing loss are incredibly common as one ages. Approximately one in three people in the United States between the ages of 65 and 74 has hearing loss, and nearly half of those older than 75 have some difficulty hearing. But there are steps you can take to protect your eyes and ears.

The high beta-carotene content of such veggies as dark leafy greens, carrots, and sweet potatoes can help keep vision crystal clear and sharp, especially improving night vision, which decreases as one ages. A diet packed with antioxidants and omega-3 fatty acids, such as in flaxseeds, can directly prevent age-related macular degeneration, according to a study in the medical journal *BMC Ophthalmology*. The antioxidant carotenoids, lutein and zeaxanthin, in those leafy greens can also keep cataracts at bay by fending off damaging free radicals in the central retina.

Goji berries are a surprising power food for the eyes, containing all of the essential amino acids along with plenty of fiber, vitamins A and C, iron, zinc, and antioxidants, including eye-supportive zeaxanthin. In a study, daily dietary supplementation with the berries for ninety days increased plasma zeaxanthin and antioxidant levels as well as lowered hypopigmentation and accumulation, which are early signs of macular degeneration.

As for hearing loss, the inner parts of the ear are sensitive and delicate, so any circulation problems can affect hearing. Such conditions as chronic smoking, high blood pressure, heart disease, diabetes, atherosclerosis, and other circulatory illnesses that are not addressed can lead to hearing loss. Common drugs, such as large doses of aspirin and certain kinds of diuretics, can also affect hearing. The cochlear, or inner ear, is a high-energy-demanding organ. The auditory system is always on and always processing sound. To process sound, it needs to be fed with a huge amount of energy molecules and adequate oxygen, delivered by proper blood circulation to the ear.

Ginkgo biloba is loaded with compounds called flavones and ginkgolides—antioxidants that help protect your inner ear hair cells and auditory canal. It is also a vasodilator, opening the tiny blood vessels and capillaries in and around your ears, resulting in less ringing and clearer hearing, as well as helping clear sinus congestion and even resolving vertigo.

For further ear protection:

- Use over-the-ear headphones instead of earbuds or in-ear headphones. Choose studio-quality, noise-canceling headphones.
- Follow the "60/60" rule when listening to music. Listen to it at 60 percent of the maximum volume for no more than 60 minutes at a time, and then take a break. Try a "hearing detox" of 5 to 10 minutes to give your ears a break.
- Exercise for hearing! Findings published in the *Journal of Neuroscience* suggest that age-related inflammation damages the capillaries and cells, and that exercising provides the best protection from that inflammation.
- Carry earplugs to use in those situations when sound is too loud, such as in movie theaters or concerts that use amplification.

Join the ranks of those who enjoy mental clarity, excellent memory recall, and overall optimal brain health as you chronologically age. As with the other body systems we will explore, there is so much you can do on your end through appropriate diet and lifestyle choices to keep you on top of your game and prevent you from "going gently into that good night" as Dylan Thomas poetically expressed.

AGE-DEFYING ADVICE: BRAIN HEALTH

Eat More:
- **Magnesium-rich foods:** greens, dark chocolate/cacao, almonds, figs, cashews, black beans, avocados
- **Anthocyanin-rich foods:** blackberries, blueberries, cherries, cranberries, eggplant, grapes, plums, red beets, red cabbage, strawberries
- **Vitamin E-rich foods:** nuts and seeds, spinach, chard
- **Omega-3-rich foods:** dark leafy greens, nuts and seeds, avocados
- **B$_{12}$-fortified foods:** nutritional yeast. Consider a supplement if you're not sure you're getting enough.

Drink More:
- **Water:** Have a cool glass of water first thing in the morning, or when feeling a little foggy, to wake up your brain.
- **Rosemary** (fresh or dried) in water or simply to sniff for a little brain boost
- **Ginkgo tea** to optimize brain circulation

Do More:
- Avoid contaminants in water, foods, food containers, and personal care products.
- Stimulate your brain via changing up your daily patterns, playing games, reading fiction, dancing, doing cross-crawl exercises, playing Ping-Pong, or juggling.
- Meditate in silence.
- Aromatherapy, especially lemon, orange, or mint, to keep senses open and mind focused
- Normalize your sleep schedule, and avoid eating late at night, exercising right before sleep, or spending too much time on your phone or tablet in bed.

Try these brain-friendly recipes that include foods and nutrients mentioned above:
- Rosemary Star Anise Tea (page 113)
- Berry Chia Bowl with Pomegranate (page 130)
- Arugula Walnut Salad with Cashew Dill Dressing (page 161)
- Stacked Avocados (page 195)
- Black Rice Sushi with Wasabi Mayo (page 222)
- Brain Health Trail Mix (page 280)

For downloadable charts of Doctor and Chef recommendations, please visit www.doctorchefresources.com.

Name: Victoria Moran
Birth Year: 1950

About Victoria: Victoria Moran is a vegan of over three decades, an obesity survivor, and the author of books, including the iconic *Main Street Vegan*. She hosts the weekly Main Street Vegan podcast and directs Main Street Vegan Academy, an in-person intensive in New York City that trains and certifies vegan lifestyle coaches and educators. Her grown-up daughter, Adair, is a lifelong vegan, stunt performer, and aerialist who inspired her mom to take up aerial yoga at age sixty-five. www.mainstreet vegan.net

Typical Daily Meals: I eat seasonally—lots of raw food when it's warm, more soups and hot cereal and comfort food in the winter. I don't snack. Eating when it's time to eat and living life the rest of the time has been key to my maintaining a 60-pound weight loss for nearly thirty-five years. Breakfast is either a smoothie or an oatmeal parfait (oatmeal with berries and other fruit, ground flax, slivered almonds). Lunch is usually a huge salad—often with steamed sweet potatoes or winter squash—and a homemade nut-based dressing. Dinner is often some variation of beans and greens (onion, garlic, mushrooms, beans, and kale, collards, Swiss chard, or some other dark leafy green with spices, such as turmeric, cardamom, garam masala). If I make a dessert, it's usually from the world of raw cuisine, such as chocolate mousse with richness from avocado instead of cream.

Typical Exercise/Lifestyle: When left to my own devices, I cycle in and out of what I call activity resistance disorder (ARD for short). During those periods, just opening the door to the gym is more than I think I can do, much less actually go in and work out. Because I know this about myself, I make regular exercise easy to do and hard to skip. My husband and I have a pact to do weight training together four days a week. I have a Fitbit and getting ten thousand steps every day is a point of honor. I take a yoga class three times a week.

Victoria says: Unless you're looking to be an Olympic gymnast, anything you want to achieve is possible at any time of life. Sometimes you just have to look a little harder. For a lot of people, going vegan and choosing whole foods takes care of everything; it's their live-happily-ever-after choice. Some of us have to look at other things, gluten sensitivity, maybe, or some genetic glitch that requires medication or other attention. I personally needed Overeaters Anonymous to get me past a binge-eating disorder before I was even able to go vegan. You [can] accommodate your own circumstances and still be a brilliant example of vibrant veganism.

THREE

AGING TAKES GUTS!: OPTIMIZE YOUR DIGESTION

When you think about antiaging, maybe you imagine losing the 15 pounds that have somehow crept on over the last decade. What you probably don't think about is healing your digestive system itself and keeping it in tip-top shape. But poor digestion is one of the most common symptoms of aging, and it's absolutely essential to correct if you want to experience a younger you.

Why? You are not what you eat, although that's part of it. You are what you eat, digest, absorb, and metabolize! For example, eating kale is wonderful, but you need to make sure your body is able to break it down and actually make use of those great nutrients you're giving it. Otherwise, you're depriving your cells and putting more stress on your body's systems, which only serves to accelerate the aging process. It can turn into a vicious cycle, but it certainly doesn't have to. Now is a good time to take your digestive health seriously!

Here's why: It turns out that most of your immune activity takes place in your gut.

This makes sense because the digestive tract is the gateway to the outside world, in that it governs what is okay and not okay to enter your body. An intricate network of activities is happening all the time right there in the center of your body, and the competency of the immune system is reliant on the health of those important digestive activities. These in turn depend on a healthy balance of resident microorganisms, which have their own important functions and reside throughout the body in what we call the microbiome.

Quite simply, the health of your digestive system is the foundation of your well-being, at any age.

Meet Your Digestive Tract

For a quick overview, here's how digestion is supposed to work: It begins in the mouth. The food you eat is first broken down as you chew it, and then is broken down further by enzymes in your saliva. Anything that compromises the chewing or salivary enzyme processes can disturb digestion.

Food must travel down a healthy esophagus and enter the stomach by proper messaging, where the brain sends a signal to for the stomach "door" to open (the lower esophageal sphincter) and for the stomach to start the release of hydrochloric acid and enzymes to further break down your meal.

When it's time, the pyloric sphincter opens to move the food into the upper part of the small intestine, the duodenum, where it is mixed with more enzymes courtesy of the pancreas and small intestine. The gallbladder and liver provide further help to break down fats. Nutrients from the food, such as amino acids and simple sugars, are absorbed into the bloodstream through the wall of the small intestine. Digestion is completed in the large intestine. There, water and minerals are absorbed into the blood to nourish cells, certain vitamins are produced if your gut flora is healthy, and finally waste is eliminated.

All of these processes are intricately organized and reliant on the health of each organ involved, the correct nutrients necessary for proper hormone messaging, and a balanced neurological system, since excess stress or tension alone can disturb digestion. The simple act of eating in a relaxed environment can increase digestive enzyme production because the body needs to reach a calm state—called a parasympathetic state of the nervous system—to allow digestive processes to occur.

Nearly 40 percent of older adults have one or more age-related digestive symptoms each year. What's going on? Here are some of the most common situations.

Indigestion and Acid Reflux

Antacids, such as Tums, Alka-Seltzer, and Maalox, are some of the most commonly used over-the-counter medicines. This is because of the widely held assumption that indigestion and reflux are caused by an overproduction of stomach acid and that the treatment is to block acid production. Makes sense, right? As it turns out, not really.

In most cases, this treatment is actually counterproductive. Most often, the issue causing maldigestion is actually *insufficient* rather than excessive stomach acid. When you lack adequate stomach acid, food does not break down enough in the stomach and reflux up into the esophagus can occur, leading to heartburn symptoms. Gastrointestinal reflux disease (GERD) is the most common upper GI disorder in older adults, which can be experienced as fullness or sore throat, not always as heartburn.

It is estimated that somewhere between 23 and 35 percent of adults over sixty-five years of age have low stomach acid. The only way to truly address indigestion is to work on improving all aspects of your digestive system, rather than block an important part of it.

Producing enough stomach acid is critical for the digestive system. Its important functions include:

- Breaking down the proteins you eat into the essential amino acids that are necessary for pretty much all physiologic function in the body

- Stimulating the pancreas and small intestines to produce the digestive enzymes and bile necessary to further break down carbohydrates, proteins, and fats
- Preventing disease, by killing pathogenic bacteria and yeast that may hitch a ride in foods you eat
- Establishing a proper environment required for the absorption of certain micronutrients, such as calcium, magnesium, zinc, copper, iron, selenium, boron, and more
- Allowing the stomach contents to empty correctly into the small intestine

Without enough stomach acid, over time, your body won't absorb nutrients properly, which can lead to osteoporosis, weakness, fatigue, cramps, anemia, and other nutritional disorders.

Six not-so-fun consequences of low stomach acid:

1. **IBS.** Undigested protein reaches the lower intestines, where it can ferment and release toxins, setting the stage for disease. This is when gas, bloating, and irritable bowel syndrome (IBS) can occur.
2. **Mineral deficiency.** As your blood becomes more acidic, it will look for minerals from anywhere in your body so as to get your blood to its more ideal alkaline state; this could

mean taking minerals from your bones.
3. **Iron or B$_{12}$ deficiency anemia**, due to lack of absorptive capabilities
4. **Rise in cortisol levels**, thereby raising blood glucose as well as adversely affecting the nervous system. Excessive cortisol secretion over time will eventually fatigue the adrenal glands and suppress the hormone DHEA, leading to premature aging.
5. **Intestinal bacterial or yeast overgrowth.** The result is a loss of important friendly bacteria, and such symptoms as nausea, diarrhea, constipation, weight loss, and a susceptibility to pneumonia.
6. **Allergies.** If foods are poorly digested, large molecules can get into the lower gut where the immune system sees them as antigens and reacts against them.

What You Can Do

A whole food, plant-heavy vegan diet requires lots of chewing, which helps stimulate enzyme and saliva production. It also provides an abundance of minerals that help maintain an alkaline pH, and increases healthy fiber. All of these benefits will help normalize both adequate stomach acid production and regulation of muscle movements, often resolving these cyclical digestive troubles by addressing the original cause!

Happily, the ability of the small intestines to absorb what you eat is not affected at all by aging, according to authors of a large study at the Gastrointestinal Center at the University of Manchester in England. Once the digestive process is firing on all cylinders, your older body's intestines are able to absorb your foods every bit as well as they did when you were young. So, when you add it all up, the biggest problem with poor nutritional absorption in the older age group is from low stomach acid. Get your stomach juices flowing!

Constipation

Constipation is the most common digestive complaint. It can be caused by . . .

- Slowed gastrointestinal muscle contractions: Due to a decrease in smooth muscle tone along a majority of the aging GI tract, food moves through the system more slowly as the contractions necessary for the movement and breakdown of food become weaker. When things slow down, more water gets absorbed from food waste, which can cause constipation.
- Calcium channel blockers for high blood pressure
- Narcotic pain relievers common after knee or hip replacement
- Iron supplements
- Inactivity
- Diuretics for high blood pressure or congestive heart failure
- Increased urination

Constipation can slow down the body's normal detoxification mechanisms, causing toxins to build up in the liver, kidneys, heart, and brain. Laxatives often prescribed to treat constipation can be addictive and may lose potency over time. With increasing age, adults tend to become more sedentary, eat and drink less, and take in much less fiber daily, all of which are habits that aggravate chronic constipation.

The most important factors in preventing constipation are drinking enough water and getting enough fiber. The good news is that there is an easy solution, because *all plants contain fiber*! Animal-based foods, including dairy and eggs, do not contain fiber; this is an important consideration for those eating higher amounts of animal products, since chronic constipation can lead to very serious digestive diseases over time.

Diverticulosis, called diverticulitis when it presents with pain and infection, occurs more frequently with age. Diverticula are small pouches that can develop in the wall of large intestine, usually on the descending side, which can cause discomfort on the lower left side of the body when small food particles become lodged in the pouches. This is a process that occurs with chronic inflammation and is often tied to years of a low-fiber diet.

Ulcers are lesions on the digestive tissue than can occur in the stomach or small intestine and may be silent or, over time, may cause pain and eventually bleeding. In aging they are often the result of chronic use of over-the-counter pain medications, which can contribute to excess bleeding.

Polyps in the colon, or colorectal polyps, are small collections of inflammatory cells often found on a routine colonoscopy. They are the result of chronic chemical or microbe-induced inflammation in the colon from poor food choices and may not initially produce any noticeable symptoms or problems, although they can grow into colon cancer over time. Risk increases after the age of fifty, and according to Johns Hopkins University, the top three risk factors include a diet high in red meats, a diet high in processed meats, and a history of inflammatory bowel disease (which is more common in animal and processed food eaters).

AGE-DEFYING ADVICE: ABDOMINAL MASSAGE

Massage can be extremely effective in helping calm and balance digestion, and can alleviate abdominal pain, constipation, and both muscular and emotional tension.

1. First, rub your hands together to create warmth, then place your palms on the center of your abdomen and take a couple of deep breaths. Notice any areas of tension.
2. Begin with a gentle clockwise motion, starting around the belly button and moving outward in concentric circles. You may use one hand or both.
3. Continue this gentle circular massage until the area feels warm and your breath deepens.
4. You may want to begin using your fingertips to specifically target areas of tension. Continue with gentle clockwise movements until you feel your muscles relax and breath deepen.

Feed Your Microbiome

As we mentioned before, your digestive tract does even more than process food. Much of your immune system's action seems to take place within the digestive system. There are lymphatic tissues all along the digestive tract, as well as a mucus layer that is protective against toxins and infectious organisms. And there is an entire dynamic ecosystem going on inside your body, known as the microbiome.

When any of these become compromised, you may become more susceptible to acute illness as well as fatigue, pain, GI distress, and generalized malaise. In fact, a growing understanding of humans' intimate relationship to the microorganisms that live within them has led to a new way of thinking about immunity, and how all systems in the body are interrelated and reliant on the health of the whole.

The trillions of bacteria and other organisms that live in your intestine and constitute most of the microbiome are built over time, starting at birth and establishing a diverse mix of organisms by around age three. Optimally, the mix of bacteria naturally changes and cycles as needed over your lifetime. You want to create a gut environment suitable for varied organisms, much like a diverse garden where the plants live in harmony and no one species takes over. *Lactobacillus* and *Bifidobacteria* both seem to play healing and balancing roles by the prevalence of these particular organisms that can be seen under the microscope in a healthy gut. Interestingly, it has been observed that by about age fifty, your microbiomes seem to want to shift back toward the mix found in your first couple of years of life, even more abundant in *Bifidobacteria*, which are now being touted as the antiaging bacteria due to their restorative and protective actions. It all happens as a natural cycle as long as things remain in balance.

In an ideal microbiome, 85 percent of the bacteria are friendly microbes working hard on your behalf to keep out any troublemakers. They are called probiotic microorganisms, which means that they are "pro life," and they work with your own cells to keep you healthy by improving your digestion, regulating your immune system, helping you absorb nutrients, enhancing your memory, and even keeping your emotions in check. These microscopic superfriends also reduce temporary inflammation, produce vitamins and enzymes, and protect you from unfriendly invaders.

Unfortunately, this normally high percentage of the good guys can decline due to various common diet and lifestyle factors. After years of exposure to the many things that wipe out the healthy bacteria in your gut—such as antibiotics (both those within food and purposely taken as medicine), processed foods, alcohol, stress, and environmental toxins and chemicals—your microbiome can become depleted, meaning that there just aren't enough of the good guys left to keep you healthy and youthful. The less healthy, greedy bacteria start to gain a foothold, and many aspects of the aging process become accelerated. When good bacteria become diminished by antibiotics and other toxins, or are not properly fed, this creates room for unhealthy microbes to take over, causing damage rather than supporting health in their effort to survive themselves. This is how insidious bacterial, viral, and fungal infections can cause major problems if unchecked over time.

Luckily, your food choices have a major impact on digestive health and your microbiome, which is quite dynamic and changing all the time. Each time you eat something, you can boost your digestive health and immunity almost immediately.

What you eat can have a tremendous effect on the composition of your microbiome, often within just a few hours of a meal. A diet high in plant-based fiber and whole foods will do wonders for your gut flora, and adding probiotic-rich fermented foods, such as sauerkraut and kimchi, whenever possible will add even more good microbes! Don't forget to include plenty of prebiotic foods, too, especially beans, lentils, and other legumes, which provide healthy plant fibers that feed and energize those resident beneficial probiotic microbes. Processed, sugary foods and anything containing emulsifiers, pesticides, artificial sweeteners, or GMOs tend to deplete good bacteria. The right gut bacteria not only help resolve most of the common IBS symptoms, such as gas, bloating, and pain from intestinal maldigestion, but will also help protect you from environmental toxins, including heavy metals, by preventing excess gut permeability.

As with everything in life, the key to a healthy microbiome is balance. And the secret to achieving this balance lies in understanding what factors affect your beneficial organism colonies, so you can make microbe-friendly choices. Take charge of your own personal inner ecosystem by doing what you know can make the biggest impact: increasing high-fiber, nutrient-dense plant foods!

Also, just as digestive processes and enzyme production are optimized when your nervous system is experiencing a calm, happy state, your microbiome is also influenced by your mental and emotional health. Stress makes your gut more permeable—or accessible—to unwanted bacteria, antigens, and toxins. Once these bad guys get in, they trigger an immune response that in turn depletes your microbiome of good bacteria. In addition, dopamine, the brain chemical that is in charge of feelings of reward and pleasure, is largely made in the gut, and is one of the main reasons that mood is so closely connected to digestive health. So, practice daily mindful meditation, yoga, exercise you enjoy, and have a little fun every day to both keep stress at bay and keep your dopamine flowing.

Will Eating More Plants Help You Lose Weight?

Many people find it harder to lose weight after around age forty and beyond. There are several reasons for this: hormonal changes, loss of lean muscle mass, redistribution of fat stores, and slowed metabolism.

Many people report losing a few excess pounds as well as having significantly increased energy shortly after adopting a whole food, plant-based diet. As a matter of fact, plant foods innately do have particular qualities that promote healthy weight maintenance. First of all, fiber! Fiber slows digestion, keeping you satiated longer. It also treats constipation and bloating by promoting movement of digested materials through the lower intestines for excretion.

The nutrient density of plant foods tends to keep your energy buzzing. You will likely feel more satisfied and have fewer cravings, since you are not starving your body of its energy needs. The extra energy you have may help you increase and maintain your motivation for exercise and choose more active rather than sedentary lifestyle behaviors.

What Does the Evidence Show?

An article in the 2011 *New England Journal of Medicine* discussed a study on weight loss in a large group of relatively healthy adults over four-year periods of time. With a focus only on foods eaten and not other lifestyle factors, weight gain was most strongly associated with the intake of potato chips, sugar-sweetened beverages, unprocessed red meats, and processed meats; and the largest weight losses were associated with the intake of vegetables, whole grains, fruits, and nuts.

It was noted that the higher fiber content and slower digestion of the whole plant foods promoted satiety, and their increased consumption would also lessen the tendency for eating more highly processed foods. The researchers also found, not surprisingly, that as people aged, those who consumed processed foods and routinely sipped sugary drinks or alcohol gained the most weight with age. So did those who watched the most television. (Not only a sedentary activity, watching television actually promotes more unconscious snacking and also influences food choices both during viewing and at other times.)

This highly publicized study went on to conclude that yes, overall, individuals consuming plant-based diets tend to have lower body mass index (BMI) than those consuming conventional, non-plant-based diets. It also suggested the adoption of a plant-based diet as an effective first-line recommendation for weight loss, in addition to its known benefit for chronic disease prevention and treatment.

Five Simple Things You Can Do to Lose Weight

1. **Have an apple a day!** According to a simple study done by the Federation of American Societies for Experimental Biology, researchers found that people who ate at least one apple a day lost more weight than those who did not. The high fiber and water content of apples may have something to do with this.

2. **Eat legumes:** the more you eat, the more you lose weight! It's true, according to research in the *American Journal of Clinical Nutrition*. People who ate just ¾ cup of beans, peas, chickpeas, or lentils a day lost half a pound a week without changing their diet or exercise habits. Legumes are full of fiber and protein, keeping you satisfied for hours.

3. **Stick with whole foods.** Many popular food additives are linked with weight gain and obesity, according to a study done by Georgia State University. Emulsifiers, which are added to most processed foods for texture and to extend shelf life, are one of the worst offenders as they interfere with good gut bacteria, which is also connected to weight gain. Artificial flavorings, artificial sweeteners, preservatives, and even food packaging have also been linked in research to obesity.

4. **Eat breakfast.** There must be a reason that nearly 100 percent of people on the National Weight Loss Registry—a database of people who've lost at least 40 pounds and kept it off for a year or more—report eating breakfast every day. A healthy, nutrient-dense morning meal will keep you satiated as well as kick the day's metabolism into gear.

5. **Get your sleep.** Getting fewer than seven hours of sleep made people eat an average of 500 extra calories the next day, according to research done by the National Institutes of Health. Exhaustion interferes with your hormones in several ways, which can all lead to weight gain. Examples are excess cortisol with adrenal stress and thyroid depression with insulin resistance as a result of imbalances in circadian rhythms, or sleep/wake cycles.

To sum it up, while there are many factors that play into maintaining optimal body weight, there is much you can do to support your body's functional abilities every day, rather than succumb to the challenges you encounter in aging. By embracing a plant-based diet with a focus on nourishment, many people have attained their ideal weight without falling into the yo-yo diet trap. Choosing to treat your body to plant nutrition, the fuel that is proven to keep your metabolic motor running most efficiently, is a perfect place to start!

AGE-DEFYING ADVICE: DIGESTIVE HEALTH

Eat More:

Fiber: especially skins of fruits, legumes, and whole raw or cooked veggies

Fermented foods: Miso, unsweetened vegan yogurt, kimchi, tempeh, sauerkraut, kombucha, and kefir are examples.

Prebiotic foods: Bananas, onions, garlic, asparagus, apples, oats, jicama, and Jerusalem artichokes are great prebiotic sources.

Whole grains: to ensure adequate amounts of both soluble and insoluble fiber

Healthy fats: Avocados, nuts, and seeds promote digestive tract healing and lower inflammation; be sure to limit or avoid inflammatory animal fats and hydrogenated oils, which can create more damage.

Tissue-healing foods: okra, plantains, cabbage, sweet potatoes, oats, squash, pumpkin

Drink More:

Hydration: Drinking water is the best medicine for constipation, heartburn, and indigestion.

Herbs, such as licorice root, ginger, chamomile, mint, and fennel, all support digestive processes as well as heal damage to gut tissue. Taking these in tea is a perfect way to directly soothe digestion as well as create a calm inner environment conducive to good digestion.

continues

---

continued from previous page

Do More:

To optimize digestion and stimulate enzyme action: start meals with bitters, such as ginger, apple cider vinegar, or a slice of green apple; chew completely; slow down, take deep breaths, give thanks.

Use natural household cleaners and cosmetics that won't wipe out friendly microbes. Discontinue using antibacterial soaps. Absorption of chemicals, such as triclosan, phthalates, and parabens, through your skin may ultimately affect your gut microbes. Check out the Environmental Working Group's Guide to Healthy Cleaning website for more information on nontoxic cleaning products (www.ewg.org /guides/cleaners/content/findings).

Do something that brings you calm every day. This may be walking, deep breathing, yoga, meditation, or other relaxation activities.

Try these digestion-friendly recipes with foods and nutrients mentioned above:

Digestive Support Tea (page 122)

Savory Grits (page 134) with Smashed Avocado Toast Supreme (page 127)

Kundalini Kitchari (page 154)

Steamed Supreme (page 176)

Sweet and Spicy Plantains (page 191)

Coconut Yogurt (page 262)

Name: Miyoko Schinner
Birth Year: 1957

About Miyoko: Miyoko Schinner is founder and CEO of Miyoko's Kitchen, an award-winning line of artisan dairy alternatives sold in thousands of stores across the country. A vegan for thirty years, Miyoko missed the "cheese experience" and spent years perfecting recipes to satisfy that craving. Miyoko is the author of five cookbooks, including the best-selling *The Homemade Vegan Pantry*. She cohosted three seasons of *Vegan Mashup*, a cooking show that aired on PBS stations. Along with her husband, she founded Rancho Compasión, a farm animal sanctuary in Northern California. www.miyokoskitchen.com

Typical Daily Meals: Lots of veggies and fruits (sometimes exclusively veggies and fruit for breakfast), legumes, grains (rice, quinoa). Although I'm a chef capable of rich and fancy foods, I enjoy eating very simply on a daily basis. I feel so much better when I eat a basic diet of fruit, veggies, grains, and legumes, and minimize oil. I do enjoy wonderful plates of pasta and the occasional dessert, but my body is happiest when eating pure, whole foods meals.

Typical Exercise/Lifestyle: In addition to shoveling manure and other sanctuary duties, I run, lift weights, and do my own lighter version of CrossFit. I used to do CrossFit pretty seriously, but due to time, energy, and other constraints, I mostly make sure I am active every day with some sort of physical activity. At sixty, I'm still able to outperform many people half my age.

Miyoko says: Don't find reasons for not being able to do something. Find reasons for doing something, then do it.

FOUR

GET STRONGER: BETTER BONES, JOINTS, AND MUSCLES

Your body is the house you'll reside in for a lifetime. So, how do you keep your structural integrity?

It turns out that osteoporosis, arthritis, weakened muscles, and bone fractures do not have to come automatically with more birthdays. We know that no one wants to believe that frailty is inevitable, and we hope that you will soon realize that you can become stronger and more agile at any age! It really is never too late to take good care of your structural body. Thankfully, a plant-based diet is high in antioxidants, which prevent tissue breakdown, and micronutrients, which help tissues repair themselves. Throw in enough amino acids—the building blocks of proteins—to provide the raw materials, and you have the dietary essentials for a strong, healthy, ageless body that will serve you for years to come. Then, all you have to do is make basic physical exercise a daily priority. "Use it or lose it" has

never been truer—make it your age-defying mantra!

Your Bones Support More Than You Think

The skeleton, of course, provides your body with structure, and enables you to move around in the world. But your bones do even more! Bones actually act as a storage space for calcium and other minerals until they are needed for biochemical processes. While calcium helps keep bones strong, it is also needed for muscle contraction, nerve impulse transmission, and blood clotting.

Bones are considered active organs since they can change every day throughout your life, constantly breaking down and building back up in a process called remodeling. Over time, the breakdown slowly overtakes the building of new bone, and bone mass will begin to decline. This occurs at different ages for women and men, mostly due to the role of estrogen, which decreases in menopause.

By around age sixty-five to seventy, the rate of bone loss becomes the same for men and women, at which point they become more susceptible to developing osteoporosis, or weakened bone strength. The best time to build bone density through diet and exercise is during years of rapid growth, such as childhood, adolescence, and early adulthood. Although everyone will lose bone with age, people who developed a higher peak bone mass when young are better protected against osteoporosis and related fractures later in life. That said, remember that it is never too late. Incorporating a nutrient-rich, plant-based diet as well as strength-building habits into your life even well into the susceptible age have proven to make a huge difference in both preventing and managing those signs of bone loss.

Maintaining healthy bones depends on the harmonious interaction of amino acids; vitamins C, D, and K; and the minerals calcium, magnesium, potassium, and phosphorus in the body, so it's crucial to have an adequate intake of all these nutrients. You'll also want to avoid smoking and drinking too much alcohol; your bones will thank you. Certain medications can cause mineral loss from the bones. Some include corticosteroids, chemotherapy drugs used in hormone-dependent cancers, long-term thyroid medicines, and any medication that can cause mineral depletion, such as some blood pressure medications, certain psychiatric medicines, and even acid-blocking drugs. If

you need to take these, be sure to be even more on top of your plant protein and mineral intake and bone-healthy habits.

Arthritis

Arthritis is the number one cause of disability in the United States. The time is now to protect your joints, keeping them supple and pain-free.

Although arthritis can occur at any age, it is estimated that half of adults over the age of sixty-five suffer from some form of it, according to the Arthritis Foundation. Osteoarthritis is a degenerative condition that is the result of increased wear and tear on joints. Rheumatoid arthritis is an autoimmune disorder that produces inflammatory joint symptoms throughout the body. Both rheumatoid and osteoarthritis are connected to excess inflammation and oxidative stress.

Despite how prevalent arthritis is, conventional treatment options have not been very impressive. For example, prednisone, a corticosteroid drug used for decades to control inflammation, is a notorious culprit in bone mineral density loss. Prednisone stops the function of osteoblasts, which are bone-building cells. When that happens, the body takes the calcium it needs out of the bone, which, over time, can result in weakened bones that increase a person's risk for fractures. This activity further exacerbates the bone loss caused by oxidative stress and hormonal changes in aging.

Oxidative stress results from an imbalance between excessive environmental stress as a result of an overload of toxic by-products of metabolism causing cellular damage, and the capacity of the cell to build up an effective antioxidant response. It sounds complex, but luckily there's a remedy that's simple. For example, vitamin C—found in high amounts in almost all fruits and veggies—has been shown to exert its antioxidant powers enough to normalize bone mass and osteoblast activity. Antioxidants protect against oxidative stress, which in turn protects against inflammation. Over time, destructive inflammatory chemicals directly drive bone resorption, which is basically taking calcium away from the bones and interfering with the body's natural ability to repair bones. Vitamin C helps slow that resorption and promote repair mechanisms instead. Thankfully, this vitamin is easily accessed and absorbed in a high-quality, varied plant-based diet.

Your best bet to stave off arthritis? Eating low-inflammatory complex carbohydrate foods and herbs and spices; also, high-antioxidant fruits and veggies are the cornerstones of a diet that will keep your joints healthy. Some key "superfoods" to keep in mind in this area include:

Turmeric: a natural pain reliever and anti-inflammatory. Other spices and herbs, such as ginger, cinnamon, thyme, cayenne, oregano, and basil, all have anti-inflammatory properties.

Omega-3 fats: Sources include dark green leafy vegetables, flaxseeds, chia seeds, hemp, and walnuts. These can help balance out an excessive inflammatory response.

Sulfur-containing foods, such as onion, garlic, asparagus, broccoli, and cabbage. These foods contain a form of sulfur, methylsulfonylmethane (MSM), that reduces joint inflammation and helps rebuild tissues.

Natural enzymes in raw fruits: Examples are bromelain and papain in pineapple and papaya, respectively. In addition to these foods' improving digestion, the proteolytic enzymes contained in them help break down and control inflammatory proteins, which aids in healing and pain relief.

Fermented foods, such as sauerkraut, kimchi, vegan yogurt (almond-, coconut-, cashew-, or soy-based), tempeh, and miso. These keep the gut healthy, which minimizes total body inflammation, and also optimize the intestinal environment for properly digesting and absorbing nutrients.

And then, get moving! Those suffering from joint inflammation tend to pursue less physical activity, yet movement is actually the best way to both improve joint function and relieve chronic pain in the long run. A lack of activity then creates more risk for other chronic diseases, such as heart disease and diabetes, lowered bone density and risk for injuries, and increased risk for both anxiety and depression.

The body wants to move, the muscles and joints want to do their job, and healthy blood circulation depends on a certain amount of physical activity to avoid stagnancy. Movement makes the whole system happy! Simply walking on a regular basis can bring about noticeable change. With arthritis, choose exercise that is easy on joints, such as swimming, water aerobics, and gentle stretching.

Furthermore, the strength of bones is stimulated by resistance work. The bones that form your jaw and teeth are also dynamic. So, as you strengthen your bones, you are also helping to maintain the strength in your teeth. Chewing is great exercise for keeping the jaw strong and the teeth protected. Another reason to chomp on veggies on a daily basis!

Muscles: It's Never Too Late to Tone Up

People tend to lose muscle mass as they age—*sarcopenia* is the term for degeneration

---

AGE-DEFYING ADVICE:
PROTECT YOUR TEETH

The health of your mouth is a reflection of the health of your body. Osteoporosis is often the underlying cause of tooth loss. In addition, studies have linked gum inflammation with cognitive decline.

Keeping the oral cavity moist and stimulating saliva flow are important because saliva acts as a natural cleanser and reduces the likelihood of cavities. Saliva, which contains necessary minerals, is critical to preventing mineral loss in tooth enamel. Some tips for protecting your oral health:

- Reduce gum irritation by rinsing and flossing after you eat, to clean away food particles located in those hard-to-reach places.
- Be conscious of teeth grinding or jaw clenching, which can contribute to gum recession.
- Brighten your smile and neutralize the acid found in plaque by consuming garlic, ginger, citrus fruits, and apples.
- Take a break between snacks and meals to give salivary glands, teeth, and jaws the proper rest they need.

- Brush or swish with some coconut oil before eating to prevent food from sticking to your teeth. Coconut oil also helps neutralize harmful bacteria and supports tooth enamel.
- Organic neem oil has antimicrobial properties that can prevent dental and gum diseases. Apply a few drops of neem oil to your dental floss before using, or put neem oil or powder on your toothbrush before brushing.
- Organic green tea extract may slow tooth decay and help freshen breath. Green tea extract is available in supplement form.
- Make sure you get plenty of vitamin C! It can reduce gum inflammation and repair soft tissues.
- Xylitol is a natural sweetener extracted from woody fibrous plant material that helps treat cavities and prevent tooth decay by stopping bacteria from sticking to teeth. You can try replacing sugar in your coffee, tea, or cooking with xylitol, or chew gum that contains it.

THE ULTIMATE AGE-DEFYING PLAN

of muscle as a result of aging or nutritional deficiency. It can happen sooner than you think. For most people, the process begins in their 30s and 40s, with a loss of up to 8 percent per decade until around age 70, after which the loss increases to 15 percent per decade.

What happens when your muscles decline? Changes that occur with sarcopenia in aging include:

- **Slowed metabolism.** Decrease in resting metabolic rate results in a loss of lean-muscle mass and decreases in overall physical activity. Resting metabolic rate is the amount of energy needed to perform your body's basic function, and a measurement of how many calories your body burns when it is at rest.
- **Frailty syndrome.** Characterized by groups of such symptoms as weakness, fatigue, weight loss, lowered physical ability, poor balance, and lowered speed of motion. While this is commonly seen as a geriatric problem, it can be seen at any age, particularly in those who have undereaten for years in an effort to be thin and in turn have nutrient deficits along with significant fat stores and low muscle mass.
- **Fatty infiltration.** This happens when muscle fibers are replaced by fat (adipose tissue). This significantly decreases muscle strength and can lead to loss of mobility. Unfortunately this process has become increasingly common at younger ages; however, it is

highly responsive to regular exercise, which can also speed up metabolism. It's never too late!

There's a reason people are more susceptible to falls and fractures as they get older. Keep in mind that the processes of sarcopenia and osteoporosis occur nearly simultaneously. If you're losing bone mass, weakened muscles probably aren't far behind, and vice versa. Loss of lean muscle mass, strength, and mobility are all critical factors in aging, which are further compounded by typical changes in nutritional and hormonal status. Falls and fractures in the elderly are usually attributable to loss of muscle mass, with the hip sometimes fracturing even before the fall takes place. (Small fractures can occur and go unnoticed. Like a crack in a windshield, the cracks can accumulate and grow until stability decreases to the point that a minor fall can then result in a complete fracture of the bone.) Not surprisingly, the degree of fatty infiltration in muscles has been found to increase the risk of hip fractures.

Skeletal muscle, which is attached to bones for movement, is different from smooth muscle found in the inner body around organs and blood vessels. As an organ system, the skeletal muscle system plays an important role in overall wellness. Skeletal muscles represent up to 40 percent of the total body mass and contain 50 to 75 percent of all body proteins. Skeletal muscle acts as an endocrine organ by secreting hormones that regulate insulin metabolism and stimulate healthy protein synthesis through muscle building. Having healthy muscle mass essentially protects you from diabetes because it creates a need for insulin to move glucose out of your blood and into tissues for muscle building. Other hormones secreted by muscle, called myokines, are known to be brain-protective, antitumor, and anti-inflammatory. "Nourishing, building, and strengthening this complex organ system by building lean muscle mass is one of the most fundamental ways to increase vitality," says naturopathic physician Tyna Moore, ND, DC.

Again, we come back to "use or lose it." Making an effort to build muscle mass at any age has major benefits for the whole body. Muscle strength can be the answer to chronic degeneration. It can help reverse tissue atrophy and loss of integrity, inflammation, obesity, blood sugar dysregulation, hormonal decline and related decreased libido, brain atrophy, and a decline in immunity.

The simplest and fastest route to avoid or reverse sarcopenia is by lifting heavy things regularly. Strength training through lifting weights will accomplish this. Of course, safe practices, such as proper alignment, are important. The guidance of a personal trainer can help ensure safety and success.

Resistance training even appears to reverse the aging process at the cellular level, by stimulating repair to the mitochondria, the cells' power source, from the damage caused by inactivity. Another immediate response to strength training is pain reduction. Clinical studies in patients with fibromyalgia, neck pain, back pain, and joint pain consistently support strength training as an effective pain reliever. Even though working out may be the last thing you want to do when you're in pain, some strength training will be much more beneficial in the long term than resting.

Yet another exciting benefit of strength training? It also appears to strengthen the immune system. One small study looked at ten female multiple sclerosis (MS) patients who participated in an eight-week program of twice-weekly progressive resistance training. The results suggest that progressive resistance training may produce positive changes in circulating immune proteins that can benefit individuals with MS, and should be looked at more closely in larger studies. Older people who do some form of regular physical conditioning exercise have shown to better maintain a healthy immune system. They tend to suffer from less acute illnesses and recover faster from infections like colds and flu.

Overall, the antiaging effects of strength training rely on its ability to stimulate the body's maintenance and repair pathways. Therefore, proper training as well as adequate recovery and refeeding, with nourishing plant foods, is where the magic lies in successful strength training.

Good sources of the nine essential amino acids required for growth and maintenance are quite varied: sea vegetables, leafy greens, watercress, parsley, broccoli, spinach, seeds (such as pumpkin, hemp, chia, sesame, sunflower), nuts (such as cashews, almonds, Brazil nuts), legumes (such as soy, lentils, chickpeas, peas), chlorella, avocado, figs, olives, berries, whole grains (such as quinoa, amaranth, rice, sprouted whole wheat [if tolerated], oats), pumpkin, sweet potatoes, beets, raisins, asparagus, mushrooms, and more. Getting a wide variety of these foods will ensure that you are taking in all nine amino acids on a regular basis.

Top Nutrients for Better Bones, Joints, and Muscles

Vitamin D is needed to absorb calcium, reduce its excretion in the kidneys, and direct it into bone. A vitamin D deficiency can begin the process of osteomalacia, which is the softening of bones.

How to get more vitamin D: supplements and sun exposure

Protein: You don't want to neglect the importance of providing the building blocks of all tissues from adequate protein.

How to make sure you're getting enough: You can use dietician Ginny Messina's

---

WHY DO YOU SHRINK WITH AGE?

This section may make you want to check your posture. It seems that, on average, people do begin to lose ¼ to ½ inch in height every decade after age 40 to 50. In addition, research from the Baltimore Longitudinal Study of Aging found that women lost an average of 2 inches between the ages of 30 and 70 (and just over 3 inches by age 80), while men lost a little more than 1 inch by age 70 (and 2 inches by age 80). Of course these numbers average out a wide variability, and some people do not lose height at all.

What is it all about? Well, there are a few reasons for this, most involving the health and maintenance of the structures of the spine. Discs between the vertebrae in the spine can become dehydrated and compressed. With loss of bone density, the spine can become more curved, and vertebrae can collapse, leading to painful compression fractures. In addition, things like muscle loss in the torso resulting in stooped posture and the gradual flattening of the arches of the feet can make also make you slightly shorter.

Of course, genetics plays a big role, as does the level of strong bone you built when you were young. But doing what you can now to protect your bones and muscles will help slow shrinkage by keeping your structure aligned and strong. An older Belgian study published in *Gerontology* found that people who did moderate aerobic exercise throughout their life had less height shrinkage than those who were sedentary all their life or who stopped exercising after age 40. Specific exercise techniques, such as yoga for aging, Pilates, and the Alexander technique, can effectively reprogram the body into better posture and alignment (these techniques can also provide tremendous chronic pain relief).

So, don't despair, keep doing simple weight-bearing exercises; get a little daily sunshine; load up on plenty of the mineral- and protein-rich plant foods that we have discussed here; take in ample amounts of liquid, in the form of water, soups, pure juices, and fruits; keep alcohol to a minimum; and quit smoking, and you just may be able to hold on to that ½ inch!

---

formula: multiply your healthy body weight by 0.4 to see how many grams of protein to aim for. (For example, if you weigh 140 pounds, you should aim for 56 grams of protein per day.) Easy to get with a variety of legumes, grains, nuts, seeds, and veggies. As a guideline, a serving (3.5 ounces) of edamame, tofu, or tempeh has 10 to 19 grams, a cup of cooked lentils has 18 grams, an ounce of nutritional yeast has 14 grams, an ounce of hempseed has 10 grams, amaranth and quinoa have 8 to 9 grams per cup cooked, nuts typically have around 7 grams per ounce, and such veggies as broccoli, spinach, asparagus, artichokes, or sweet potatoes usually provide 4 to 5 grams per cup cooked.

B vitamins all play a role in bone health and most are easily found in a plant-based diet. However, B_{12} is less available in plants and can become deficient in all aging individuals due to lowered absorption in the gut, so supplementing is a good consideration regardless of diet, and essential if your diet is purely plant based. Vitamins B_2, B_6, and B_9 (folate) are also needed particularly in the formation and function of osteoblasts, which are the bone-building cells. (See page 17 for more on B vitamins.)

Vitamin C prevents bone loss through its role in the synthesis of connective tissue as well as keeping the blood more alkaline for mineral balance.

How to consume more vitamin C: Some good sources are papaya, bell peppers, citrus, broccoli, Brussels sprouts, cauliflower, strawberries, kiwi, and kale. Recommended amounts usually refer to supplementation during times of increased need, and can range from 500 to 1,000 milligrams or even much higher. Because vitamin C is water-soluble and quickly excreted through the kidneys, there is no real danger in taking an excess amount, besides potential digestive discomfort as the body releases it.

Calcium is stored in bone matrix to provide strength; needed in balance with other nutrients for true bone structure (like bricks need mortar).

How to consume more calcium: collards, kale, bok choy, (calcium-precipitated) tofu, tempeh, figs, tahini, blackstrap molasses, almond butter, okra

Phosphorus is also important in balance with calcium to build strong bones. The kidneys will filter out most excess, and it is very easy to get enough because all plants contain it.

In recent years, some controversy has unfolded about health risks involved with excessive dietary intake of phosphorus from high consumption of soft drinks containing phosphoric acid and processed foods containing phosphate stabilizers, emulsifiers, anticaking agents, and acidity regulators. A diet based on whole natural foods rather than processed foods is likely to avoid excessive phosphorus risks. High levels of phosphorus will lead to a need for more blood calcium, potentially decreasing calcium loss in the urine, increasing calcium absorption from foods (indirectly, via activation of vitamin D), and pulling calcium from the bones. Soft drinks can contain added phosphoric acid in amounts of 400 to 600 milligrams per can or bottle, enough to cause damage especially with a daily habit.

Magnesium: Up to 60 percent of your magnesium is concentrated in your bones and the remaining is found in soft tissue and blood. The constant high demand for magnesium in so many biochemical processes can lead to a depleted supply in cells. As a result, cells are forced to pull what limited magnesium concentration is found in a delicate balance out of bone formations. Low levels of blood magnesium affects heart rate, nervous function, and can lead to chronic headaches and muscle spasms.

How to consume more magnesium: greens, beans, avocados, dark chocolate, seeds, and dried fruits

Potassium balances out acidity in the blood to prevent calcium loss. A plant-based diet high in potassium will result in less acidic urine, which signifies a healthy acid-alkali balance in the body.

How to consume more potassium: legumes, avocados, beet greens, spinach, chard, sweet potatoes

Vitamin K needed for the activation of protein in bones and for adequate bone mineral density.

How to consume more vitamin K: leafy green veggies, natto, broccoli, cabbage, green tea, green peas

Omega-3 fatty acids reduce inflammation in the body, helping reduce pain and joint swelling and lowering the risk of osteoporosis and rheumatoid arthritis. They help promote healing and growth with strength training. Healthy fats also help provide sustained energy for exercise. They are needed in the absorption of necessary fat-soluble vitamins, such as vitamins A, D, E, and K.

How to consume more omega-3s: flax, hemp, pumpkin, and chia seeds; avocados, walnuts, and leafy greens. Tip: Try buying your nuts and seeds raw and toasting them yourself for optimal freshness and to improve digestion. (The exceptions are chia, hemp, and ground flaxseeds, which should always be eaten raw. Flaxseeds should be freshly ground and kept in the freezer between uses.)

Trace minerals, such as zinc, copper, molybdenum, manganese, iodine, and chromium, can be obtained by adding plenty of herbs and spices, and sea vegetables, such as arame, wakame, and nori, to your cooking. These are essential for proper tissue health. Minerals work collaboratively in the body, so the more mineral variety and density you take in from foods that come straight from the earth, the better off you will be. Also, obtaining them in plant form, rather than as supplements, will be more balanced to prevent any overconsumption or deficiencies.

AGE-DEFYING ADVICE:
BONE, JOINT, AND MUSCLE HEALTH

Eat More:

Nuts and seeds, which have plenty of protein, minerals, and anti-inflammatory healthy fat. Maintain a reasonable intake, such as a handful, as a guide, or a small amount sprinkled onto a salad or veggie bowl.

Green leafy veggies, which contain a wide range of bone-supportive nutrients, such as calcium, vitamin K, boron, magnesium, omega-3s, and potassium. Eat these in abundance.

Vitamin C–rich fruits and veggies, such as kiwi, citrus, berries, cherries, mangoes, papaya, pineapple, guava, melons, peppers, onions, broccoli, cauliflower, Brussels sprouts, cabbage, spinach, tomatoes, squash, sweet potatoes, and okra. Supplement for extra C if needed.

Soy, which has a phytoestrogen effect in maintaining bone, and is also high in calcium. Always go organic.

Beans and legumes, which are top sources of lean protein, with plenty of fiber and an array of necessary tissue-building minerals

Whole grains, especially iron- and protein-rich quinoa and amaranth

Celtic or Himalayan sea salt, for healthy mineral electrolyte balance

Trace minerals, such as zinc, copper, molybdenum, manganese, iodine, and chromium, for optimal tissue healing. Cook with plenty of herbs, spices, and sea vegetables, such as arame, wakame, or nori.

Drink More:

Mineral water, from a natural spring source for additional mineral balance, including potassium and magnesium. Mineral profiles will be different depending on the source, so check labels.

Herbal teas and infusions, which can be a great way to increase minerals and overall tissue nourishment to increase building and repair and lower inflammation. Some mineral-rich medicinal herbs to try are oat straw, nettle, red clover, alfalfa, horsetail, and dandelion. Either singly or in combination, use 1 tablespoon of dried herb per 8-ounce cup and steep for 3 to 5 minutes. You can also find these in prepared blends in tea bags.

Do More:

Walking daily, for at least 20 to 30 minutes

Stretching, morning and evening

Mini trampoline (rebounder)

Safe weight-bearing exercises; for example, stand on one foot for 3 minutes and other foot for 3 minutes at a time

Weight lifting. Start small with 2- to 5-pound weights; if you can easily do at least 20 reps, add more weight as you can safely handle.

TheraBand exercises: There are numerous videos and resources online.

Swimming, walking in water

Get daily sun exposure for plenty of vitamin D!

Try these movement-friendly recipes with foods and nutrients mentioned above:

Nourishing Tonic (page 122)

Ancient Sunrise (page 135)

Sunny Kale Salad (page 162)

Salad in a Jar (page 157) with Turmeric Tahini Dressing (page 172)

Himalayan Lentils and Greens (page 214)

Raw Choco-Cherry Bombs (page 281)

FOUNTAIN OF YOUTHER

Name: Ellen Jaffe Jones
Birth Year: 1952

About Ellen: Ellen Jaffe Jones is an inspiring motivational speaker on the US Vegfest circuit and at other venues, a certified personal trainer, running coach, vegan lifestyle coach, and healthy cooking class instructor. Ellen became a media consultant for the Physicians Committee for Responsible Medicine, where she began teaching cooking classes that hatched the idea for her first book, *Eat Vegan on $4 a Day*. She has currently placed in 130 5K or longer races for her age group and has done two marathons and a dozen half marathons since 2006, "just" on plants. www.vegcoach.com

Typical Daily Meals: Breakfast: slow-cooked oats with berries, flax/hemp seeds, and sliced almonds or walnuts. Lunch: Ginormous salad (one of the perks of working at Fit2Run is it has a smoothie and food bar that is a vegan dream). Dinner: Whole grains, such as quinoa, brown or wild rice, millet, or wheat berries, with lots of cooked veggies, sometimes the kind premixed at the store; soup during cold weather, such as miso/seaweed or veg/bean combo. I eat whole food plants. Low-fat, stir-fried, or sautéed veggies. An occasional premade frozen burrito or mostly vegetables-showing veggie burger.

Typical Exercise/Lifestyle: I try to run 3 miles at least every other day. I've read tons of books on senior fitness and running, and have written my own, *Vegan Fitness for Mortals* . . . because not all of us are designed, meant, or want to run 100 miles at a time. [At races] sometimes I joke, I win my age group because I show up. Working fitness into my daily routine is crucial. I also do a series of core exercises to stay strong, such as planks and baby crunches, along with high-intensity sprints to work on speed. Having a strong core is crucial to keeping a strong back.

Ellen says: Running and a vegan diet are magical. Now that I work in the running industry, I get multiple people every day saying things like, "My god, you are two years older than me and you look twenty years younger!" I've been asked to show my driver's license. People ask if I dye my hair. Every day, someone does a double take when they find out my age or I tell them, which I often do. Remaining fit keeps you positive and focused in an increasingly crazy and disconnected world.

FIVE

PROTECT YOUR HEART FOR THE LONG RUN

Let's get to the heart of the matter. Your heart is essentially what gives you life! In everything you do, beat by beat, your physical heart is working to keep you going, circulating oxygen and nutrients in the blood to keep your organs healthy, so that you may experience all the joy, connection, and warmth that you feel in your emotional heart. The trouble is that for many people, their heart is struggling to keep up with their unbalanced lifestyle.

Heart disease has a direct impact on longevity—it is still the number one cause of death in both men and women in the United States and worldwide. Heart disease starts with cholesterol-heavy plaques developing in the walls of the arteries that supply the heart (the coronary arteries). This disease process is called atherosclerosis. These ragged plaques encroach upon the blood flow channel of the coronary arteries and can trigger the formation of blood clots—which then stop blood flow to the heart muscle.

This injury can result in ischemia, arrhythmias, angina, and congestive heart failure, which are all forms of heart disease. Many people live with these diseases for years, but often they are not well controlled despite potent medications. These conditions are what lead to heart attacks, strokes, or embolism, which are all tragic consequences of some form of inadequate blood flow through the blood vessels.

Hypertension is consistent high blood pressure over time. It's often called the "silent killer" because it may not cause symptoms until it's too late. It is important to have your blood pressure checked regularly.

Arrhythmias are irregularities in heartbeat rate or rhythm, from changes in electrical impulses, which can cause too fast or too slow a heart rate. They can affect blood delivery to where it is needed and cause an array of symptoms, such as lightheadedness, dizziness, and feelings of flutter in the chest. There are many causes, which include structural abnormalities, long-term exposure to stimulants, and unmanaged emotional stress, along with the most common—and reversible—cause: clogging of the heart arteries from atherosclerosis. The abnormal rhythms are often treated with medications, but the whole food, plant-based diet presented in this book can melt away atherosclerotic plaques and restore blood flow to the injured cells that may be generating those abnormal rhythms.

Heart failure, also known as congestive heart failure, occurs when the heart is no longer able to pump adequate amounts of blood to meet the body's needs.

Angina: regular episodes of tightness in the chest due to reduced blood flow to the heart, usually with physical exertion. It can manifest in severe pain to arm, shoulders, and neck that can last from 1 to 15 minutes and is a sign of severe restriction of blood flow to the heart muscle.

Even without an exercise component, a plant-based diet can reduce angina attacks by more than 90 percent within twenty-four days. This has been shown in many studies since the 1970s, according to a report at nutritionfacts.org.

Ischemia is a restriction of blood supply to tissues of the heart or other organs. This is an early sign of low blood flow that can cause angina and lead to a heart attack or stroke.

Embolism: obstruction of an artery by a substance, usually either a blood clot, a fat globule, or an air bubble inside the artery. Emboli can affect blood flow to the brain (stroke), lungs (pulmonary embolism), or heart, impeding the organ's function.

Heart attack: a clot causing sudden blockage in a coronary artery supplying blood to the heart muscle, which may or may not cause pain and distress, and which often results in heart muscle damage.

Stroke: a sudden interruption of oxygenated blood to the brain, sometimes causing loss of speech, weakness, or paralysis and often leading to loss of brain cells damaged by deprivation of oxygen and glucose.

What increases your risk of heart disease?

- **Chronological age:** Heart disease risk begins to rise after age 55, as blood vessels can begin to stiffen and a lifelong buildup of plaque in the arteries starts interfering with the flow of blood.
- **Sex:** Men get heart disease about 10 years earlier than women do. Women are generally protected by estrogen until after menopause, when their heart disease risk begins to match that of men.
- **Family history:** Your risk of heart disease is higher if your father or brother was diagnosed with it before age 55, or your mother or sister before age 65.

- **Blood pressure:** Blood pressure above 120/80 mm Hg over time ages your heart.
- **Cholesterol:** The higher your cholesterol level, the older your heart.
- **Smoking:** Any smoking raises the risk of heart attack, even if it's only once in a while. It's time to quit if you haven't already. Exposure to secondhand smoke can be dangerous, too.
- **Weight:** Being overweight or obese puts extra demands on your heart.
- **Diabetes:** Diabetes or prediabetes puts you at greater risk for heart problems because high blood glucose can damage blood vessels to the heart and contribute to atherosclerosis.

Fortunately, we can say with confidence that heart disease can be both prevented and reversed by choosing whole plant foods as the basis for most every meal. Thanks to pioneering physicians Dean Ornish, Caldwell Esselstyn, Neal Barnard, Joel Kahn, Kim Williams, and a growing number of others there is often an alternative to bypass surgery that is simple, lifelong, and has only positive side effects!

In fact, there is one big heart disease risk factor you can absolutely control through your diet: your cholesterol. Let's take a closer look.

Cholesterol

Yes, the topic of cholesterol can be one of the most confusing in nutrition right now.

You may have read or heard conflicting things. Is cholesterol good for you? Bad for you? Should you eat it? Avoid it? Let's set the record straight.

First of All, What Is Cholesterol?

Cholesterol is a waxy, fatlike substance needed to maintain the integrity and fluidity of the membrane structure of all cells, especially in the brain. Your body also needs it to produce hormones, vitamin D, and enzymes.

Cholesterol travels through your bloodstream in small packages called lipoproteins, which are made of fats on the inside and proteins on the outside. Two kinds of lipoproteins carry cholesterol throughout your body: low-density lipoproteins (LDL) and high-density lipoproteins (HDL). A high LDL level—what you may have heard referred to as "bad" cholesterol—can lead to a dangerous buildup of cholesterol in your arteries, and even affect the brain.

"Unhealthy patterns of cholesterol could be directly causing the higher levels of amyloid known to contribute to Alzheimer's, in the same way that such patterns promote heart disease," says Bruce Reed, MD, a study researcher and a codirector of the UC-Davis Alzheimer's Disease Center. A higher HDL level—the so-called "good" cholesterol—is helpful because it carries cholesterol from other parts of your body back to your liver, which then removes the excess cholesterol from your body.

While cholesterol is essential in the diet for important processes such as the production of important hormones, creation of bile for fat digestion, cell membrane structure, and proper brain cell signaling, it does not mean that more is better, or that we can ignore the well-established dangers of excess cholesterol from eating animal fats. Current understanding is that it is not the cholesterol that is "bad" or "good," but that the lipoprotein carriers (HDL and LDL) can be susceptible to differing amounts of damage, turning on the inflammatory processes. This, in our opinion, places the emphasis back on the importance of diet—preventing excess inflammation in the body through a whole food, nonprocessed, noninflammatory diet and lifestyle, rather than simply looking at cholesterol levels.

Why Do You Need Cholesterol?

Did you know that your body is capable of manufacturing all the cholesterol it needs? In fact, each cell synthesizes cholesterol through a complex process.

This cholesterol is vital to strengthening the membranes of each and every cell in the body. It is also important in the production of many hormones in the body, including estrogen, progesterone, cortisone, and aldosterone. These steroid hormones help the body manage stress and balance sodium and water in the body, not to mention regulate sexual function.

Cholesterol is so important that the body can make it out of anything—fats, carbohydrates, or proteins. You don't have to eat cholesterol to make cholesterol, but you do need to eat real foods. Animal products, including meats and dairy, contain cholesterol

itself from the animal, as well as saturated and even trans fats, which stimulate your liver to make even more. Eating these is a surefire way to raise both cholesterol levels and dangerous inflammation in the body.

Trans-fatty acids (natural in animal fats and synthetic in many processed store-bought foods) as well as elevated levels of blood sugar can interfere with normal cholesterol metabolism. For some people, tropical oils, such as palm oil, palm kernel oil, and coconut oil, also can trigger the liver to make more cholesterol. Be particularly careful of packaged and processed oils, which are susceptible to rancidity and therefore not able to be used in the body. Some people can handle a little oil, especially if it is on the low end of the processed spectrum. *Cold-pressed*, *virgin*, and *unrefined* describe oils that are closer to their natural form. Highly refined vegetables oils should be avoided along with animal fats. While some recipes in the book do call for small amounts of the less-processed oils, all the recipes have a completely oil-free option.

Why Medications Are Not the Answer

Statin medication to reduce total cholesterol has been the most prevalent preventive treatment for both heart disease and dementia. A 2011 study found over 32 million Americans are taking a statin drug. But statins are not without some serious drawbacks. The side effects are numerous while the efficacy and safety of these drugs continue to be questionable, despite their prevalence.

It is important to keep in mind that statins are not benign drugs, as they are associated with a host of side effects, including muscle aches and pains, neuropathy, diabetes, and cancer. Moreover, their effectiveness in preventing heart attacks and strokes has been extremely low! Many cardiologists are now "going rogue" by instead promoting low-fat, plant-based diets, including whole grains, as the answer for preventing and reversing heart disease, while avoiding potential negative effects from long term statin use.

Here's the thing. Your body's cholesterol synthesis pathway doesn't just make cholesterol. Branches of this same pathway are responsible for metabolizing a wide variety of other molecules, including vitamins A, E, and K, and coenzyme Q (CoQ10), an important antioxidant the body makes for energy use and muscle maintenance, among other things. Statins block all of these. In fact, you may have noticed a sudden interest in CoQ10 supplementation, which increased when statins came along and created widespread deficiency.

Statin drugs also cross the blood-brain barrier and can therefore reduce the cellular production of lipoproteins there. Essentially, statins do not allow brain cells to produce the cholesterol they may need, and are suspected to be another risk factor for dementia and brain decline.

Healing Your Heart Through Diet

It is important to not only avoid the potential for oxidized cholesterol by lowering inflammation, but also to help support your body's natural way of eliminating excess fat and cholesterol through the liver. Because your body produces cholesterol, it is not necessary to acquire it at all from food. Keep in mind that while saturated fats and trans fats are troublesome in and of themselves, they are also dangerous because they both increase the dangerous LDL cholesterol.

Many experts agree that the closer you get to a whole food, plant-based diet, the better. Just by cutting down on animal foods (which have no fiber), you may lower your cholesterol 5 to 10 percent. If you go a step further and adopt a vegetarian diet, your cholesterol level may drop 10 to 15 percent. Eating vegan may get you down 15 to 25 percent, and consuming a minimally processed, plant-based diet may decrease your cholesterol levels by 35 percent or more.

The amount of confirming studies on this subject can fill an entire book. One that stands out is Dr. Esselstyn's arrest and reversal study in which he clearly showed coronary artery blockages dissolving after only a few weeks on his strict whole food, plant-based protocol. It is quite dramatic to view the slides that show the before and after effect on the arteries! The current mainstream model for diagnosing and treating heart disease is built around the authoritative Framingham Heart Study, started in 1948, which originated the term *risk factor* as one of the first studies to look at prevention. This study has been used to create a popular "risk calculator" that most mainstream cardiologists use to guide treatment decisions, such as prescribing statin medications or hypertensive drugs to reduce blood pressure. According to Framingham, the number one risk factor for cardiovascular disease is chronological age in and of itself. This is what brought about recommendations such as daily aspirin for people over a certain age. But according to cardiologist Dr. Joel Kahn, "Framingham just isn't adequate anymore." He insists, "It doesn't address inflammatory markers, environmental stressors, and all the other factors we know about. We've stalled because of the complexity of cardiovascular disease."

Beyond cholesterol, such factors as low blood levels of omega-3 fatty acids, elevated C-reactive protein (a marker of inflammation in the body), excess insulin, deficiency in nitric oxide, low levels of vitamin K and of vitamin D, hormone imbalance, and excess homocysteine are also important in assessing overall heart disease risk. Kahn says simply, "Live well, eat well, exercise well, sleep well, and sweat a bit."

Here are some dietary steps you can take:

Do everything possible to support healthy *nitric oxide* levels. Nitric oxide is critical to healthy arterial function. The top way to increase nitric oxide is by increasing leafy greens, such as chard, kale, spinach, and arugula, and green herbs, such as cilantro, basil, parsley, and dill, in your diet. Studies show that increasing blood levels of L-arginine, found in many plant foods, such as pumpkin seeds, sesame seeds or tahini, almonds, peanuts, soybeans, and beets, can also benefit nitric oxide levels. Remember to avoid roasted and salted nuts and seeds, and that a small amount is plenty enough. Arginine is converted to nitric acid, which will cause blood vessels to relax and dilate, dramatically increasing blood flow through

them. Just a small increase in diameter translates into a huge improvement in blood flow. For example, if you double the radius of a vessel, your blood flow is sixteen times as great!

To help boost nitric oxide, Dr. Kahn first recommends lifestyle modifications, such as getting more exercise and juicing. Green tea and pomegranate extract are both beneficial as well.

Lower your homocysteine. More recently, there has been a focus on preventing atherosclerosis (clogging of the arteries) and heart disease by lowering blood plasma levels of the amino acid homocysteine. This can usually be accomplished by increasing the intake of vitamins B_6, B_9 (folate), and B_{12}. Another nutrient to consider is choline from plant-based sources, which, as it is metabolized into betaine, can help lower homocysteine. Such B vitamin–rich foods as cauliflower, avocados, sunflower and sesame seeds, pinto beans, blackstrap molasses, B_{12}-fortified plant milks, and nutritional yeast may be considerations for helping to keep homocysteine in balance. Keep in mind, however, that high levels of choline, as found in animal products, energy drinks, and choline supplements, can also be metabolized into trimethylamine oxide (TMAO), which can damage arteries. Sticking with plants won't do this.

Get more vitamin D. A number of studies have linked low blood levels of vitamin D with increased arterial stiffness and endothelial dysfunction, more fatal strokes, and even a higher risk of fatal cancer among patients with cardiovascular disease.

Researchers at Copenhagen University Hospital and the University of Copenhagen reviewed data from studies of more than ten thousand Danes and compared those with the lowest levels of vitamin D (less than 15 ng/mL) to those with the highest levels (more than 50 ng/mL). What they found is that those with low levels of vitamin D (versus the optimal level) were 64 percent more likely to have a heart attack. Plus, they had a 40 percent higher risk of ischemic heart disease, a 57 percent increased risk of early death, and an 81 percent higher risk of dying from heart disease.

Vitamin K is a fat-soluble vitamin necessary for proper blood clotting. It is also an antioxidant that can help slow the process of atherosclerosis. A deficiency in vitamin K has been associated with increased calcium deposition and coronary artery calcification. Leafy greens, such as kale, chard, and spinach, provide lots of vitamin K and should be enjoyed daily (and some authorities say several times a day!) for optimal health and disease prevention.

Magnesium is responsible for the function of muscle contraction and heart rhythm. As previously mentioned, magnesium assists in regulating nerve impulses by relaxing smooth muscles, such as those around arteries. More reasons to consume plenty of dark leafy greens, as well as moderate amounts of sesame and pumpkin seeds, avocados, almonds, figs, and the darkest chocolate you can find.

Hydrate. Simply drinking water pumps up the liquid volume of blood, which reduces the risk for blood clots.

Antioxidants are your radiation armor. Have an extra-large dose of leafy greens, a green smoothie, or more colorful veggies before traveling by plane, receiving any radioactive medical scans, and doing vigorous exercise at high elevations or areas with a lot of pollution, to help keep oxidative damage in check.

Eat heart-healthy superfoods. The following foods may be especially protective:

- **Hawthorn berry** is now being studied clinically for its ability to normalize heart arrhythmias. The whole berries made into a tea or syrup are a delicious way to add extra nourishment to your heart while supporting its regular rhythms.
- The thick skin of all **berries** and also **grapes** is specifically protective by strengthening the blood vessel lining and by keeping platelets from becoming overactivated.
- **Ginger, garlic, and turmeric** can increase circulation and block cholesterol uptake in the gut. These three are all well-known anti-inflammatory and antioxidant foods.
- **Cacao** contains flavonoids that can decrease LDL, increase HDL, and reduce platelet stickiness. It is also a great source of magnesium, which is important in calming spasms in smooth

muscle, improving blood vessel health and heart rhythms.

Green tea contains a powerful antioxidant called EGCG, which has been a popular subject of numerous recent studies on several health benefits, including cardiovascular and metabolic health. Drinking green tea seems to help prevent heart disease by helping lower LDL and triglycerides.

Hibiscus tea is known to lower chronically high blood pressure. In a Tufts University study, drinking hibiscus tea (3 cups daily) lowered participants' systolic blood pressure by 7 points in six weeks on average, matching or outperforming many prescription medications.

Four More Ways to Protect Your Heart

1. **Exercise:** Regular exercise results in a strong heart and open blood vessels, which equal optimal blood flow. Dr. Dean Ornish, who has a powerful program for preventing and reversing

---

HIGH BLOOD PRESSURE AND THE SODIUM-POTASSIUM CONNECTION

Sodium is an essential mineral for life, but most people consume too much. The typical daily intake is about 3,300 mg, yet your body needs only about 200 mg of sodium a day. Most of the excess comes from salt added to processed foods, beverages, and restaurant meals. Too much sodium can result in high blood volume and is known to be a major risk factor for hypertension.

It's wise to limit sodium, but it might be wiser still to eat a high-quality diet rich in potassium, which blunts sodium's negative effects. The more potassium you eat, the more sodium you pass out of your body through urine. Potassium also helps relax blood vessel walls to lower blood pressure. The easiest way to throw your sodium-potassium ratio off kilter is by consuming a diet of processed foods, which are notoriously low in potassium while high in sodium.

Symptoms of low potassium include water retention, raised blood pressure, heart irregularities/arrhythmias, muscular weakness and muscle cramps, continual thirst, constipation, and confusion or irritability. If experiencing any of these, ask yourself, *Am I eating enough plants?* The best way to keep your potassium levels in the right range is to get it from foods, which are balanced with other minerals. Potatoes, bananas, avocados, leafy greens, nuts, apricots, and mushrooms are high in potassium. You can also switch up your salt. Processed table salt contains 97.5 percent sodium chloride. The rest is man-made chemicals. Instead, we recommend natural unprocessed salt, which contains about 84 percent sodium chloride. The remaining 16 percent is naturally occurring trace minerals. In particular, Himalayan salt is much higher in potassium and lower in sodium compared to other salts. Himalayan salt contains 0.28 percent potassium, compared to 0.16 percent in Celtic salt, and 0.09 percent in regular table salt.

heart disease, suggests increasing one's general level of activity and making exercise a part of daily life. Include at least 20 minutes of daily aerobic exercise.

2. **Spend time barefoot on the earth.** According to cardiologist Dr. Stephen Sinatra, simply regrounding your body by making direct contact with the bare earth has many profound benefits to our health, including heart health. This may be as simple as walking barefoot in the grass, on the beach, or in dirt or mud. The "Earthing" theory is that the earth's surface contains free electrons that are continually replenished through natural processes, and your body naturally absorbs these particles when you make physical contact with the ground. Dr. Sinatra explains that chronic inflammation, the cause of many chronic diseases including heart disease, may be the result of an electron deficiency from lack of connection to the earth.

   At least a dozen studies have shown significant physiological benefits of having direct contact with the earth: decreased symptoms of inflammation, lowered stress and increased calmness in the body through moderation of nervous system activity and stress hormone secretion, improved blood pressure and circulation, and a reduction in chronic pain.

3. **Connect with your pulse.** Without counting, take a few minutes to notice the quality and rhythm of your pulse. Simply checking in and feeling your pulse can have a calming and normalizing effect. Check out the book *HeartMath Solution* that explores heart intelligence and the ability to intuitively use your own biofeedback to calm stress responses. The HeartMath Institute is now dedicated to teaching and developing tools for people to understand and interact with their heart intelligence as a powerful way to regain heart strength and health.

4. **Meditation/visualization:** Along with healthy plant foods and exercise, some form of stress management is essential to keeping the heart in balance. Meditation is a simple way to incorporate a few minutes of calm into your day. The latest research confirms that people who practice meditation are significantly less likely to have a heart attack or stroke or die within five years. You can find guided meditation recordings that use visualization to help get you started. Alternatively, you can take five minutes any time of day to practice a few rounds of deep but easy breathing, keeping your attention focused on the nostrils where your breath is going in and out. Doing some form of this regularly reduces stress and anxiety, which can lower heart rate and blood pressure while reducing overactivity of stress hormones, such as cortisol.

For more information on ways to keep your heart healthy, we also recommend Dr.

Dean Ornish's work. He has been a pioneer in revolutionizing the way to think about health and disease, by having the courage to stand by a simplified, holistic, pharmaceutical-free approach to prevent and reverse heart disease. His program has demonstrated much success over many years, and has opened the door for further research in the area of disease reversal through lifestyle changes.

The beat goes on! Day by day, through the foods you choose, you can bring health and vitality to the organ that brings life to all your other organs. As you see, regardless of your current state of heart health, there is much you can do to protect your heart to keep it strong for life.

AGE-DEFYING ADVICE:
CARDIO HEALTH

Eat More:
Antioxidant foods with plenty of potassium, magnesium, fiber, and healthy fats: berries, greens, oats, broccoli, cauliflower, dark chocolate, beets, sweet potatoes, apples, avocados, walnuts, figs, chia seeds, ground flaxseed, pumpkin seeds, garlic, ginger

Drink More:
Have a cup of green or herbal tea, such as hibiscus, hawthorn, ginger, turmeric, or cinnamon.
Consider trading an alcoholic beverage for a high-quality mineral water with a spritz of lemon or lime.

Do More:
Exercise. Do what you enjoy, and do it every day. Mix up such activities as walking, biking, hiking, swimming, yoga, or group sports to keep your heart healthy.

Walk barefoot outside for at least 30 minutes whenever possible.
Enjoy some sunshine often. Even sitting out on the patio counts.
Do 5 to 20 minutes of guided meditation or simple calm regulated breathing.
Connect to your pulse.

Try these heart-friendly recipes with foods and nutrients mentioned above:
Berry Chia Bowl with Pomegranate (page 130)
Oil-Free Roasted Red Pepper Dressing with a large mixed green salad or steamed greens (page 170)
Wilted Collard Salad (page 166)
Santorini Okra Tomato (page 177)
Braised Kale with Shallots and Slivered Almonds (page 185)
Jackfruit Taco Filling (page 216)
Salt-Free Seasoning (page 253)

THE ULTIMATE AGE-DEFYING PLAN

FOUNTAIN OF YOUTHER

Name: Joel Kahn, MD
Birth Year: 1959

About Joel: Dr. Joel Kahn trained in interventional cardiology and stopped thousands of heart attacks in their tracks. A preventive health expert, he opened the first heart disease reversal clinic in the Midwest (www.kahnlongevity center.com) and began to write, lecture, and do education TV. He opened Green-Space Café in Ferndale, Michigan, with his son Daniel and wife, Karen, which offers whole food, plant-based (WFPB) high-quality foods and drinks, now an expanding chain and food truck. He is the author of five books and a public television special (*The Whole Heart Solution*). www.drjoelkahn.com

Typical Daily Meals: WFPB lunch of salads, beans, grains, vinegars, ferments, sprouts. Snack of walnuts, whole fruit. Dinner at GreenSpace Café, such as grilled cauliflower steak.

Typical Exercise/Lifestyle: Practice yoga daily with 5 Tibetans flow. Daily Kirtan Kriya meditation. Often daily infrared sauna. Rotate treadmill, rowing, kayaking, SUP, spin class cardio.

Joel says: My motto is "Extreme in diet, moderate in exercise, abundant in love." My decision forty-plus years ago to adopt a WFPB diet has transformed my health, my energy, my career, and my future. It has made me a kinder person, more mindful, more patient, and more connected to family and friends. Put plants in your life, your heart . . . and your brain and you will live a life fulfilled and of meaning.

SIX

KIDNEY HEALTH IS KEY

You may be surprised to know that changes in kidney and urinary function are some of the first signs of aging. Inadequate nutrient and water intake can stress the kidneys, the amazing organs that permit the body to clean the blood of wastes and to absorb, use, and regulate fluids and minerals. Keeping your kidneys healthy is just another great reason to nourish your body with pure water and nutrient-dense plant foods throughout the day, every day.

Kidney Stress and the Urinary System

The kidneys are two kidney bean–shaped organs found in your lower midback, behind the lower lobes of your lungs. And they are hardworking! Among their many important functions, their chief role is to filter and cleanse the bloodstream, eliminating through the urine the fluid and by-products of foods or medicines that your body does not need. The kidneys filter the waste produced by normal body processes, such as protein breakdown, while maintaining the balance of acids and bases and other chemicals (electrolytes, heavy metals, etc.) needed in your blood and tissues. In addition, the kidneys play important roles both in controlling blood pressure and in the production of red blood cells.

Your kidneys are normally more than capable of meeting your body's demands for blood filtration, red blood cell production, acid-base regulation, and blood pressure control. Older kidneys, however, may not be as resilient as younger ones, especially if they have been stressed by conditions, such as chronic high blood pressure, diabetes, chronic NSAID (anti-inflammatory drug) ingestion, or atherosclerosis. The result may be a higher risk of fluid imbalances, buildup of waste products, and a decreased efficiency in removing drugs and other potential toxins from the body. The kidneys can usually withstand the extra demands placed on them for quite a while without causing noticeable symptoms, so be sure to take good care of them through healthy diet and lifestyle choices before any symptoms manifest.

Because the urinary system is working alongside the lungs, skin, and large intestine as other organs of elimination, the health of one is dependent on the health of each system. They are all being influenced daily by such things as hydration levels, food choices, medications, and environmental exposures. The amount of fluid and waste released into the bladder for excretion may depend on how much is released through the other elimination pathways in the breath, sweat, and gastrointestinal system.

The health of the lower sections of the urinary pathway—the ureters, bladder, and urethra—is important because they facilitate the final elimination of what the kidney has filtered out. The bladder, a muscular organ that stores urinary waste to be excreted, also deserves some attention as it, too, can become stressed over time. If the bladder's normal function becomes challenged in some way from structural displacement, muscle weakness, or nerve damage, there may be an incomplete elimination of urine, causing the kidney to become overburdened and a risk for infections to occur.

The Speed Walk to the Nearest Restroom

Okay, we are going to bring it up. A situation most people have experienced at times, whether they want to admit it or not . . . *Why am I peeing so much?*

Overactive bladder (OAB), the frequent urge to urinate, is a problem for both men and women. It's possible to have overactive bladder at any point in your life, but it's especially common in older adults. The prevalence of OAB in people younger than fifty years of age is less than 10 percent. After the age of sixty, the prevalence increases to 20 to 30 percent. But why?

The following are some of the most common underlying causes and risk factors associated with OAB symptoms:

Weak pelvic muscles: The pelvic floor muscles are like a sling that holds up the bladder. For women, a pregnancy and childbirth can often lead to a stretching and weakening of the vital pelvic floor muscles. When pelvic floor muscles are compromised, the bladder can move out of place. The opening of the urethra can stretch, causing urine leakage. Men can have weakened pelvic muscles as well from strain or improper alignment.

To strengthen your pelvic muscles, be sure to engage your core when lifting anything heavy. You can also practice a set of movements commonly called Kegel exercises, which involve pulling up rhythmically on the pelvic floor (all the muscles around the lower pelvic area) with the lower abdominal muscles as you exhale, and keep pulling up on the squeeze until you need to take a breath. This can be done very discreetly, any time of day. If you are doing a Kegel correctly, you should not have any muscles on the outside of your body visibly contracting. A strong pelvic floor muscle should be able to hold a contraction for ten seconds. Do three sets of these ten-second holds and then rest. Repeat five or six times daily.

Tissue atrophy: In women, lower estrogen levels during menopause can cause urethral tissue to become thinner, less resilient, and less elastic, leading to reduced sphincter control. Phytoestrogens in the diet seem to have a mild estrogenic activity, and therefore may theoretically help soften these symptoms when estrogen levels decrease. Research shows promise in the use of phytoestrogens for several menopausal symptoms. Although meta-analysis reveals that more conclusive direct studies need to be done to understand the exact mechanisms at play when eating them as compared to concentrated herbal supplementation.

What we do know is that the isoflavones and lignans (types of phytoestrogen compounds) found in certain foods have strong antioxidant benefits that can certainly curb the oxidative damage to these tissues, protecting them from the effects of aging. You can get phytoestrogens from eating organic soy in the form of whole soybeans (edamame), miso, tempeh, and tofu. Other sources are flaxseeds, oats, lentils, sesame seeds, and sweet potatoes.

Extra weight or obesity: Carrying around extra pounds is linked to OAB and urine leaks, since excess weight puts more pressure on the bladder. And as we know, a common side effect of maintaining a whole food, plant-based diet is a permanent loss of excess weight.

Fluid buildup: Those who are sedentary or have heart disease may develop fluid buildup in their legs during the day. At night, this fluid causes them to need to empty their bladder frequently. If you have fluid retention in your legs that's causing an active bladder overnight, try walking around more throughout the day. When sitting, flex your calf muscles and raise your legs to waist level to help move that fluid along.

Diuretic medications: Diuretics are very commonly prescribed for high blood pressure. These medications cause your body to get rid of water and salt faster through the urine. As a result, this can cause the bladder to fill up faster and possibly leak. Natural diuretic foods will flush the water and salt at a much more manageable rate than medications. Think: celery (also known to lower blood pressure), cucumber, lemon juice, asparagus, grapes, watermelon, and pineapple.

Benign prostatic hyperplasia (BPH), which means simply enlargement of the prostate gland. It is called benign because it is not cancerous; however, while it is very common, it is not pleasant, nor is it normal. The prostate starts out about the size of a walnut. By the time a man is forty, and if he has been eating the standard American diet laden with animal protein, saturated fats, and meats from animals raised with growth-promoting hormones, the prostate may have grown slightly larger, to the size of an apricot. By age sixty, on the same fast-fuel regimen, it may be the size of a lemon. When this happens, the bulky prostate can press against the undersurface of the bladder and encroach upon the urethra. This can seriously slow down or actually completely block urine flow. Some men may feel as if they need to pass urine all the time or are awakened during sleep with the sudden need to pass urine.

A prostate specific antigen (PSA) test, given to men over the age of fifty is most often a measure of inflammation in the prostate and often correlates with symptoms of BPH. Top nutrients and herbs for prostate health include zinc and beta-sitosterol (both found in pumpkin seeds and pecans), green tea, lycopene (tomato, pink grapefruit, watermelon), and vitamin D. Nettle leaf and saw palmetto especially have been used medicinally in cases of inflamed or enlarged prostate. You'll want to check with a naturopathic physician or other health professional familiar with using these kind of natural healing agents if you experience more serious urinary symptoms or receive blood tests that warrant more aggressive treatment. The aforementioned foods and herbs all have reputations for helping provide proper nourishment as well as reducing inflammation to keep "the man's gland" in top shape.

Bladder or kidney stones: Uric acid accumulation can cause stones along with painful inflammation. You are more likely to have uric acid stones if you have: low urine output from chronic dehydration; a diet high in animal protein, especially red meat; a hefty alcohol habit; a history of gout; or inflammatory bowel disease.

Cherry juice is known to reduce uric acid levels, effectively reducing the risk of stones. The whole fruits or pure unsweetened pressed juice could be a consideration for those prone to gout from excess uric acid. Calcium deposits from supplementation can cause calcium stones to chemically precipitate as crystals in the urinary tract, which then seed infections in the kidney and bladder.

Irritability or chronic inflammation within the bladder or urethral tissues can be caused by chronic food sensitivities. Pay attention to any potential food reactions, such as burning or increased frequency, especially at night. If there is any serious suspicion that a particular food is irritating the bladder, refrain from eating it for two to three weeks and see whether the symptoms subside. If they do, reintroduce a small amount of the "test" food, and if bladder irritability reappears, then do not eat that food for a year. Re-challenge (assuming you want that food in your diet, at all) in one year to see whether the sensitivity has persisted or, as often happens, disappeared.

Stay hydrated to prevent toxin accumulation and stone formation. Sugar and artificially sweetened beverages have also been connected with stone formation.

Please see our recommendations on page 67 for herbs and supplements that can help soothe irritation and repair damage to the urinary tract. And remember to make sure you drink plenty of water, plus more! Healthy urination is a good thing, and many of these kidney-related problems stem from dehydration.

As we have mentioned (see page 58), most Americans consume far too much sodium and far too little potassium, putting strain on not only the heart, but also the kidneys. We reiterate this important topic here as a reminder that making a few changes in food choices can greatly help shift the balance, lowering the risk for kidney disease as well.

Here are some foods that will keep the kidneys purring:

Berries, which contain those blood vessel protecting phytonutrient chemicals to support kidney and urinary circulation. Cranberries specifically contain D-mannose sugar, which has a slippery property that keeps bacteria from adhering to bladder walls, preventing urinary tract infections. Cherries are known to decrease uric acid in the body.

Cultured foods will balance the microbiome in the urinary tract as well as the digestive tract, helping prevent the potential for microbial infections and to lower overall inflammation.

Omega-3 and omega-6 fatty acids, to keep the immune system in healthy balance: cold-pressed, raw, unrefined olive, nut, and seed oils, walnuts, flaxseeds, evening primrose oil, and black currant oil. (Dr. Klaper recommends no more than 1 teaspoon TOTAL of liquid oil—of all kinds—per day. Also, keep high-fat nuts and seeds to a reasonable amount, such as a small handful per day.)

Phytoestrogenic foods: apple, cherries, olives, plums, carrots, sweet potatoes, tomatoes, peanuts, soy foods, brown rice, barley, oats, wheat. According to research on soy specifically, these can have a protective effect on kidney function.

Foods rich in zinc, selenium, and vitamin E: squash seeds, almonds, sesame seeds, tahini, kelp, Brazil nuts, pumpkin seeds

Other urinary tract–friendly foods: anise, tangerine, cherries, figs, litchis, sunflower seeds, mangoes, sea vegetables

Herbal medicines: Additionally, the following herbs have a well-established history for protecting, soothing, and healing the urinary tract. Herbal teas are fantastic at both increasing water absorption and/or promoting gentle diuretic properties when needed, as well as providing tissue supportive minerals in a gentle way. It is best to consult with an experienced practitioner to make specific recommendations for your needs.

- **Buchu** (*Barosma betulina*)
- **Cleavers** (*Galium aparine*)
- **Corn silk** (*Zea mays*)
- **Horsetail** (*Equisetum arvense*)
- **Marshmallow root** (*Althea officinalis*)
- **Usnea** (*Usnea barbata*)
- **Dandelion leaf** (*Taraxicum officinale*)
- **Saw palmetto** (*Serenoa repens*)
- **Nettle** (*Urtica dioca*)

- **Hibiscus** (*Rosa sinensis*)
- **Uva Ursi** (*Arctostaphylos*)

All of your body's systems are interdependent and weave together like an intricate, rich tapestry. The health of each part determines the health of the whole. It behooves you to bring mindfulness and attention into your daily life in such a way that you are nurturing and supporting them all.

AGE-DEFYING ADVICE:
KIDNEY AND URINARY HEALTH

Eat More:
Hydrating foods that contain plenty of fiber, digestible protein, phytoestrogens, minerals, healthy fats, probiotics, and natural anti-inflammatory compounds: thick-skinned berries, tofu, yams, seeds, whole grains, cabbage, sauerkraut, vegan yogurt, cucumbers, celery, citrus, melons, and avocados

Drink More:
Water! If continuously thirsty, consider adding electrolytes from lemon juice, berries, or even a tiny pinch of sea salt to water to increase absorption.

Herbal teas: dandelion leaf, nettle, saw palmetto, hibiscus

Pure berry juices: pressed, unsweetened cranberry, cherry, or blueberry juice in small amounts

Simple high-potassium veggie juice: one carrot, a stalk of celery, two bunches of spinach, some parsley, and a little water.

Do More:
Hydrotherapy: Hot foot baths and alternating hot/cold water to pelvic and low back areas will stimulate circulation away and back, helping to promote proper kidney flushing.

Exercise: walking daily; aerobic exercise for 20 minutes 3 times a week; practicing proper alignment and core engagement with lifting, Kegel exercises, squats

Yoga for strengthening and stretching pelvic floor muscles: chair pose, downward dog, child's pose, legs up the wall

Stop smoking: Cigarette smokers have a two to three times' higher risk of bladder cancer than nonsmokers.

Anti-inflammatory supplementation: Bromelain, quercetin, and turmeric/curcumin can be found singly or in combination when extra support is needed to reduce inflammation. Check with an experienced practitioner for specifics.

Try these kidney-friendly recipes that include foods and nutrients mentioned above:

Hydration Station (page 115)
Lemon Dill Asparagus Spears (page 175)
Herb-Roasted Tofu (page 220)
Sweet and Spicy Pumpkin Seeds (page 257)
Tomato Cucumber with Pine Nuts (page 158)
Pepita Pesto with Avocado (page 265)

FOUNTAIN OF YOUTHER

Name: Cherie Soria
Birth Year: 1947

About Cherie: Cherie Soria is the founder and codirector of Living Light Culinary Institute and author of four books, including *Angel Foods*, *Raw Food Revolution Diet*, and *Raw Food for Dummies*. She is often referred to as the mother of gourmet raw vegan cuisine. She has been the inspiration of thousands of raw food chefs around the world!

Typical Daily Meals: (all organic) Green smoothies, green juice, full-meal salad, steamed quinoa, oatmeal, and/or lentils, raw nuts and seeds, fresh fruits

Typical Exercise/Lifestyle: Running, hiking, core and weight training

Cherie says: Invest in your health; you'll never regret it! It's never too late to change your life and become the person you could have been.

SEVEN

LOOK YOUNGER: SECRETS OF SKIN HEALTH

Who doesn't want smooth, glowing, vibrant skin? The condition of your skin is not only vital to your appearance, but also your overall health and well-being. Healthy skin maintains a balance of fluids. Highly sensitive, it acts as the body's first line of defense against microbial infections or injury, and it eliminates toxins from the body. The many important functions of the skin include:

- Regulation of body temperature
- Acting as a barrier to prevent loss of essential body fluids and to protect organs from toxins.
- Excretion of wastes through sweat
- Synthesis of vitamin D, a necessary hormone, stimulated by the sun's rays falling on the skin
- Sensation, transmitted through skin nerves, to make you aware of heat, cold, vibration, or injury

As people age, their skin tends to get drier and lose firmness. As a result, crow's feet, wrinkles, and sagging set in. As the skin's moisture is depleted, it becomes less effective as a protective barrier, and its other functions diminish as well. In a similar way, people may notice their hair losing the natural moisture and fullness it once had. Years of exposure to sun, cigarette smoke, alcohol, and other damaging factors can make it harder to recover its luster.

Healthy skin and hair are the result of a healthy body. By eating a diet rich in nutrients that improve overall health, such as antioxidants, healthy fats, and fiber, more youthful skin and lustrous hair are possible at any age. In particular, foods in a plant-based diet are good sources of both vitamin C and lysine. These are big collagen boosters, promoting a plump, youthful suppleness to skin, as well as maintaining elasticity to prevent wrinkles. Lots of recipes in this book contain these skin-nourishing nutrients; see page 80 for recipe suggestions containing collagen-boosting and moisture-protecting nutrients.

Here's how to put your best face forward and keep your suit of armor beautiful and strong!

Inside Your Skin

Did you know that your skin is actually an organ? Like other organs, the skin is constantly working to provide support and protection through its capacity to eliminate and absorb, and can be supported to function properly with basic nutrition and self-care practices. As the largest organ of elimination, the skin acts in concert with the liver as an excretory of toxins. Skin rashes and breakouts can be a result of the body trying to eliminate toxins through the skin rather than the digestive system. Always look to support liver and gastrointestinal health when trying to improve skin health! See Chapter 3 on digestive health for some more insight and self-care tips.

The outermost layer of the skin, the epidermis, is always renewing itself by growing new skin cells and migrating them up to the surface. The cells of the deeper layer hold in moisture, preserve your body heat to protect you from temperature extremes, and repair tissue damage. The structures at the upper surface secrete a film of fluids, water, and lipids through sebaceous and sweat glands embedded in the dermis, keeping skin supple and protecting it from infection.

Your skin is the largest interface between your body and its environment. It is continually influenced by the "internal"—your anatomical, physiological, and biochemical changes—as well as the "external"—exposure to such things as temperature, sunlight, and pollutants. Pressure from, say, clothing that fits too tight or sitting in the same position for long periods of time, can cause skin breakdown through abrasion from irritating fabrics and unsupportive chairs, beds, or workstations.

Smoking introduces multiple chemicals into the body that produce oxidative damage and contribute to the effects of aging. Excessive sun exposure can predispose the skin to future skin damage, such as the development of premalignant lesions. Regular exposure to UV rays over time causes the skin to produce more melanin pigment and to thicken as a protective effort. This is when hyperpigmentation, or darkened spots on the skin, can occur.

With such variable factors affecting skin through the course of life, it is not surprising that drastic changes can occur in the nature, texture, and integrity of skin with age.

The aging process affects skin at every layer. Aging of the skin is associated with skin thinning, atrophy, dryness, wrinkling, and delayed wound healing. These undesirable effects are exacerbated by declining estrogen levels in postmenopausal women.

Collagen is the most abundant protein in your body, especially type 1 collagen. Mostly found in the deeper layer of skin called the dermis, it's what helps give your skin strength and structure, along with replacing dead skin cells. In simplest terms, it's the "glue" that helps hold all the tissues in your body together. Elastin is another protein that essentially provides elasticity to help tissues resume their shape after being stretched. It works together with collagen throughout the body to maintain softness and stretch in tissues, and is also affected by damage over time.

Decreased collagen production can cause signs of aging, such as wrinkles, sagging skin, and joint pains, due to weaker or decreased cartilage. Lifestyle factors, such as eating a diet high in sugar, smoking, dehydration, and excess amounts of sun exposure can contribute to depleting collagen levels. Collagen-related diseases most commonly arise over time from a combination of genetic defects, nutritional deficiencies, and digestive problems affecting production of collagen.

Aging skin can have slower turnover, division, and differentiation of keratinocytes and fibroblasts, which are skin cells that work together to both heal and strengthen as well as stimulate new skin cell growth. This slowing of their actions can lead to reduced wound healing and natural exfoliation. Changes in blood flow close to the skin's surface also play an important role in skin changes, as reduced blood delivery to these tissues compromises hydration and nutritional exchanges with skin cells.

The good news? You can slow and possibly even reverse skin damage associated with the aging process with a simple prescription: proper hydration, antioxidant action through plant foods, and exercise. Hydration is so incredibly important and so easy to let fall by the wayside. Just optimizing water intake and absorption can make wrinkles disappear! And as you will see, the antioxidant phytochemicals that plants are famous for will go to work to directly protect your skin from environmental oxidative damage. Both aerobic exercise and hydrotherapy can help improve surface vasculature and blood circulation. Weight management, as well as cardiovascular and endocrine health all positively influence skin health, by supporting oxygenation, nutrient exchange, and detoxification of skin cells. Regular exercise promotes the proper structure and function of collagen and improves lymphatic drainage to remove toxins, as well as relaxation and balance, further protecting the skin from the detrimental effects of stress.

Having all these areas of health in balance is what will truly ensure that your skin has plenty of oxygen and nutrients to both repair and heal continually, and to do its work as a powerful detox organ.

What to Eat for Better Skin

The best foods for your skin function are those that help improve gut health and contain the nutrients needed to support the biochemistry of detoxification. Focus on foods that contain the following:

Fiber, which improves gut health. Fiber removes toxins, including unhealthy fats, yeasts, and other microorganisms through the digestive tract so they do not contribute to skin blemishes or rashes.

Healthy fats, needed to protect cell membranes, decrease inflammation, and also help maintain moisture.

Foods with high water content, to ensure adequate hydration and absorption. These include cucumbers, lemons, limes, tomatoes, melons, strawberries, celery, grapefruit, carrots, broccoli, zucchini, grapes, and lettuce. Moisture is, of course, the key for keeping skin looking plump and youthful, which is why staying hydrated is one of the best ways to improve the appearance of your skin.

Foods high in minerals, such as zinc, silica, sulfur, and copper, and in **antioxidants**, including beta-carotene, vitamins C and E, and others with specific skin-protective actions. More about these:

Chlorella is an algae food in supplement form that contains the highest amount of chlorophyll. It contains beta-carotene, known to stimulate collagen production and prevent premature aging, and is also rich in fiber, which supports digestion and detoxification. By improving detoxification, chlorophyll also helps reduce inflammation and promote digestive health, which in turn leads to brighter and healthier skin.

Silica-rich foods, including oats, leafy greens, onions, bananas, starchy root vegetables, nopal cactus (prickly pear), cucumbers, and almonds, have been shown to improve skin health. Silica helps the skin retain moisture, which is important for a smooth, youthful appearance. Silica forms compounds called glycosaminoglycans, which make up the skin's connective tissue and bind to water molecules in the skin to prevent moisture loss. One glycosaminoglycan you may be familiar with is hyaluronic acid, found in many antiaging skin injections, creams, and treatments. It helps skin cells retain moisture and also facilitates the passage of nutrients into the skin and the removal of waste products. Eating silica- and other mineral-rich foods can provide the precursors necessary for your body's natural hyaluronic acid production.

Cilantro and parsley support phase II liver detoxification, which is the process to eliminate toxins from your body. Liver support is crucial for preventing toxins from being eliminated through your skin and causing breakouts.

Coconut oil contains lauric acid, a natural antifungal, which can help protect the health of the digestive tract from pathogens that can compromise gut microbiome balance, such as yeast. Use in moderation if you are looking to reduce saturated fats in your diet. (And it can do double duty—coconut oil on your skin makes a great body moisturizer, antimicrobial protectant, and chemical-free eye makeup remover.)

Celery is an amazing skin food because of its high fiber and high water content. It also contains a gut- and skin-supportive antioxidant nutrient called lutein, which is said to be protective against colon cancer.

Cacao is a rich source of flavanols, which are phytonutrients that have been shown to improve skin elasticity and protect against UV exposure.

Pumpkin is rich in beta-carotene, which is the precursor to vitamin A, or retinol. Many over-the-counter topical skin creams use derivatives of vitamin A to help stimulate new skin cell production, eliminate acne, and fade dark acne scars. Eating food sources of beta-carotene will provide these same benefits, but in a more powerful way by healing from the inside out.

Beta-carotene is the pigment that gives orange and red plant foods their colors, so also consider **yellow and orange peppers, squash, sweet potatoes, apricots, tomatoes, and carrots**. Studies support the efficacy of the intake of green and yellow vegetables to slow and/or reverse the appearance of fine lines and wrinkles.

Biotin, or vitamin B_7, is important in skin and hair health and readily available on a plant-based diet. Leave the eggs to the hens and choose almonds, walnuts, cauliflower, or carrots instead to increase your nutrient benefit!

Want to reduce wrinkles? It's all about collagen! The following foods are especially beneficial for boosting collagen production:

Foods high in vitamin C, such as citrus, berries, greens, kiwi, and bell peppers, have many beneficial effects in combating sun damage, a.k.a. photodamage, by helping collagen production for the repair of the damaged skin, while promoting a decrease in elastin production, which is often overproduced in response to photodamage. Vitamin C also increases the production rate as well as DNA repair of new connective tissue cells called fibroblasts, which can both decrease with age.

As an antioxidant, vitamin C protects against toxins found in your air, food, and water supply that contribute to breaking down collagen and damaging the skin's inner layer. Vitamin C also helps with skin cell repair and regeneration, which is why it's commonly added to topical skin-care products.

Dark-colored fruits, such as berries, grapes, plums, and prunes. These contain anthocyanidins, which are natural plant pigments that have powerful antioxidant properties.

Berries also contain a nutrient called ellagic acid, which has been shown to prevent collagen breakdown from UV damage to protect against the signs of aging. Like citrus fruits, berries are rich in vitamin C, which as you now know, helps link specific amino acids together for collagen formation.

Tomatoes are rich in the antioxidant lycopene, which also protects the skin from sun damage and helps with collagen synthesis while also preventing collagen breakdown.

Foods high in zinc, such as pumpkin seeds, kidney beans, chickpeas, spinach, walnuts, cashews, and almonds. Zinc regulates essential enzymes, and aids in the transport of vitamin A from the liver to the skin. Zinc also helps speed up wound healing, and maintain healthy cell membranes, which makes it a must-have nutrient for skin health. Pumpkin seeds are one of the best plant sources of zinc, which is essential in the enzyme activity for collagen synthesis. Studies have also shown taking zinc

supplements may help slow down the rate of collagen breakdown, suggesting zinc-rich foods may do the same.

Avocados provide antioxidant vitamin E that helps prevent collagen breakdown, as well as healthy fats that improve the health of skin cells. One study adding avocado oil to your diet showed a significant increase in soluble collagen.

Foods high in sulfur, such as garlic and onions, and cruciferous vegetables. Sulfur is a trace mineral that helps synthesize and prevent the breakdown of collagen. Garlic and its close cousins shallots, leeks, chives, and onions are some of the best dietary sources of sulfur, so don't forget to add them as well to your recipes liberally, along with broccoli, cauliflower, cabbage, and Brussels sprouts.

Chia seeds are an excellent plant-based source of omega-3 essential fatty acids, which slow aging by building healthy skin cells and providing moisture to the skin, creating a smooth, supple appearance from the inside out.

Green tea. The catechins in *Camellia sinensis* extracts have been well researched and documented, specifically epigallocatechin gallate (EGCG) for its potent antioxidant, and specifically anticancer benefits. Researchers have extended green tea's antioxidant benefits to include protection against the damage caused by cigarette smoke, pollution, stress, and various toxins.

AGE-DEFYING ADVICE:
KEEP YOUR SKIN PH BALANCED

There's another factor that can improve your skin's appearance—improving its natural pH. "The skin's barrier, which is known as the acid mantle, is responsible for keeping in lipids and moisture while blocking germs, pollution, toxins, and bacteria," explains Patricia Wexler, MD, a New York City dermatologist. "To work its best, the acid mantle should be slightly acidic, at a 5.5 pH balance. When it's too alkaline, skin becomes dry and sensitive; you may even get eczema. You may also experience inflammation, which inhibits the skin's ability to ward off matrix metalloproteinases, the enzymes that destroy collagen and cause wrinkles and sagging."

According to a 2010 study published in the *British Journal of Dermatology* that tracked women's skin over an eight-year period, women with an alkaline stratum corneum (the skin's outermost layer) developed more fine lines and crow's-feet—and were more prone to sun damage—than those with more acidic skin.

What can you do to rebalance your skin pH in favor of more acidity? Probiotics' benefits for the gut directly translate to the skin. This is why many skin-care protocols will recommend taking a probiotic supplement and eating probiotic foods as a first step. Probiotic foods, such as miso, sauerkraut, high-quality vegan yogurt, and kimchi, eaten on a regular basis, will both eliminate microbial skin reactions and help normalize pH. You can check the pH of the water in your home and experiment with ways to balance out a higher pH. For example, whereas face and body soaps are often more alkaline, causing more skin dryness, natural remedies, such as argan oil, apple cider vinegar, and oats, can help balance out pH, which aids in preventing that water loss. Facial masks made with avocado, papaya, or tomato can help lock in moisture. Of course, all these also have other nutrient properties that protect skin from several angles.

AGE-DEFYING ADVICE:
A SKIN CARE REGIMEN FOR A YOUTHFUL GLOW

Follow these simple self-care practices and prepare to astound!

Exfoliation, via skin brushing: Use a natural-fiber brush or loofah and brush toward the heart to remove dead skin cells and encourage new skin growth. This also promotes healthy circulation and detoxification. Visit www.doctorchefresources.com for a skin brush tutorial video.

continues

continued from previous page

Hydrotherapy: Alternating hot and cold creates a pumping action to bring fresh blood and nutrients to the area being treated. These can be accomplished through compresses on one area of the body or a complete immersion of the entire body. With the complete immersion, the hot brings the blood away from the internal organs, and the cold moves the blood toward them. This is the way that the skin is used to help optimize circulation in the body and assists in wound healing as well.

Oil massage: Any type of massage will further stimulate healthy circulation. Following the skin brushing and/or hydrotherapy with an oil massage helps lock in the moisture and keeps the skin protected.

Regular sweating: Through steam, sauna, or exercise, sweating assists the skin in its normal detoxification processes by removing toxins. (Be sure to remove makeup before exercising or getting in the sauna.)

Castor oil packs: Castor oil packs prevent skin congestion by optimizing the function of the liver. Castor oil may also be used for spot treatments on skin as it draws immune cells to the area that needs to be healed, while also creating a protective barrier. See www.doctorchefresources.com for pack instructions.

Make your own facial care: Pumpkin, vegan yogurt, ground oats, papaya, coconut oil, avocado, matcha green tea powder, rose water, lavender, and chamomile are all good choices. See www.doctorchefresources.com for some facial care recipes and tutorials.

Argan or avocado oil for face and hair: Rich in vitamin E, fatty acids, beta-carotene and carotenoids, and phytosterols, argan oil appears to be a good option for a variety of skin types.

Hair Loss and Going Gray

Since hair is an extension of your skin, your luxurious mane can also feel the stress of time. Hair follicles actually tend to get smaller over time, which can certainly contribute to both thinning and fragility. Oil glands also shrink, resulting in less natural moisture. These changes compound hormonal changes that result in both hair dryness and a lower rate of growth. While these are expected to some degree, they are also manageable with good nutrition and care.

Besides nutritional deficiencies, most of hair damage with age is the result of damage from chemical-laden products and heat-styling techniques that strip the hair of natural oil and nutrients. The same nutrients for skin health are also important in hair health. Along with a healthy intake of vitamins, minerals, and healthy fats, anything you can do to protect your hair from damage, help strengthen it, and provide moisture are important. Hydrotherapy (as simple as alternating hot/cold when washing hair) and massaging the scalp can help stimulate follicles and oil glands. Include some argan oil for added benefit. From the Moroccan argan tree, this mild oil is rich in antioxidants as well as healthy fats that both protect and repair hair damage.

As far as graying goes, when your hair goes gray, you are losing the pigment melanin. Some percentage of loss of melanin is due to simple individual genetic profile. The rest is caused by loss of nutrients, environmental damage, and stress over time. Oxidative stress from smoking and an inflammatory diet has been linked with premature graying, as have deficiencies in vitamin B_{12}, iron, as well as thyroid and adrenal function.

One theory on graying of hair is that it is caused by changes in mineral intake or absorption, according to a 2012 study in the *Biological Trace Research Journal*. Copper has been one of interest because of its known role in the production of melanocytes, which are the cells that produce melanin to give both skin and hair their pigment. Copper deficiency seems to be linked to premature graying. Good sources of copper are nuts and seeds, particularly black sesame and nigella seeds.

So, while your diet may not have you forgoing the hair dye just yet, you can improve the overall health of your locks simply by including the foods and nutrients mentioned in this chapter.

A Note on Nails

Nails also require both proper nutrient intake and adequate blood flow to stay healthy and strong. The state of your nails can often say a lot about your overall state of health. Nail dryness, splitting, discoloration, and changes in shape can all be signs of more serious disease.

Much of the damage to nails comes from exposure to chemicals, toxins, and high pH water and detergents that can all lead to tissue damage, dryness, and microbial growth. So, protecting your hands with gloves, and giving them a little love after a long day of working or cleaning, can go a long way. Keeping nails trimmed as well as replenishing lost moisture will allow them to maintain their integrity, working as a protective barrier against infection and damage as well. Of course, the same nutrients mentioned for skin and hair will in turn keep nails beautiful and shiny as well. Visit www.doctorchefresources.com for a healing hand salve recipe and tutorial.

It's radical but true: your food choices can play a role in the reflection you see in the mirror. If you make the right choices, you may just see a younger version of yourself looking back at you!

AGE-DEFYING ADVICE:
SKIN HEALTH

Eat More:

Healthy fats, such as avocados, greens, nuts, and seeds, to keep skin supple and hydrated

Fiber, such as beans, whole grains, pumpkin, and celery, for healthy digestion and detoxification

Cultured foods, such as sauerkraut, kimchi, vegan yogurt, and miso, for microbiome balance

Anti-inflammatory/liver-supportive foods and herbs, such as garlic, onion, beet, ginger, turmeric, cinnamon, basil, oregano, cilantro, parsley, thyme, astragalus, nettle leaf, and dandelion

Fruits and veggies with a high water content, mineral balance, and collagen-boosting vitamins A, C, and E, such as kiwi, pomegranate, tomatoes, cucumbers, berries, citrus fruits, melons, grapes, carrots, celery, okra, zucchini, pumpkin, greens, and peppers

Drink More:

Half your body weight in ounces of pure water as a minimum

Hydrating elixir: Juice of ½ lemon, 1-inch slice of fresh ginger, and a pinch of cayenne pepper in a cup of cold or warm water daily

Green tea for antioxidant protection

Cultured beverages, such as kombucha and coconut kefir

Do More:

Exfoliation: skin brushing with a natural brush, loofah, or dry towel

Hydrotherapy: alternating hot and cold shower rinses to stimulate circulation and flushing

Oil massage

Cool hair rinses/scalp massage

Regular sweating

Castor oil packs; see www.doctorchef resources.com for instructions.

Make your own facial cleansers and masks

Argan or avocado oil for face and hair

Proper, safe sun exposure

Keep nails trimmed, clean, and moisturized

Try these skin-friendly recipes with foods and nutrients mentioned above:

Kale Kiwi Avocado Juice (page 117)

Berry Good Breakfast Bowl (page 129)

Roasted Red Pepper Soup with Fennel (page 144)

Lemony Herbed Cauliflower Roast (page 211)

Ruby Kraut (page 259)

Name: Babette Davis
Birth Year: 1950

About Babette: Babette is a vegan chef, fitness expert, and motivational speaker. She runs a successful restaurant, Stuff I Eat, and participates in health summit events around the country. Chef Babette recently guest starred in the new HBO hit comedy series *Insecure*. Her passion lies in inspiring individuals who may not otherwise be acquainted with healthier lifestyles due to environmental and economic barriers. She will be releasing her first book, *Cash In On Cashews*, the first book in her Crave Series, which focuses on the versatility of the amazing cashew nut.

She fuels her body with the nutrients to allow her to continue the active lifestyle and body she proudly displays at the age of sixty-seven. It is her passion to help others embrace health and start today no matter how old they are. www.chef babette.com

Typical daily meals/snacks: I am a very light eater. I spend most of my day snacking but my snacks are full of nutrients, which help fuel my cells and prevents me from being hungry.

Typical daily exercise/lifestyle: Push-ups, planks, and cardio (I love the spin bike).

A typical day for me looks something like this: 2:30 a.m.—Rise

4:00 a.m.—Get dressed and head to work

4 a.m.–noon—Prep food for my restaurant

5 a.m.—Fresh juice: My go-to is green apples, ginger, cilantro, and a splash of lemon. I usually add a pinch or two of cayenne pepper.

1 p.m.-2 p.m.—Go home and work out

2 p.m.—Snack: raw nuts and seeds

3 p.m.—Nap: sooooo important

4 p.m.—Snack: kombucha

7 p.m.—Dinner: a salad or stir-fry with quinoa

7 p.m.-9 p.m.—Kick back and watch CNN or MSNBC or a movie, social media

9 p.m.—Beauty rest for the evening

My lifestyle is simple. Less is more. I am REAL, ORGANIC, RAW!!! I don't try to be anything other than who or what I am. I am a mother and grandmother. I am a student of life. I am constantly learning and growing. I love nature and animals. I love to garden. I'm a hippie at heart. I am a work in progress. I never claim perfection as I believe we all have room for improvement.

Chef Babette says: Life is not complete unless you move. Our journeys are constant and our transitions are infinite, our health is merely a vehicle to enjoy all that's in between.

EIGHT

FEEL YOUNGER: LESS STRESS, MORE ENERGY

A plant-based diet can keep you moving when age tries to slow you down. As we've seen, fruits, veggies, nuts, and whole grains are easy on the digestive system, which means the nutrients you eat use less energy to process. They are also absorbed efficiently and completely, which means more energy reserves for use elsewhere, such as dancing, lifting weights, chasing around toddlers, or running a marathon.

Eating plant-based can also have a positive influence on your endocrine system, which manufactures your hormones. Hormonal changes are a big topic in aging, but what are we really talking about? With age, hormone receptors tend to function less well. Slowed receptor responses affect a wide range of normal body functions, since receptor sites are where biochemical signaling occurs. Receptor proteins are essentially the eyes and ears of cells, telling the cells how to respond based on what is happening in the bloodstream. Changes in normal signaling can lead to such symptoms as fatigue, mood changes, weight gain or loss, immune system imbalances, cognitive declines, insomnia, dry skin, and hair loss, which are often blamed on aging. Let's explore ways that you can improve and restore your body's messaging through optimal nourishment to your cells and in turn to all areas of your life.

What Your Hormones Do for You

Your endocrine system consists of a group of glands and organs that control various body functions by producing hormones. Hormones are chemical substances that affect the activity of another part of the body. In essence, hormones serve as messengers, coordinating activities throughout the body. The endocrine system controls your metabolic functions, such as the production of energy and the absorption and transport of necessary nutrients.

But as you get older, hormone production can get off kilter. Levels of most hormones decrease with aging (though others may increase), and endocrine function can decline with age because hormone receptors become less sensitive. This is mostly due to oxidative damage to cells when overwhelmed by toxic reactive molecules, changes in circulation, nutrient deficiencies, and emotional or environmental stress.

The pattern of age-related changes in each endocrine system is unique. Both hormone levels and the responsiveness of the target organs can become altered. For example:

Aging can lead to a mild carbohydrate intolerance and an increase in blood glucose in healthy, nonobese individuals, as cell receptors become less responsive to insulin. This process starts when the body becomes overloaded with the sugars and fats from processed, pro-inflammatory foods. At first, more insulin is released than is needed, causing blood glucose to go down too fast and symptoms of hypoglycemia, such as dizziness, shakiness, and anxiety in between meals. The strong need for glucose then stimulates the adrenals to produce more cortisol, which increases blood sugar. This mechanism eventually hampers the ability of insulin to do its job of sending glucose to the tissues where it is needed. This is what then turns into insulin resistance, a precursor to type 2 diabetes. An even more prevalent current theory revolves around excessive fats in the diet that become stored in muscle and liver cells. This intracellular lipid inhibits the enzymes needed for normal glucose metabolism.

Insulin resistance may cause tiredness or a feeling of overfullness after meals, or weight gain. It may also have no symptoms at all until blood work shows elevated glucose over time.

In a similar fashion, when normal metabolism is hindered in some way, organs can respond less well to thyroid hormones, resulting in symptoms of thyroid disease, such as fatigue, weight gain, dry skin, and intolerance to hot or cold.

A focus on whole unprocessed foods, healthy regular exercise, and stress management is what is necessary to normalize metabolism, and in turn reset healthy hormonal patterns that have gone awry.

The reproductive system naturally becomes altered by endocrine cell death, resulting in decreased estrogen and testosterone levels in women and men. In women, the decline in estrogen levels leads to menopause. In men, testosterone levels usually decrease gradually. Symptoms can be fatigue, low muscle tone, low sex drive, hair loss, and mood changes, such as depression or irritability.

Many health issues are the result of either inadequate or excessive hormone secretion.

On the other hand, nutrition, medicinal herbs, and appropriate lifestyle changes can help regulate these imbalances, leading to profound improvements in health. For example, getting enough magnesium is necessary for producing insulin, as mentioned, the hormone involved in the essential process of getting glucose (fuel) into your cells when needed.

By understanding a little about how the hormonal system works and how to protect the delicate cycles that it relies on, you can continue to enjoy balanced living even through the expected ups and downs of daily life.

Reproductive Hormone Health

Estrogen and Progesterone
Women's reproductive capacity naturally declines in the late fourth to fifth decade of life due to decreases in hormones estrogen and progesterone. Menopause is often accompanied by such effects as an increased risk of osteoporosis, challenges with mood, and a greater potential for cardiovascular and cerebrovascular diseases. The most common complaints during this time that lead to seeking treatment are hot flashes, insomnia, anxiety or depression, and loss of skin elasticity. It is important to understand natural ways to support the body's adjustment to normal hormonal changes by looking at how individual symptoms manifest.

Eating for Menopause
Of course, focusing on fiber-rich whole veggies, fruits, grains, beans, and plenty of water should be the basis of a menopause supportive diet to keep any negative effects of hormonal changes to a minimum. A few specifics to keep in mind:

Eat cruciferous veggies for healthy estrogen. The compounds 3,3'-diindolylmethane (DIM) and indole-3-carbinol (I3C), found in cruciferous vegetables, both favorably affect estrogen metabolism and help optimize a healthy ratio of the different types of estrogen. They also help promote the liver's detoxification functions, helping remove excess hormone and chemical hormone disruptors. Eat broccoli, cabbage, cauliflower, collards, kale, kohlrabi, mustard greens, turnips, Brussels sprouts, and chard.

Optimize DHEA. DHEA, the precursor to both male and female sex hormones, can help curb cortisol excess and keep the brain functioning optimally. Healthy fats will ensure its production, as well as will stress management, exercise, vitamin C, magnesium, ginseng/eleuthero root, and maca powder.

Calcium: Calcium should be balanced with other minerals for proper bone health. Plant sources of calcium include leafy greens, bok choy, almonds, tahini, broccoli, chia seeds, beans, lentils, and peas.

Phytoestrogens: These are plant chemicals that are similar in structure to estrogen and can gently modulate or balance estrogen activity. Eat organic sprouted tofu, edamame, tempeh, miso, sweet potatoes, mung beans, and sprouts.

Testosterone
Beginning around age thirty, a man's testosterone levels begin to decline, and they continue to do so as he ages. Low testosterone levels are related to such conditions as cardiovascular disease, osteoporosis,

Alzheimer's disease, and diabetes. In addition, testosterone is responsible for healthy neurological function and improved psychosocial and behavioral dynamics.

Evidence suggests that testosterone and sperm levels are decreasing in men across the globe. This suggests that some factor other than age must be contributing to the declines in testosterone over time. Environmental toxicity and chemicals known as endocrine disruptors (EDCs; see page 90) are likely some of the largest culprits. A wide range of chemical exposures, including prescribed drugs, such as statins, can adversely impact testosterone production in men. At the same time, abnormal estrogen levels can increase due to widespread exposures to estrogen-mimicking compounds in processed food, water, and environmental pollutants.

In addition to avoiding these EDC contaminants, exercise routines that include higher physical intensity with challenging weight loads stimulate endocrine physiology and create metabolic demand for testosterone and sperm. Even personal goal setting and competitive sports promote healthy motivation and achievement, which seems to positively affect testosterone production. And, by the way, studies suggest that regularity of sexual activity is inversely related to mortality. This means that the more sex you enjoy, the longer you live!

A healthy libido is a sign of vitality for both men and women, and is supported by all of the lifestyle factors we have discussed in this chapter, such as the specific whole plant foods that support hormone and mood balance, exercise, sunshine, stress management, and of course, all the elements of the NOURISH system.

AGE-DEFYING ADVICE:
EAT GRAPES FOR MORE ACTIVE SPERM

Want to increase fertility? Men can eat a bunch of red grapes daily to give their guys a boost: the skins contain resveratrol, which makes for hardier sperm. Chinese researchers found the equivalent of 500 mg—roughly the amount in 5 to 10 grams of grape skins—was enough to both raise testosterone levels and improve sperm's ability to swim. Resveratrol, known as a neuroprotector and potent antioxidant, is found in thick-skinned berries and cacao as well.

Stress and Adrenal Health

Avoiding life stress is impossible, and actually not a healthy way to go, since emotional expression is essential to your being. A certain amount of stress motivates and moves you continually. What is important is the way you move through challenges in your life. This is a huge component in self-care and healthy aging, as unmanaged emotional stress can also lead to the inflammatory and oxidative processes that promote cell damage.

The adrenal glands are walnut-size organs that sit on top of the kidneys and are responsible for the production of several regulatory hormones, including male and female sex hormones. Although small, the adrenals are responsible for many very important functions in the body. They are vital to cortisol regulation, overall metabolism, keeping inflammation at bay, and energy levels.

When it comes to stress response, the health of the adrenals is a top priority, as they govern the secretion of cortisol. Cortisol's action allows you to keep going when you need extra energy, by stimulating the production of glucose. Its goal is to restore homeostasis after exposure to some form of stress, by increasing the energy available to the cells.

Excess cortisol leads to biochemical problems since it reduces the immune response, impairs brain cognition and memory, slows thyroid function, disrupts healthy bone formation, and causes abdominal fat storage, which stresses the heart, all in an effort to keep you going. Cortisol's action is in opposition to the rest and calmness that is actually necessary for your body to repair, heal, digest, and detoxify. In excess, it tends to overpower the other adrenal hormones. This can happen easily in the culture of constant motion that most people live in day to day. So, it takes a real effort to find the necessary balance.

Interestingly, with aging, the hypothalamus and pituitary gland, which make up the endocrine command center in the brain, can become less sensitive to negative feedback from cortisol. That means that these regulatory glands become less able to receive the signal to stop making cortisol, possibly due to years of constant demand for it. When this happens, more cortisol than is needed will flood the body when a perceived stress occurs, making it harder to recover from stressors and also slowing the time it takes to develop an immune response to illness. Women may begin to secrete more cortisol in response to stress than do men.

Maintaining healthy circadian rhythms is the best way to keep the adrenals functioning properly and the hormones it is in charge of in a good balance. The circadian rhythm is a natural cycle that tells our body when it is time to do things like sleep, rise, or eat, ideally creating very regular routines throughout the day by following environmental cues, such as sunlight, darkness, and temperature. It is considered the body's

internal clock, and is important in regulating many physiological processes. Cortisol and melatonin have important roles in circadian balance. Such herbs as licorice root, ashwaghanda, rhodiola, and holy basil can be very helpful in times of stress when the adrenal hormones are in great demand. Also adequate levels of vitamin C, B vitamins, and magnesium are necessary for optimal adrenal health and function.

Caffeine, alcohol, and lack of sleep can exacerbate a cortisol imbalance. Consider trading these for a high-nutrient meal, a smoothie, or a snack with plenty of B vitamins and magnesium, an Epsom salts bath, and some adrenal supportive herbal tea to relax in the evenings.

Another hormone of note that is produced in healthy adrenal glands is aldosterone, which functions mainly to stabilize the blood pressure by strictly regulating fluid and mineral balance in the blood. Like other hormones, it relies on a normal circadian rhythm to function properly. When the adrenals become stressed, aldosterone can also be oversecreted, leading to blood pressure dysregulation. This is why those with high stress and adrenal fatigue can have low blood pressure and salt cravings, due to electrolyte imbalance and fluid depletion.

Less Daytime Fatigue, Better Sleep at Night

Melatonin is the hormone that the body secretes when it's time to sleep. It is regulated by signals in the environment that support sleep, such as darkness, a quiet environment, a cool temperature, and the length of time that you have been awake. One way to promote melatonin production at night is to make sure you are exposed to natural light early in the day. This is a great example of just how connected you are to your natural environment: noticing how the sun brightens to signal the morning, and the light gradually goes down at night, can help regulate circadian rhythms. Loud noises, bright indoor lighting, and staying up too late can disrupt that natural rhythm that your body needs.

Optimizing sleep by supporting proper melatonin production can be a foundation for aging well. Melatonin production can be supported through general preventative practices, such as good nutrition, lowering excess inflammation through healthy lifestyle choices, balancing circadian rhythms with routines, and regular nourishing exercise.

Melatonin and its metabolites are potent antioxidants with anti-inflammatory, hypotensive, cell communication–enhancing, potentially cancer-fighting, brown fat–activating (brown fat increases resting metabolism), and blood lipid–lowering effects, thereby protecting tissues from a variety of insults. Melatonin also increases human growth hormone and helps protect your mitochondria, directly reducing the risk for Parkinson's disease, Alzheimer's, and other dementias, as well as heart failure and muscle weakness. By supporting overall hormone balance, melatonin is powerful medicine made directly by your body to optimize reproductive health, cognition, mood, blood sugar regulation, weight management, and

bone metabolism, while improving overall antioxidant status and lowering blood pressure.

Tart cherries, orange bell peppers, walnuts, and flaxseeds can be considerations for a light evening snack since they are known to help with melatonin production.

Breathe

When it comes to fighting fatigue, oxygen is just as important as food. Simply breathing in oxygen allows your cells to produce more energy. The oxygen diffuses across the cell membranes of your lung tissue into your bloodstream, where proteins called hemoglobin in the red blood cells pick it up and deliver it to your tissues. The more oxygen in your body, the more efficient your metabolism. Improving your oxygen intake and assimilation is critical to maintaining your energy level and is important in preventing disease and signs of aging.

Movement helps bring oxygen to cells and also invites the need for more oxygen, which is part of why exercise feels so good, like quenching a deep thirst. Muscular activity accelerates the rate of oxygen usage, as do essentially all biochemical processes. Exercise and physical effort require the body to take in large quantities of oxygen, and can condition the body to function with more efficiency. It is important to breathe adequately during exercise so as to accomplish this conditioning without causing stress from exhaustion.

You may notice tiredness if your breathing is irregular in some way. Many people either hyper- or hypoventilate throughout the day without realizing it. It is helpful to become aware of your breathing patterns, and to spend a few minutes daily practicing breathing exercises to help normalize the rhythm. You can start by taking a few minutes to simply becoming aware of your breath as it enters and leaves your nostrils. Then, notice how your breath interacts with your body, bringing fresh oxygen in. Feel it moving through your throat, lungs, and abdomen. Simply notice without judgment and allow the breath to move into a calm rhythm. Let this be an enjoyable and relaxing exercise that you can do for yourself at any time. You will see that it will replenish and stabilize your energy level in the long run.

Are Environmental Contaminants Affecting Your Hormones?

Many industrial chemicals known as endocrine disruptors (EDCs) find their way into people's backyards and inside their homes. They can be found in foods, food preservatives, pesticides, storage containers, cosmetics, cleaning products, fragrances, furniture, and even tap water:

Bisphenol A (BPA) is a hormone disruptor that can imitate estrogen and other hormones in your body, causing harm by interfering with the production, secretion, transport, action, function, and elimination of natural hormones. Make sure your plastic and canned food and beverage containers are BPA-free and wash your hands after handling thermal paper receipts from stores. Plastic water bottles are a major source.

Parabens are also estrogen-mimicking chemicals used as preservatives in many personal care products, such as shampoos, conditioners, and lotions. Check for parabens near the end of the ingredient list, usually as methylparaben or propylparaben.

Polychlorinated biphenyls (PCBs) are hazardous chemicals that were once used in oil industries and electrical equipment. They have been discontinued due to their known neurotoxic effects and cancer risks, but many still remain in the environment. They have been detected in the fatty tissues of fish and other animals.

Dioxins form during many industrial processes when chlorine or bromine are burned in the presence of carbon and oxygen. They can disrupt the delicate ways that both male and female sex hormone signaling occurs in the body. Products, including meat, fish, milk, eggs, and butter, are most likely to be contaminated, so you can cut down on your exposure simply by eating fewer animal products.

Atrazine is an herbicide that is widely used to kill weeds on farms (it's used on the majority of corn crops in the United States, as well as a number of other food crops), and consequently it's a pervasive drinking water contaminant. It has been linked to delayed puberty, breast tumors, prostate inflammation, and cancer. Buy organic produce and get a drinking water filter certified to remove atrazine.

Perchlorate, a component in rocket fuel, contaminates conventional produce and milk products, according to Environmental Working Group and government test data. When perchlorate gets into your body, it competes with the nutrient iodine, which the thyroid gland needs to make thyroid hormones. A reverse osmosis filter will reduce perchlorate in drinking water. Eat organic and reduce any potential effects by making sure you are getting enough iodine in your diet through iodized salt and organic sea vegetables.

Perfluorinated chemicals (PFCs) are the chemicals used to make nonstick cookware. These can affect thyroid and sex hormone levels. One particularly notorious of these compounds called PFOA has been shown to be completely resistant to biodegradation. This is why you want to skip most nonstick pans. There are now hardened ceramic pans and pots that are virtually inert and are thus much safer.

Organophosphate pesticides are pesticides that target the nervous systems of insects. Despite many studies' linking organophosphate exposure to effects on brain development, behavior, and fertility, they are still used commonly today. Eat and grow organic!

Hormones in animal products: Conventional beef cattle are treated with estrogen to make them grow bigger faster, and dairy products are a source of estrogen from cows' own estrogen production. Dairy cows are often pregnant when they're milked, and this leads to higher levels of estrogen in the milk and subsequent dairy products. The bovine hormones, meant to stimulate cell growth in cows, can actually confuse human metabolism, leading to such diseases as obesity, diabetes, and even certain cancers. Avoid animal products, and you won't ingest them!

Foods That Help Balance Your Hormones

Healthy fats: Healthy fats are the building blocks of all hormones. They also help lower inflammation and keep excess cortisol under control. Seed cycling—a regular rotation of pumpkin, flax, sesame, and sunflower seeds—will help ensure a balance of all the healthy essential fatty acids. This is an easy naturopathic hack used historically to help balance hormones in all stages of life. See www.doctorchefresources.com for a handy chart.

How to consume more healthy fats: unprocessed nuts and seeds, avocados, fresh or dried coconut

Crucifers and sulfurous vegetables: Cruciferous veggies such as broccoli, cabbage, and Brussels sprouts, as well as garlic, onion, beets, and other dark green leafy veggies, are also known as "sulfur foods" for the generous amount of that element they contain. They are liver-supportive foods, which is important because a healthy liver is essential for healthy hormone balance. The liver is involved in both hormone production and the recycling and removal of toxins that can interfere with hormone health. Cruciferous veggies also contain the antioxidant indole-3-carbinol, known to fight cancer by regulating estrogen.

How to consume more sulfur-containing and liver-supportive foods: garlic, onions, broccoli, cabbage, Brussels sprouts, beets, dark green leafy veggies

Fiber: Fiber is important for healthy digestion and is part of the last step in removing toxins, including excess hormones, from the body.

How to consume more fiber: quinoa, flaxseeds, beans, thick-skinned veggies, sweet potatoes, squash, berries

Amino acids: The essential amino acids play major roles in the biochemical balance of all hormones, by modulating hormonal production through specific signaling.

How to consume more amino acids: quinoa, lentils, chickpeas, black beans, peas, green tea (green tea contains the amino acid L-theanine, which controls stress hormones and helps with melatonin production)

Cultured foods: Remember that a healthy microbiome is the cornerstone of all body balance and is strongly connected to the way the neurological system responds to stress. Probiotics can help ensure proper signaling among all hormonal systems. They also help destroy and remove hormone disrupting environmental toxins.

How to consume more cultured foods: miso, coconut yogurt, sauerkraut, kimchi

Minerals, such as selenium, iron, iodine, and magnesium, are also major structural and functional components of all hormones.

How to consume more minerals: leafy green veggies, Brazil nuts, kelp, mushrooms, seeds

AGE-DEFYING ADVICE: ENDOCRINE HEALTH

Eat More:

Healthy fats: avocados, coconut, nuts, and seeds

Seed cycling: Regularly rotate eating pumpkin, ground flax, sesame, and sunflower seeds. Eat as a snack, or add a daily tablespoon of these to meals.

Liver-supporting foods: beets, greens, garlic, onions, herbs and spices, cruciferous veggies

Minerals: iodine, zinc, selenium, magnesium found in green leafy veggies, Brazil and other nuts, sea vegetables, root vegetables, mushrooms, beans, and whole grains

Herbs, such as ginger, turmeric, and ginseng root, for anti-inflammatory effects and stress hormone balancing

Drink More:

Purified spring water, to avoid endocrine-disrupting chemicals

Calming herbal teas to balance adrenals. Licorice, lemon balm, holy basil, chamomile, oat straw, rhodiola, and ashwaghanda are great choices. Consider mushroom-infused coffee or herbal coffee replacements if caffeine is challenging adrenals.

Do More:

Hydrotherapy: Epsom salts bath in evenings, cool blast to adrenal area in morning shower

Castor oil packs: See www.doctorchefresources.com for info and instructions.

Get some sunshine for vitamin D!

Promote melatonin secretion at night: Dim the lights, shut down your computer and cell phone, keep your room dark with light-blocking curtains, and start winding down at a similar time every night to create a regular rhythm.

Avoid endocrine-disrupting chemicals in plastics and household products, and eat organic produce as much as possible. Check the Environmental Working Group website's water filter guide (www.ewg.org/tapwater/water-filter-guide.php), and consider using an indoor air filter if you suspect contaminants in your home.

Try these endocrine-friendly recipes with foods and nutrients mentioned above:

Maca Pepita Elixir (page 118)

Tofu Rancheros (page 137)

Miso Roots Soup (page 142)

Roasted Cauliflower and Broccoli (page 181)

Black Gomasio Crusted Tofu (page 215)

Superfood Chocolate Bark (page 284)

Name: Lani Muelrath
Birth Year: 1952

About Lani: Lani Muelrath, MA, is an award-winning health educator, inspirational speaker, and the author of three best-selling books. Lani has been vegetarian/vegan for forty-five years and has been teaching in health and wellness for over four decades. She has been practicing mindfulness meditation for over twenty-five years. She is the author of *The Mindful Vegan: A 30-Day Plan for Finding Health, Balance, Peace, and Happiness*, *The Plant-Based Journey*, and *Fit Quickies*. www.lanimuelrath.com

Typical Daily Meals: Breakfast is typically whole grains, nuts, plant-based milk, a mountain of berries or other fruit, and good grainy toast with nut butter and jam. Sometimes I'll make waffles or biscuits. For lunch, I'll prepare a big salad and a robust sandwich with avocado, tomato, and homemade hummus. In the winter it's often instead a substantial bowl of soup full of squash, vegetables, and beans or lentils. Dinner is typically brown rice or other whole grain or pasta or potatoes or squash with tofu or tempeh, or beans, and a big plate of colorful steamed vegetables or stir-fry and one of the assortment of sauces I like to make.

I've found the best way to stay naturally healthy and at your naturally healthy weight is to eat when hungry. So, I keep real food at the ready: fruit, such as apples or a big bowl of grapes; nuts and seeds; rice and beans; toast and nut butter; whole-grain crackers and veggies with hummus—even leftovers are good for keeping you well fed and energized, mentally and physically.

Typical Daily Exercise/Lifestyle: Typically I am up early, and after morning meditation and a soy cappuccino, it's time to step out the door for a walk to the lake before returning for breakfast. After lunch we usually get out into nature again with our mountain bikes for another outdoor adventure. Evening is time to relax, unplug, and restore with reading, a movie at home, another short meditation.

Lani says: The cultivation of a mindfulness meditation practice has been pivotal for me in creating a life of greater kindness, compassion, and ease. For example, after struggling with food, weight, and eating for several decades, when I decided to abandon dieting practices and eat mindfully instead, I dropped more than 40 pounds twenty years ago, which has been sustained to this day.

Awakening to the vegan lifestyle is a tremendous door opener to living a happier, healthier life. Yet in concert with that, cultivating some practice that helps you stay more intimately connected with your innate qualities of peace, compassion, and equanimity will serve you tremendously. Mindfulness practice and mindfulness meditation practice—which I teach in *The Mindful Vegan*—have served people for thousands of years in this capacity. If you have some practice that strengthens these elements in you, by all means keep with it or pick it back up again. If you are looking for something to support you in this regard, mindfulness meditation is my highest recommendation for living more mindfully and making the biggest difference.

part two

AGE-DEFYING VEGAN RECIPES

Over 175 delectable, plant-based recipes for health and longevity—using seven main ingredients or less!

The path to an ageless body and mind starts with the food you eat. The recipes in this book are packed with nutrients from ingredients that support longevity, brain and heart health, skin health, and the youthful glow everyone seeks. And they are delicious—with something for everyone! The style here is "vegan fusion," a type of cuisine that celebrates culinary contributions from around the world.

We've kept it simple: The age-defying recipes in this book feature great flavor from only seven main ingredients (excluding salt and pepper, cooking oil, and optional ingredients). Every ingredient counts! Keeping the ingredients to a minimum allows you to crush your meal prep as a quick and easy chef extraordinaire.

The recipes in each chapter are listed roughly in order from lightest to heaviest.

Use these recipes as a starting point for creating your own versions and specialties based on your preferences and whatever ingredients are on hand and available locally. Once you have understood the simple concept of a Template Recipe (page 98), you will discover how easy it is to create hundreds and even thousands of variations to please every palate.

All of the recipes list the approximate amount of time you will be doing actual prepping of ingredients (Prep Time). They also list the amount of time required to cook the food (Cook Time). We also list time for such things as marinating, soaking, and cooling down. Total Time is what the recipe will take from start to finish. If total time is less than the other times added up, that means you can prep some of the ingredients while other items are cooking. Serving sizes and total yields are listed in volume ounces, not weight ounces, unless otherwise noted.

The time you spend preparing food can be a calming and healing experience for you. Do what you can to create a clean and peaceful environment. Play your favorite music, decorate the table with flowers, and let your creative juices flow. Use your time in the kitchen as an opportunity to cultivate mindfulness and gratitude. Leave your cares at the door, and focus on the present-moment experience of preparing the food. Be aware of the colors, textures, and aromas of the ingredients. Using all of your senses helps your body to better absorb nutrients. Think lovingly of the people for whom you will be preparing the food. They will notice it!

NINE

BASIC COOKING TECHNIQUES

Are you new to vegan cooking? *Please download our convenient Recommended Kitchen Gear and Vegan Pantry Essentials checklists at www.doctorchefresources.com.*

If you aren't already eating a plant-based diet, we want to make it as easy as possible for you to get these healthful foods into your routine. In this chapter, you'll find some core tools for your vegan culinary toolbox. Knife cuts, techniques for cooking grains and beans, how to create the perfect roasted tempeh, how to press tofu, how to water sauté, and how to grill like a boss! These are just some basic guides. Cooking, like life in many ways, comes down to practice and trial and error. Keep a positive attitude and be gentle with yourself as you evolve as a cook. We believe in you! You will be a rock star in no time.

7 Tricks for Making Meal Prep a Snap

Here are some more ways to get the most out of your meal preparation:

1. **Spice blends save time.** Stock up on as many of the blends as you can. This way, you are measuring only once but getting the benefit of several ingredients. Check out the Global Spice Blend recipes in this book (pages 249–252), or see what creative blends are available at your local market. Garam masala, pumpkin pie spice, and Chinese five-spice powder are typically easy to find and they are guaranteed to deliver on flavor.
2. **Use high-flavor ingredients.** Use ingredients that pack a big flavor in a small package to quickly take food to the next level. For example, *nutritional yeast* will give food a nutty, cheesy flavor (plus a dose of B vitamins and protein). *Wheat-free tamari*, a soy

sauce derived from the miso-making process, provides an umami flavor and can help flavors pop when you add just the right amount). *Chipotle powder* instantly delivers smokiness and heat, which can invigorate your palate big time! Discover your favorites . . . maybe it's a hot sauce; a condiment, such as truffle oil; or an aged balsamic vinegar.

3. **Frozen foods are your friend.** While fresh is always best, many need to rely on frozen foods to whip up quick and nutritious meals on the go. Consider using frozen veggies, such as spinach, mixed vegetables, broccoli, okra, and corn. For fruits, stock up on berries for your morning smoothie. Even prepared vegan frozen meals, such as pizza or bowls, can serve your needs in a pinch. If you have time, you can add fresh veggies and herbs to take it up a notch. Keep these frozen gems on hand to be there when you need them.

4. **Think Template Recipes:** This will expand your creativity in the kitchen. By breaking a recipe down into its components, know that you can alter any one of them to create a whole new recipe. Even when you leave every other part of the recipe the same, altering one component creates a new flavor profile for the entire dish.

   The supercool thing is that once you learn how to view recipes as templates, it helps you break out of the "what's for dinner?" trap. In the past, while thumbing through a cookbook, you might have passed over a recipe if you did not have the ingredients listed. However, once you view recipes as a template, you can see the underlying formula, and make substitutions based on what you have on hand. For more info on Template Recipes, and how one dish can turn into hundreds and thousands, please visit www.doctorchefresources.com.

5. **Zen out.** To simplify the preparation and cleanup of the dishes you are preparing, try to minimize the equipment. See whether you can cook your veggies in the same pot as the pasta, use the same bowl for different recipes, and so on. Also, before beginning any preparation, create a clean work area and gather all your necessary ingredients and kitchen gear.

6. **Be prepared.** To help cut down on preparation time, set aside an hour or so on one of your least busy days for advance prepping. Having prepped ingredients on hand makes it easier to create meals on the go. You can cut vegetables and store them in a glass container in the fridge. Make a Salad in a Jar (page 157); cook a squash, grain, or pot of beans. You can then use these foods in recipes over the next few days. Consider preparing a pot of rice or quinoa in a rice cooker in the morning and using it for the evening meal.

7. **Food is medicine.** Each time you eat something, ask yourself whether that food will serve as fuel to "turn back the clock" and optimize your health and nutrition. To help get plant-based foods in the rotation, take what you are eating and think "plus one":

What one thing can I add to my plate to add a bit more nutrition to what I am eating? Maybe it's adding a few fresh berries to your cereal, or sprinkling some sunflower seeds or chia seeds on your vegan yogurt, or adding a handful of fresh arugula the next time you break out a frozen vegan pizza.

A big caveat on this one. Please don't be hard on yourself if you fall short of your goals. Stand up, wipe the chocolate cake crumbs off your face, and get back in the game! Be gentle with yourself as you progress toward your vision of where you would like to be in your diet and life!

Basic Knife Cuts

Refer to this section as you prepare the recipes if you have any questions about how to cut the ingredients.

Mince: The finest that can be cut by hand, to mince is to chop a food into very small pieces. Used with garlic, ginger, fresh herbs.

Dice: Slightly larger than mince, ¼-inch uniform pieces. Good for carrots, onions, zucchini, potatoes, peppers.

Chop: Larger than diced; usually ½ inch in diameter. Try with carrots, zucchini, potatoes, beets, peppers, onions, eggplant, tomatoes.

Slice: Many types are possible: thin or thick, half-moon shape, rings, or diagonal. Works with onion, cabbage, cucumber, zucchini, carrots, eggplant, peppers, beets, tomatoes.

Chiffonade: Thin ribbon strips of herbs, such as basil, mint, or sage. To chiffonade, form a stack of a few leaves of the herb, roll like a burrito, and cut thin slices to form the ribbons.

Cube: Chopped into uniform squares. Can vary in size. Try with carrots, eggplant, zucchini, beets, jicama, potatoes.

Julienne: Long, thin strips (à la matchsticks) about ⅛ inch wide. Used with carrots, zucchini, peppers. Try using different-colored bell peppers, such as red, orange, and green.

Shred: Cut into thin strips, either by hand or using a grater or food processor. Try carrots, beets, zucchini, jicama, cabbage.

> **TIMELESS TIPS**
>
> **If You Don't Have Fresh Herbs**
> If a recipe calls for fresh herbs and all you have is dried, you can substitute 1 teaspoon of dried herb for every tablespoon of fresh herb called for in the recipe.
>
> **Key Conversions**
> If you find yourself needing to multiply or reduce recipes, you will find the following formulas very helpful:
> 1 tablespoon = 3 teaspoons
> 4 tablespoons = ¼ cup

Cooking Grains

Follow these steps and you will always have perfectly cooked grains.

1. Rinse the grain thoroughly and drain the excess water.
2. Bring the measured amount of grain and liquid (either vegetable stock or water) to a boil. You may wish to add a small amount of sea salt. (The advantage of adding the salt at this stage, rather than after the grain is cooked, is that the salt flavor will be more uniformly distributed. Also, stirring the salt into cooked grains can create a mushy texture.)
3. Cover with a tight-fitting lid, lower the heat to low, and simmer for the recommended time. As the grain is being steamed, do not lift the lid until the grain is finished cooking. Cooking times may vary, depending on altitude and stove cooking temperatures. The grain is generally done when it is chewy and all the liquid is absorbed.

Enhance the flavor of your grain dishes by adding such ingredients as minced garlic or ginger, diced onion, a couple of bay leaves or kaffir lime leaves, or crushed lemongrass while cooking. If you wish to use a rice cooker, Miracle and Instant Pot put out a stainless-steel version. Steer clear of aluminum or nonstick rice cookers.

Grain Cooking Chart

Grain	Liquid per cup of grain	Approx. cooking time	Approx. yield
Amaranth: Ancient grain of Aztecs, higher in protein and nutrients than most grains	2½ cups	25 minutes	2½ cups
Barley, pearled: Good in soups and stews. Contains gluten.	3 cups	45 minutes	3½ cups
Buckwheat: Hearty, nutty flavor. When toasted, it's called kasha and takes less time to cook. Also used as a breakfast cereal.	2 cups	15 minutes	2½ cups
Cornmeal: Made from ground corn—a staple of Native Americans; use in corn bread or grits.	3 cups	20 minutes	3½ cups
Couscous: A North African staple made from ground semolina. Contains gluten.	1½ cups	15 minutes	1½ cups
Farro: An ancient variety of wheat with a nutty flavor that is high in fiber, iron, protein, zinc, niacin, and folate. Wonderful as the base for risottos. Contains gluten.	2¾ cups; drain excess if necessary	30 minutes for whole grain, less for pearled and semipearled	2 cups
Kamut: An ancient variety of wheat that many with wheat allergies are able to tolerate. Contains gluten.	3 cups	1 hour	3 cups

Grain	Liquid per cup of grain	Approx. cooking time	Approx. yield
Millet: A highly nutritious grain that is used in casseroles, stews, and cereals. Especially tasty with flax oil.	2½ cups	20 minutes	3 cups
Oats: A versatile grain that is popular as a cereal, for baking, and for milks. Look for certified gluten-free varieties if needed.			
Steel-cut	3 cups	30 to 40 minutes	3 cups
Groats	3 cups	1 hour	3 cups
Rolled	3 cups	10 minutes	3 cups
Quick	2 cups	5 minutes	2 cups
Polenta: A type of cornmeal; used in Italian cooking. To cook, bring liquid to a boil. Lower the heat to a simmer and whisk in the polenta, stirring until done.	3 cups	10 minutes	3 cups
Quinoa: Ancient grain of the Incas. High in protein and nutrients. Has a delicate, nutty flavor.	2 cups	20 minutes	2½ cups
Rice: Rice has a high nutrient content and is a staple in many of the world's cultures. Basmati rice has a nutty flavor and is used in Indian cooking.			
Brown basmati	2 cups	35 to 40 minutes	2¼ cups
White basmati	1½ cups	20 minutes	2 cups
Brown long-grain	2 cups	45 minutes	3 cups
Brown short-grain	2 cups	45 minutes	3 cups
Wild	3 cups	1 hour	4 cups
Jasmine	1¾ cups	20 minutes	3½ cups
Sushi	1¼ cups	20 minutes	3 cups
Rye: A staple grain throughout Europe. Used as a cereal or ground to make breads, including pumpernickel. Contains gluten.			
Berries	4 cups	1 hour	3 cups
Flakes	3 cups	20 minutes	3 cups
Spelt: An ancient form of wheat. It contains more protein and nutrition than wheat.	3½ cups	1½ hours	3 cups
Teff: From Ethiopia, the smallest grain in the world, and the main ingredient for *injera* flatbread	3 cups	20 minutes	1½ cups
Wheat: A primary bread grain. Bulgur is used in Middle Eastern dishes, such as tabbouleh. Cracked may be used as a cereal. Contains gluten.			
Whole	3 cups	2 hours	2¾ cups
Bulgur	2 cups	15 minutes	2½ cups
Cracked	2 cups	25 minutes	2½ cups

Before you cook dried legumes, pick over them thoroughly, removing any stones or debris.

Dried legumes, except split peas, should be soaked before cooking, and they can take some time to soften, which is why many people soak their legumes overnight. If you forget to soak them overnight, a quick method is to bring the legumes and four times the amount of water to a boil, remove from the heat, cover, and allow to sit for a few hours.

Soaking improves digestibility and reduces gas. Other methods for improving digestibility include adding some fennel seeds, a handful of brown rice, or a few strips of the sea vegetable kombu (rinse well before using) to the legumes while cooking.

After soaking or boiling legumes, discard the soak water, place the beans and the measured amount of vegetable stock or filtered water in a heavy-bottomed pot, bring to a boil, cover, lower the heat to a simmer, and cook until tender. Do not add salt to the cooking liquid; it can make the legumes tough. Legumes are done cooking when they are tender but not mushy. They should retain their original shape.

Please see the following legume cooking chart. Note that the times in the chart are for cooking dried legumes. Reduce the cooking time by 25 percent when legumes are soaked.

LEGUME COOKING CHART

Legume	Liquid per cup of legume	Approx. cook time	Approx. yield
Adzuki/aduki beans: Tender red bean used in Japanese and macrobiotic cooking	3¼ cups	45 minutes	3 cups
Anasazi beans: Means "the ancient ones" in Navajo language; sweeter and meatier than most beans	3 cups	2 hours	2 cups
Black beans (turtle beans): Good in Spanish, South American, and Caribbean dishes	4 cups	1¼ hours	2½ cups
Black-eyed peas: A staple of the American South	4 cups	1¼ hours	2 cups
Chickpeas (garbanzo beans): Used in Middle Eastern and Indian dishes. Pureed cooked chickpeas form the base of hummus.	4 cups	3 to 4 hours	2 cups
Great northern beans: Large white beans	4 cups	1½ hours	2 cups
Kidney beans: Medium-size red beans. The most popular bean in the United States, also used in Mexican cooking.	4 cups	1½ hours	2 cups
Lentils: Come in green, red, and French varieties. A member of the pea family used in Indian dal dishes and soups.	3 cups	20 to 45 minutes	2¼ cups

Legume	Liquid per cup of legume	Approx. cook time	Approx. yield
Lima beans (butter beans): White beans with a distinctive flavor and high in nutrients			
Regular limas	3 cups	1½ hours	1¼ cups
Baby limas	3 cups	1½ hours	1¾ cups
Mung beans: Grown in India and Asia. Used in Indian dal dishes. May be soaked and sprouted and used in soups and salads.	3 cups	45 minutes	2¼ cups
Navy beans (white beans): Hearty beans used in soups, stews, and cold salads	4 cups	2½ hours	2 cups
Pinto beans: Used in Mexican and Southwestern cooking. Used in soups and as refried beans in burritos.	4 cups	2½ hours	2 cups
Soybeans: Versatile, high-protein beans widely used in Asia. May be processed into tofu, tempeh, miso, soy milk, soy sauce, and soy cheese.	4 cups	3+ hours	2 cups
Split peas: Come in yellow and green varieties. Do not need to be soaked. Used in soups and Indian dals.	3 cups	45 minutes	2¼ cups

Working with Tofu

Tofu is sold in a number of different forms, including superfirm, extra-firm, firm, soft, and silken. There is even a sprouted tofu, which is said to be easier to digest. Each form lends itself to a particular type of food preparation. (The recipes in this book specify which form of tofu is required for the dish.)

Silken: Blend and use to replace dairy products in puddings, frostings, dressings, creamy soups, and sauces.

Soft: Use cubed in soups or pureed in sauces, spreads, or dips.

Medium and firm: Use scrambled, grated in casseroles, or cubed in stir-fries.

Superfirm and extra-firm: Use grilled or baked as cutlets, or cubed and roasted. It may also be steamed and used in steamed vegetable dishes.

Leftover tofu should be rinsed and covered with water in a glass container in the refrigerator. Change the water daily. Use within 3 or 4 days. Firm and extra-firm tofu may be frozen for up to 2 months. Frozen tofu, once defrosted, has a spongy texture that absorbs marinades more than does tofu that has not been frozen.

How to press tofu: Some recommend pressing tofu to remove excess water, create a firmer tofu, and help the tofu absorb marinades more effectively. Pressing is generally not needed for the superfirm and many extra-firm varieties. If you would like to press your tofu, place the block of tofu on a clean surface, such as a plate, baking sheet, or casserole dish. Place a clean plate on top of the tofu and weigh down with a jar or other weight. Allow it to press for 15 to 45 minutes, draining the liquid periodically. You can also purchase a tofu press at one of the websites listed in the Resources (page 307).

To make tofu cutlets: Slice a block of extra-firm tofu into thirds or fourths. If you wish, you can then cut these cutlets in half to yield six or eight cutlets per 14-ounce package. You can also cut the tofu diagonally to create triangular cutlets. Cutlets can be marinated and then roasted or grilled.

To make tofu cubes: To make medium-size cubes, slice the tofu as you would for three or four cutlets. Then, make four cuts along the length and three cuts along the width of the tofu. You can make the cubes larger or smaller by altering the number of cuts.

Working with Tempeh

Tempeh is a cultured soy product that originated in Indonesia, and tastes best when thoroughly cooked before consuming. Tempeh is high in protein, and has a heavier, coarser texture than tofu. It usually has a mild, slightly fermented flavor. Its color is usually tan with a few dark gray spots.

Many different varieties of tempeh are created by mixing the soybean with grains, such as millet, wheat, or rice, together with sea vegetables and seasonings. There are many brands of tempeh on the market. Some of our favorites are the Tofurky brand and the Soy Boy brand. It is typically available in an 8-ounce package. Several varieties come in a thick, square block; others, as a thinner rectangle. Some recommend steaming the tempeh before using in recipes, to remove the bitterness and help it absorb marinades more effectively. To do so, place a steamer basket in a large pot with about 1 inch of water over high heat. Cover, bring to a boil, and add the tempeh to the steamer basket. Lower the heat to medium and cook, covered, for 10 minutes. Store leftover tempeh in a sealed glass container in the refrigerator for up to 3 days.

To make tempeh cutlets: You can slice the square block in half to create a thinner block and then cut it in half or into triangles. The longer block may also be sliced into thinner cutlets. These cutlets may then be cut into cubes.

Roasting Tofu and Tempeh

Tofu and tempeh cubes can be marinated, roasted, and then stored for a couple of days in a glass container in the refrigerator, to be used in salads, stir-fries, or on their own as a snack. With tofu, it is best to use extra-firm or superfirm varieties, for optimal texture.

To roast tofu and tempeh cutlets, and cubes, follow these three simple steps:

1. Preheat an oven or toaster oven to 375°F. Cut the tofu or tempeh into cutlets or cubes as mentioned earlier.
2. Place the cutlets or cubes in a marinade of your choosing. A simple marinade can consist of a spritz of tamari, a small amount of olive oil, and a small amount of water. Allow them to sit for a few minutes and up to overnight. If marinating overnight, store in an airtight container in the refrigerator. If you follow an oil-free diet, you can omit the oil and add vegetable stock or additional water.
3. Place on a well-oiled baking sheet or casserole dish. Roast until golden brown, 15 to 20 minutes, stirring the cutlets or cubes occasionally to ensure even cooking. Because brands and oven temperatures differ, check periodically to attain your desired level of doneness. If making cutlets, you can flip them after 10 minutes. Try a convection oven or use a BROIL setting, for a crispier crust. If using the BROIL setting, the cutlets and cubes will cook faster than roasting.

Grilling

Grilling creates a smoky, deep, and rich flavor. Try grilling tempeh and tofu cutlets, as well as many vegetables, such as portobello mushrooms, corn, onions, baby bok choy, carrots, bell peppers, asparagus, zucchini, coconut meat, or eggplant. You can even grill fruit, such as pineapple slices, peaches, apples, or pears.

For added flavor, place the food in a marinade (see page 255) from a few minutes to overnight before grilling. Baste or brush lightly with oil, brushing occasionally and grilling until char marks appear and the food is heated thoroughly, flipping periodically. If using a gas grill, avoid placing food over a direct flame.

Another grilling option is to use a stovetop grill. Kitchen supply stores sell cast-iron and nonstick pans that are flat, straddle two burners, and have a griddle on one side and a grooved side for grilling. The flavor is similar and you get the signature char marks.

Steam or Water Sautéing

Steam or water sautéing may be used if you wish to eliminate the use of heated oils in your diet. Water or vegetable stock is used instead of oil in the initial cooking stages for dishes that are sautéed. Place a small amount of water or vegetable stock in a heated pan, add the vegetables, and follow the recipes as you would if using oil. Add small amounts of water at a time, if necessary, to prevent sticking. Lemon or lime juice may also be mixed in with the water, for added flavor.

Toasting Spices, Nuts, and Seeds

Toasting brings out a deeper flavor of ingredients. There are two main techniques for toasting:

1. *Dry sauté pan.* For this method, place a dry sauté pan over high heat and allow the pan to heat up. Add the food to the pan and cook until the food turns golden brown, stirring constantly. This method is good for spices, grains, and small quantities of nuts or seeds. If you wish, you can use an oil sauté for seeds or nuts by placing a small amount of high-heat oil, such as sesame, in the pan before adding the seeds or nuts.
2. *Oven.* Preheat your oven to 350°F. Place the food on a dry baking sheet and leave in the oven until golden brown, stirring occasionally and being mindful to avoid burning. This method is best for nuts, seeds, and shredded coconut. Nuts become crunchier after cooling down. As mentioned earlier, if you have more time, you can enhance the flavor even more by roasting at lower temperatures for longer periods of time. For instance, nuts roasted at 200°F for 45 minutes have a richer, toastier flavor than those roasted at a high temperature for shorter periods of time.

Soaking Nuts and Seeds

Soaking nuts and seeds is one of the main techniques in vegan raw food preparation. Soaking improves their digestibility and makes more nutrients available. Even soaking for just 15 minutes will produce some benefit, so don't hesitate to soak if you're short on time.

Rinse the nuts or seeds well and place them in a bowl or jar with water in a ratio of 1 part nuts or seeds to 3 or 4 parts water. Allow them to sit for the recommended time before draining, rinsing, and using in recipes.

Seed and Nut Soaking Times

Nut	Soak Time
Almonds	4 to 6 hours
Brazil nuts	4 to 6 hours
Cashews	1 to 2 hours
Hazelnuts	4 to 6 hours
Macadamia nuts	1 to 2 hours

Nut/Seed	Soak Time
Pecans	4 to 6 hours
Pine nuts	1 to 2 hours
Walnuts	4 to 6 hours
Pumpkin seeds	1 to 4 hours
Sesame seeds	1 to 4 hours
Sunflower seeds	1 to 4 hours

Natural Sweeteners

Eating refined white sugar and high-fructose corn syrup will age you fast. Their consumption is linked to many health problems, including emotional disorders, obesity, diabetes, and tooth decay. According to William Duffy's classic book *Sugar Blues*, it is believed that because refined sugars are missing the nutrients that are contained in naturally sweet whole foods, the body is drained of its own store of minerals and nutrients in its efforts to metabolize the sugar.

But you don't have to give up sweets altogether. Instead, try cooking with naturally occurring and minimally processed sweeteners. You can replace traditional white sugar with raw cane sugar or organic sugar at a one-to-one ratio without making any changes to your recipes. You can also replace the white sugar with any of the sweeteners that follow. These sweeteners are superior to white sugar, but since they are all concentrated, please use in moderation.

The following chart indicates how much of a sweetener is needed to replace 1 cup of white, refined sugar. The chart also indicates how much liquid to delete from the recipe to maintain its consistency if the sweetener is a liquid.

Sweetener Chart

Sweetener	Replace 1 cup of refined sugar with	Reduce liquids by
Agave nectar: A natural extract from this famous Mexican cactus, with a low glycemic index. When possible, purchase the raw variety, which is less processed than the cooked varieties.	¾ cup	⅓
Barley malt syrup: Roughly half as sweet as honey or sugar. Made from sprouted barley and has a nutty, caramel flavor. (Contains gluten.)	¾ cup	¼
Blackstrap molasses: This syrup is a liquid by-product of the sugar-refining process. It contains many of the nutrients of the sugarcane plant, including iron and calcium. Has a strong, distinct flavor.	½ cup	¼

(Continues)

Sweetener (Continued)	Replace 1 cup of refined sugar with	Reduce liquids by
Brown rice syrup: A relatively neutral-flavored sweetener that is roughly half as sweet as sugar or honey. It's made from fermented brown rice.	1 cup	¼
Coconut crystals: This air-dried coconut nectar creates a nutrient-rich granulated sugar that is our recommended sugar for the recipes in this book. It has a dark, rich flavor with a lower glycemic index than cane sugar. Manufactured by Coconut Secret.	1 cup	0
Coconut nectar: A mildly flavored sweetener manufactured by Coconut Secret that is a wonderful replacement for agave nectar. It has a low glycemic index and is loaded with vitamins, minerals, amino acids, and other nutrients.	¾ cup	⅓
Date sugar: A granulated sugar produced from drying fresh dates.	⅔ cup	0
Fruit syrup: The preferred method of sweetening involves soaking, then blending raisins and dates with filtered water to create a sweet syrup. Try ½ cup of raisins with 1 cup of water and experiment to find your desired sweetness.	1 cup	¼
Lucuma powder: A raw, low-glycemic sweetener with a slight maple flavor. Comes from the lucuma fruit, grown in the Peruvian Andes.	1 cup	0
Maple syrup: Forty gallons of sap from the maple tree are needed to create 1 gallon of pure maple syrup. It is mineral rich and graded according to color and flavor. Grade A is the mildest and lightest; Grade C is the darkest and richest. Good for baking.	¾ cup	¼
Stevia (powdered): Stevia is a plant that originates in the Brazilian rainforest. The powdered form is between 200 and 400 percent sweeter than white sugar. It is noncaloric, does not promote tooth decay, and is said to be acceptable for diabetics and those with blood sugar imbalances. For baking conversions, please visit www.ehow.com/how_2268348_substitute-stevia-sugar-baking.html.	1 teaspoon	0
Sucanat: Abbreviation for "sugar cane natural." It is a granular sweetener that consists of evaporated sugarcane juice. It has about the same sweetness as sugar. It retains most of the vitamins and minerals of the sugarcane.	1 cup	0
Xylitol: A naturally occurring sugar substitute found in the fibers of fruits and vegetables, such as berries, corn husks, oats, plums, and mushrooms. Originally extracted from birch trees in Finland in the nineteenth century. Said to promote dental health and to be a safe sweetener for diabetics because of its low glycemic index.	1 cup	0
Yacón: This tuber is a distant relative of the sunflower. From the Andean region of South America, mineral-rich yacón syrup has a dark brown color and is used as a low-calorie sweetener.	¾ cup	⅓

DIY Date Syrup

You can make this fruit-based sweetener to replace maple syrup, agave nectar, or other concentrated sweeteners.

MAKES ABOUT 1 CUP SYRUP

¼ cup pitted dates
1 cup water

Combine the dates and water in a strong blender and blend until smooth. Store in a glass jar in the refrigerator for up to 4 days.

TEN

BOUNTIFUL BEVERAGES

Lift up your glass and toast to good health, and to long life! In this section, we feature beverages that can actually help you achieve those results from what you have in your glass.

Of course, **water** is the queen of antiaging beverages. It is essential to keeping all your biochemical processes running smoothly, as well as ensuring that your joints stay lubricated and your skin retains its suppleness. Don't miss your body's many cries for water. The next time you feel a pang of hunger, try drinking a glass of water first and you will be surprised how satiating it can be. If you want to bump up your water consumption, consider adding herbs, such as rosemary sprigs, mint leaves, or fennel fronds, to your glass. Or fruit, such as lemon, lime, orange, or grapefruit slices. For a spa day, add some cucumber slices. The added flavor makes it easier to drink more water, more often. And you'll get the benefit of added micronutrients from the foods you add.

Teas are wonderful to enjoy, especially a decaffeinated tea at the end of a long day. Consider making your own medicinal teas (see page 122) or stock up on your favorite organic teas. Be sure to include a hibiscus tea, which is reputed to have a wide range of benefits for the cardiovascular, digestive, and immune systems.

Juices are one of the best sources of liquid nutrition since the nutrients are most easily assimilated into your bloodstream. Try the Hydration Station (page 115) and Citrus Cleanse (page 117).

Once you see how easy it is to create your own **plant-based milks**, you will never turn back. Check out the Pumpkin Seed Milk (page 116) to see for yourself. Plant-based milks can form the base for other drinks, such as Maca Pepita Elixir (page 118). Get your superfoods in with the Cacao Turmeric Elixir (page 120).

Smoothies have benefit of all the fiber of the whole food. They are also the simplest way to get superfoods into your diet. Partake of the Choco-Cherry Berry Smoothie (page 121), and you will be amazed that something that tastes so good can be so good for you. For a taste of the tropics, imbibe the Creamy Tropical Bliss (page 118). One of Mark and Ashley's go-to morning smoothies consists of almond or soy milk, an all-in-one superfood blend (our favorite is New Greens Sustain that Mark formulated with all-organic ingredients), hemp seeds, maca powder, chia seeds, green powder or chlorella, cacao nibs, and banana or fresh berries. Be sure to enjoy juices and smoothies within thirty minutes to optimize the nutrition.

For additional smoothie recipes, including our patented go-to smoothie Template Recipe mentioned above (as well as a video), please visit www.doctorchefresources.com.

Since beverages can be hydrating (think: teas, juices, elixirs) they are useful to optimize the health of your skin. The heavier smoothies, especially those loaded with superfoods, can nourish all your body systems—fueling your longevity and feeding your brain, heart, skin, digestive system, organs, and more!

TIMELESS TIPS: SMOOTHIE SIMPLIFICATION

1. Keep frozen fruits, such as berries, peaches, or mangoes, in the freezer for when you run short on fresh fruit, or when you want to have a cold smoothie. Consider placing peeled bananas in a container or bag in the freezer as well. These can be whole or chopped, and can be just ripe to overripe.

2. Keep a stock of superfood add-ins for your custom smoothies, including ground flaxseeds, chia seeds, cacao nibs, hemp seeds, goji berries, and/or chlorella. Ground flaxseeds are also good to have on hand to add to juices; store in your freezer to keep them fresh.

3. Once you have your favorite smoothie dialed in, consider assembling the ingredients for a batch the night before. Place all the ingredients together in a container, so you just need to combine them in a blender and blend when you are ready.

Rosemary Star Anise Tea

You can feel the healing in every sip with these flavorful ingredients from your spice rack! Rosemary is said to help with memory and concentration, while the anise and cinnamon can improve digestion and balance blood sugar.

TOTAL YIELD: 28 OUNCES
Serving Size: 7 ounces
Number of Servings: 4
Prep Time: 5 minutes
Cook Time: 15 minutes
Total Time: 20 minutes

3½ cups water
1 (6-inch) sprig rosemary
1 cinnamon stick
1 star anise
1 teaspoon coriander seeds or cardamom pods
2 slices blood orange or orange

1. Place the water in a small pot over high heat and bring to a boil. Lower the heat to low. Add the remaining ingredients.
2. Allow to simmer for 15 minutes. Strain well and enjoy!

VARIATIONS

⚘ Replace the orange slices with lemon or lime.

⚘ Add 1 teaspoon of whole cloves and 1 teaspoon of whole black peppercorns.

⚘ Add 1 tablespoon of yerba maté for more energy.

⚘ Add 1 tea bag of green tea 5 minutes before serving.

Morning Miracle

An ultrasimple beverage to start your day and for any time you want to give your immune system a boost. Ginger and cayenne help keep the blood moving, while turmeric calms any excess inflammation. Feel free to add your favorite sweetener to taste. Enjoy on an empty stomach.

TOTAL YIELD: 24 OUNCES
Serving Size: 12 ounces
Number of Servings: 2
Prep Time: 5 minutes
Cook Time: 15 minutes
Total Time: 20 minutes

3 cups water
1 (2-inch) piece fresh ginger, sliced
1 (1-inch) piece fresh turmeric, sliced
½ lemon, sliced
Pinch of cayenne pepper
½ teaspoon chlorella (optional)

1. Place the water in a small pot over low heat. Add the ginger and turmeric and cook for 10 minutes. Add the lemon and cook for 5 minutes.
2. Add the cayenne and chlorella, if using, and stir well.
3. Pour through a strainer into your favorite mug and enjoy.

VARIATIONS

⚘ Replace the lemon with lime or orange.

⚘ Add a cinnamon stick along with the ginger.

Green Dragon

Get your green on with this refreshing and energizing beverage to keep you going strong through the day. Light and hydrating apple and cucumber balance out the deep mineral-rich kale and the two super-root medicines. Enjoy a boost to your heart health, digestion, and immunity all in one.

TOTAL YIELD: 18 OUNCES
  Serving Size: 9 ounces
  Number of Servings: 2
  Prep Time: 10 minutes
  Total Time: 10 minutes

1 (2-inch) piece fresh ginger, unpeeled or peeled
1 (1-inch) piece fresh turmeric, unpeeled or peeled
3 large apples, cored
3 large kale leaves with stem
1 large cucumber, chopped
1 tablespoon freshly squeezed lime juice

Process the ginger, turmeric, apples, kale, and cucumber through a juicer. Add the lime juice and mix well. Have fun imbibing!

VARIATIONS

- Add a small handful of fresh cilantro.

- Once juiced, transfer to a blender along with the flesh of ½ avocado.

- Add 1 tablespoon of ground flaxseeds and stir well before drinking.

Bright Eyes Tonic

Wake up to this savory and sweet elixir with a kick of cayenne heat. A delicious way to receive tons of antioxidant protection. You can feel the beta-carotene, lycopene, and allicin compounds going to work right away!

TOTAL YIELD: 24 OUNCES
  Serving Size: 12 ounces
  Number of Servings: 2
  Prep Time: 10 minutes
  Total Time: 10 minutes

2 cloves garlic
4 stalks celery
1 large tomato, quartered
2 pounds carrots, tops removed
1 tablespoon freshly squeezed lemon juice
Pinch of cayenne pepper

1. Process the garlic, celery, tomato, and carrots through a juicer.
2. Add the lemon juice and cayenne and stir well before enjoying. Add more lemon juice to taste, if desired.

VARIATIONS

- Add a small handful of fresh parsley along with the tomato.

- Replace the lemon juice with ¼ cup of freshly squeezed orange juice.

Hydration Station

When the heat of summer or the exertion of exercise strikes, this is your beverage. For the next level of hydration, add the coconut water listed in the variations. High in water content as well as healthy fiber, grapes and watermelon are perfect pick-me-ups on a warm day. Bananas round out the flavor and texture, and provide electrolyte balance as well as a boost of B vitamins.

TOTAL YIELD: 16 OUNCES
> Serving Size: 8 ounces
> Number of Servings: 2
> Prep Time: 5 minutes
> Total Time: 5 minutes

1 heaping cup grapes
1 cup chopped watermelon (small pieces)
1 large banana

Place all the ingredients in a blender and blend until smooth.

VARIATIONS

- Add 1 tablespoon of ground flaxseeds or chia seeds.

- Add 1 cup of coconut water.

- Replace the watermelon with honeydew or Crenshaw melon, or with berries, such as blueberries or strawberries.

Tart Cherry and Pomegranate Tonic

Behold the heart-healthy mojito mocktail. So brightly delicious and refreshing! In general, we shy away from prepared juices, but these two powerhouses are the exception. Cherry juice is not only known for its ability to reduce pain by lowering uric acid in gout or muscle soreness, but also is one of the few known substantial sources of melatonin. Pomegranate's tiny seeds hold lots of vitamin C, with proven immunity-boosting, tissue-repairing, and cell-protecting qualities, as well as two other powerful antioxidants well known to prevent disease and reduce inflammation.

TOTAL YIELD: 16 OUNCES
> Serving Size: 8 ounces
> Number of Servings: 2
> Prep Time: 10 minutes
> Total Time: 10 minutes

Leaves from 2 sprigs mint
⅔ cup tart cherry juice
⅔ cup pomegranate juice
2 teaspoons freshly squeezed lime juice
⅔ cup sparkling water
Your choice of sweetener

1. Place the mint leaves in a pitcher or two glasses. Crush with a cocktail muddler or with your hands.
2. Add the remaining ingredients and stir well before serving.

VARIATION

- Go crazy and add a scoop vegan ice cream, for the float of your dreams.

Pumpkin Seed Milk

You, too, will realize the glory of the humble pumpkin seed, or pepita. We will give you a hint . . . they're not just for Halloween! These beautiful seeds are full of zinc, important in skin health, immunity, and hormone health, with specific benefit to the prostate gland. This is a creative and delicious way to take in necessary zinc as well as plenty of antioxidant vitamin E, magnesium, and other important trace minerals.

TOTAL YIELD: 24 OUNCES STRAINED
Serving Size: 8 ounces
Number of Servings: 3
Prep Time: 5 minutes
Total Time: 5 minutes

1 cup pumpkin seeds
3½ cups water
3 to 4 Medjool dates, pitted (optional)
Pinch of sea salt
⅛ teaspoon ground allspice or nutmeg

1. Place all the ingredients in a blender and blend until creamy.
2. Pour through a fine-mesh strainer, nut milk bag, or other fine-mesh strainer bag.
3. Store in a glass jar in the refrigerator and enjoy within 3 to 4 days.

VARIATIONS

- Feel free to add your favorite sweetener to taste (see pages 107–108), instead of the dates.

- Add 1 teaspoon of pure vanilla extract, or the seeds from 1 vanilla bean, along with pumpkin seeds.

- Replace the pumpkin seeds with the seed, nut, or combination of both you desire. Try Brazil nuts, cashews, macadamia nuts, pecans, or the old faithful, almonds.

- For an **Oat Milk**, soak steel-cut oats for 12 hours. Rinse and drain well. Add to the blender and prepare as above.

Citrus Cleanse

Looking for delicious and creative ways of including raw garlic in your diet? If not, you probably should be . . . raw garlic is a natural antibiotic that can stop a pending infection in its tracks. Start with one clove and work your way up to three. Turmeric blends well with these gorgeous citrus fruits, adding even more immunity-boosting power. Enjoy this vitamin C burst at the start of your day, especially if you are feeling under the weather.

TOTAL YIELD: 32 OUNCES
Serving Size: 8 ounces
Number of Servings: 4
Prep Time: 20 minutes
Total Time: 20 minutes

2 cups chopped pineapple
1 cup freshly squeezed orange juice
½ cup freshly squeezed grapefruit juice
1 to 3 cloves garlic
½ teaspoon peeled and minced fresh turmeric

Place all the ingredients in a blender and blend well.

VARIATIONS

- Add one banana.

- Add ½ cup of finely chopped kale.

- Add 1 tablespoon of superfoods, such as chia seeds, ground flaxseeds, or hemp seeds.

- You can also add 2 teaspoons of maca powder and/or chlorella.

- Missing your days of hanging out at the mall? Add ⅓ cup of raw cashew pieces to create a creamy Orange Julius–esque beverage.

Kale Kiwi Avocado Juice

Feel the power of green energy times four with brain-healthy avocado, skin-refreshing kiwi, blood-boosting kale, and liver-detoxifying cilantro and lime. Enjoy this refreshing juice with your favorite green salad.

TOTAL YIELD: 20 OUNCES
Serving Size: 10 ounces
Number of Servings: 2
Prep Time: 10 minutes
Total Time: 10 minutes

1½ cups apple juice
½ cup stemmed and chopped kale
2 peeled kiwis (about ⅔ cup)
½ avocado, peeled, pitted, and mashed (about ½ cup)
2 tablespoons freshly squeezed lime juice
1 tablespoon fresh cilantro
Pinch of cayenne pepper

Place all the ingredients in a blender and blend well.

VARIATIONS

- Replace the apple juice with pear juice.

- Replace the kale with spinach.

- Replace the lime juice with lemon juice.

Creamy Tropical Bliss

Nothing satisfies more than a visit to the tropics. Next best thing? Take a two-minute vacation with this divine beverage. High-in-vitamin C orange fruits and a lovely green oxygen boost are rounded out by the mighty antiviral and brain-supporting powers of coconut.

TOTAL YIELD: 32 OUNCES
Serving Size: 16 ounces
Number of Servings: 2
Prep Time: 20 minutes
Total Time: 20 minutes

1 cup coconut water
1½ cups chopped fresh or frozen mango
1 cup fresh papaya
1 fresh or frozen banana
¾ cup young coconut meat
1 teaspoon chlorella (optional)

1. Place the coconut water, mango, papaya, banana, and coconut meat in a blender and blend until smooth.
2. Transfer to glasses and garnish with chlorella, if using. If you are feeling wild, you can swirl the chlorella for a decorative presentation.

VARIATIONS

- Replace the mango and papaya with other tropical fruits, such as cherimoya, jackfruit, durian, star fruit, or your faves.

- Replace the mango and papaya with other fruits, such as peaches, pears, or berries.

- Replace the coconut water with water, fruit juice, or a plant-based milk, such as almond or cashew.

Maca Pepita Elixir

We love maca! It is one of the true gifts from nature to help strengthen our immune system. Maca is also known to support the body's DNA in creating energy, and to help balance female hormones. For both of those reasons, it can have aphrodisiac effects. Enjoy this sweet, sexy, nutrient-rich, and balancing elixir!

TOTAL YIELD: 24 OUNCES
Serving Size: 12 ounces
Number of Servings: 2
Prep Time: 10 minutes
Total Time: 10 minutes

2 cups almond milk (for homemade, see variation on page 116)
¼ cup pumpkin seeds
2 teaspoon maca powder
1 medium-size banana
2 tablespoon hemp seeds
4 to 5 Medjool dates, pitted (optional)
⅛ teaspoon ground cinnamon

Place all the ingredients in a blender and blend until creamy.

VARIATIONS

- Add 2 tablespoons of cacao nibs along with the hemp seeds.

- Replace the pumpkin seeds with sunflower seeds or pistachio nuts.

- Add 1 teaspoon of chlorella along with the maca powder.

Strawberry Delight

When you crave a sweet, creamy shake, turn to this healthy, rich alternative that won't give you the sugar crash. The cashew and dates as well as cardamom help balance blood sugar while providing a delicious base for the yummy fruits. A great way to take in highly absorbable essential vitamins and minerals as well as plenty of fiber.

TOTAL YIELD: 24 OUNCES
   Serving Size: 12 ounces
   Number of Servings: 2
   Prep Time: 10 minutes
   Total Time: 10 minutes

1¼ cups water
½ cup raw cashew pieces
1 large banana
1 cup chopped strawberries
4 Medjool dates, pitted
¼ teaspoon ground cardamom
Coconut nectar or pure maple syrup, to taste (optional)

1. Place the water and cashews in a blender and blend well.
2. Add the remaining ingredients and blend until creamy.

VARIATIONS

- Replace the strawberries with the fruit of your choosing, such as blueberries, raspberries, mango, papaya, peach, or nectarine.

- Replace the cashews with Brazil nuts, sunflower seeds, macadamia nuts, or pumpkin seeds.

- Replace the cashews and water with a plant-based milk of your choosing, such as almond, soy, hemp, or coconut.

Cacao Turmeric Elixir

With plenty of magnesium, B vitamins, healthy fat, selenium, and super phytonutrients, this creamy beverage can provide a needed burst of energy along with its healing powers. (Check out the soaking chart on page 107, if you have time to soak the Brazil nuts before making the smoothie.) Enjoy cold or warm as a late-afternoon snack.

TOTAL YIELD: 20 OUNCES
Serving Size: 10 ounces
Number of Servings: 2
Prep Time: 10 minutes
Total Time: 10 minutes

2 cups water
½ cup chopped Brazil nuts
4 Medjool dates, pitted
1½ tablespoons raw cacao powder, or 3 tablespoons cacao nibs
1 teaspoon ground turmeric
⅛ teaspoon ground cinnamon
Pinch of sea salt (optional)
Pinch of ground black pepper
Coconut nectar or pure maple syrup, to taste (optional)

1. Place the water and Brazil nuts in a blender and blend well.
2. Add the remaining ingredients and blend until creamy. Enjoy over ice, at room temperature, or as a hot beverage. To heat, place in a small pot over low heat and stir occasionally.

VARIATIONS

- For a thinner beverage, you can blend the Brazil nuts and water and strain through a fine-mesh strainer, nut milk bag, or cheesecloth. Return the strained liquid to the blender with the remaining ingredients and blend well.

- Replace the Brazil nuts with cashews, almonds, pecans, walnuts, or your favorite nut or seed.

- Add ⅛ teaspoon of ground nutmeg and/or ground cardamom along with the cinnamon.

- Add a peeled and minced (1-inch) piece of fresh ginger, one fresh or frozen banana, and/or ½ cup of fresh or frozen berries.

Berry Peach Smoothie

Celebrate the bounty of the summer season with these immunity-boosting fruits. Berries, greens, and sweet peaches keep your eyes, hair, and skin fresh, and provide a plethora of vitamins A, C, E, and K as well as B vitamins. If you want to omit the plant-based milk, you can replace it with water or ice to reach your desired consistency.

TOTAL YIELD: 22 OUNCES
   Serving Size: 11 ounces
   Number of Servings: 2
   Prep Time: 5 minutes
   Total Time: 5 minutes

1½ cups plant-based milk
1 banana
1 cup chopped fresh or frozen peach
1 cup fresh or frozen mixed berries
¼ to ½ cup arugula, spinach, or kale
Coconut nectar or desired sweetener,
   to taste (optional)

Place all the ingredients in a blender and blend until creamy.

VARIATIONS

- Superfood it up by adding 2 teaspoons of maca powder, 2 teaspoons of hemp seeds, and 1 teaspoon of chlorella.

- Add 2 tablespoons of your favorite seed or nut butter, such as almond, peanut, or sunflower.

Choco-Cherry Berry Smoothie

Creamy, rich, yummy, and decadent . . . and good for you? Sign us up! Enjoy the benefits of top superfoods cacao and goji berries, as well as mineral-rich sweetness from banana and dates, for an incredible flavor blend. Top with pomegranate arils or goji berries and enjoy as a healthful dessert or an afternoon energy boost.

TOTAL YIELD: 32 OUNCES
   Serving Size: 16 ounces
   Number of Servings: 2
   Prep Time: 5 minutes
   Total Time: 5 minutes

2 cups vanilla almond or soy milk
1½ cups fresh or frozen pitted cherries
1 large banana (optionally frozen)
¼ cup cacao nibs, or 3 tablespoons
   unsweetened cacao powder
4 to 5 Medjool dates, pitted
2 tablespoons goji berries
1 teaspoon pure vanilla extract (optional)

Combine all the ingredients in a blender and blend until creamy.

VARIATIONS

- Add ¼ cup of pomegranate arils before blending.

- Add 2 teaspoons of mesquite powder, maca powder, or chlorella.

- Replace the dates with your sweetener of choice to taste.

Bonus Recipes: Herbal Teas

You can make your own herbal teas by purchasing dried herbs and combining them to create your own blends. It's simple . . . combine the listed ingredients in a bowl and mix well. The following blends will create 2 dry ounces of tea by weight. Herb blends can be kept for several months in a cool, dark place.

To brew, you will use 1 tablespoon of dried herbs per 8 ounces of water. Bring the water to a boil, lower the heat to low, and allow the herbs to steep for 10 to 20 minutes to extract their medicinal properties. If the tea has cooled, you may reheat slowly. Strain the tea into your cup with a mesh strainer.

All the ingredients are measured by weight.

Digestive Support Tea

½ ounce licorice bark
½ ounce fennel seeds
½ ounce dried lemon balm
¼ ounce dried chamomile flowers
¼ ounce ground ginger

Nourishing Tonic

½ ounce dried rose hips
¼ ounce dried nettle leaves
¼ ounce oat straw
¼ ounce dried red raspberry leaves
¼ ounce dried spearmint leaves
¼ ounce ground ginger
⅛ ounce dried red clover leaf and/or alfalfa leaf

Calming Tea

½ ounce dried lemon balm
½ ounce dried chamomile flowers
¼ ounce dried lavender buds
¼ ounce dried rose hips
¼ ounce oat straw
⅛ ounce dried orange peel
⅛ ounce dried spearmint leaves

Adrenal Support

½ ounce ground ginger
¼ ounce dried rhodiola
¼ ounce dried ashwaghanda
¼ ounce dried astragalus
¼ ounce licorice bark
⅛ ounce dried rose hips
⅛ ounce cinnamon bark

For more herbal tea recipes and videos, please visit www.doctorchefresources.com.

ELEVEN

BREAKFAST OF THE IMMORTALS

Want energy to burn? Then, be sure to eat your breakfast! One of the surefire ways to optimize your day is to start off with a power-packed, plant-based meal. As you go through your day, remember to NOURISH yourself. Make sure that you are selecting foods that will nurture vitality in all your body systems mentioned in Part 1 to do your part on the journey of longevity.

Your meal mantra should consist of the following words: "Superfoods and Nutrient Density." Ask yourself, *How can I maximize the nutrition of this meal?* For breakfast, consider including fresh berries, or seeds, such as hemp seeds, chia seeds, pumpkin seeds, or sunflower seeds. Nuts, such as walnuts, and nut butters can also bump up the nutrition. Starting off strong with a good dose of nutrition will ensure that your brain, heart, musculoskeletal, digestive, and immune systems have what they all need to thrive throughout your day . . . protecting yourself from the inside. Start off your day with an alert and calm mind and a strong and healthy heart.

Breakfast bowls are a quick and easy method for upping the nutrition of your morning meal. Rotate through the Berry Good Breakfast Bowl (page 129), Ancient Sunrise (page 135), Chlorella Smoothie Bowl (page 131), and Berry Chia Bowl with Pomegranate (page 130).

Your breakfast can range from light to heavy, as your appetite dictates. Lighter meals can consist of a superfood smoothie from Chapter 10 and toast with tahini or nut butter, topped with nutritional yeast. You can optionally add hemp or flax oil to your toast, or other superfoods, such as cacao nibs, chia seeds, or hemp seeds. We are even known to add a dollop of vegan yogurt on our toast.

Feeling hungry? Have you ever had a full English breakfast? This can include roasted tomatoes, Mushroom Medley (page 184) or sautéed mushrooms and spinach, and baked beans over toast. Indulge further with a vegan sausage and even the Queen of England would be gobsmacked at how wonderful it is. For a video demonstration and recipes for a full vegan English breakfast, please visit www.doctorchefresources.com.

Superhungry? Consider creating the brunch of your dreams: try Superseed Baked French Toast (page 136), Tofu Rancheros (page 137), Superfood Buckwheat Pancakes (page 132), and Smashed Avocado Toast Supreme (page 127), with Herb-Roasted Potatoes (page 199) to complete the Vegan Grand Slam.

TIMELESS TIPS: BREAKFAST HACKS

1. Remember to think "plus one." Think of one thing you can do to increase the nutrition of your first meal. Is it adding a sprinkle of chia seeds on your vegan yogurt? Adding some fresh berries to your granola? Small changes to your meals can add up to big gains in vitality and longevity.

2. Think ahead. Plan your morning meal the night before so you can switch into autopilot in the a.m.—this can be a lifesaver, especially for those who aren't morning people. Soak chia seeds for your chia bowl, soak rolled oats for an overnight oatmeal (which you can optionally heat briefly before enjoying), and even crumble your tofu for your Tofu Rancheros the night before.

3. Convenience is within your reach. Stock up on store-bought granola, frozen vegan waffles, vegan pancake mix, tempeh bacon, and vegan breakfast sausages.

Smashed Avocado Toast Supreme

Avocado is a perfect morning food because it is easy to digest, filling, and provides nutrients, such as monounsaturated fats, folate, and magnesium, that get the brain and nervous system off to a great start. It is also a nice base for adding veggies packed with vitamins and minerals to keep you going all morning. Enjoy with the toppings mentioned, or top with Magical Mushroom Medley (page 184), for an extra-savory snack.

TOTAL YIELD: 2 SLICES TOAST, 4 OUNCES SMASHED AVOCADO

    Serving Size: 1 slice toast, 2 ounces smashed avocado
    Number of Servings: 2
    Prep Time: 5 minutes
    Cook Time: 5 minutes
    Total Time: 10 minutes

2 slices vegan bread (try gluten-free or your favorite)

1 medium-size avocado, peeled, pitted, and mashed

2 teaspoons freshly squeezed lime juice

1 teaspoon nutritional yeast

¼ cup baby arugula

6 thin slices cucumber

6 cherry tomatoes, halved

1 teaspoon Black Sesame Gomasio (page 253), or 2 pinches chipotle powder

Pinch of sea salt (optional; omit if using gomasio)

1. Toast the bread.
2. Top with the smashed avocado, lime juice, nutritional yeast, arugula, cucumber, cherry tomatoes, and gomasio. Dig in!

VARIATIONS

- You can stir together the avocado, lime juice, and nutritional yeast in a bowl before adding to the toast.

- Replace the bread with vegan rice cakes or crackers.

- Replace the cucumber and lime with other veggies, such as cabbage, bell pepper, or red onion.

- Add 1 teaspoon of your favorite Global Spice Blend, such as Indian, Mexican, or Moroccan (pages 249–252), to the avocado while smashing.

Superfood Granola

Save on cost and avoid unnecessary sugar and preservatives by making your own simple and high-nutrient, gluten-free granola. Oats and superpowered hemp and chia seeds provide a nice high-protein, high-fiber, energy-boosting base. Add more superfoods, such as goji berries or cacao nibs, after cooking. Enjoy with fresh seasonal fruit and an optional dollop of vegan yogurt (for homemade, see page 262).

TOTAL YIELD: 32 OUNCES
   Serving Size: 8 ounces
   Number of Servings: 4
   Prep Time: 10 minutes
   Cook Time: 40 minutes
   Total Time: 50 minutes

DRY

1½ cups rolled oats
¾ cup flour, such as a gluten-free flour blend (for homemade, see page 254), or spelt, whole wheat pastry, or unbleached all-purpose
¼ cup hemp seeds
2 tablespoons chia seeds
1 teaspoon pumpkin pie spice
⅛ teaspoon sea salt

WET

¾ cup almond milk (for homemade, see variation on page 116)
¼ cup pure maple syrup, coconut nectar, or date syrup (for homemade, see page 109)

1. Preheat the oven to 350°F. Place the dry ingredients in a bowl and mix well. Place the wet ingredients in another bowl and mix well. Add the wet to the dry and mix well.
2. Spread out the mixture on a parchment paper–lined baking sheet and bake for 20 minutes. Remove from the oven and stir once. Return the pan to the oven and bake until golden brown and crisp, about 20 minutes. Store in a glass container for up to a week.

VARIATIONS

- Add 1 teaspoon of pure vanilla extract to the wet ingredients.
- Experiment with different plant-based milks.
- Add ¼ cup of uncooked millet, quinoa, or amaranth to the dry ingredients.

Berry Good Breakfast Bowl

Berries are where it's at! Berries improve digestive health, balance blood glucose, and protect your blood vessels, allowing proper nutrient and oxygen delivery to all organs, including the eyes and brain. The more creative ways you can think of to include berries in your diet, the better off you will be. Enjoying them alongside other fruits, tahini, yogurt, and seeds creates a full bowl of all essential nutrients. Blackstrap molasses adds a nice dose of iron, while cacao adds magnesium and B vitamins. We love to include them in the mix.

TOTAL YIELD: 32 OUNCES
Serving Size: 16 ounces
Number of Servings: 2
Prep Time: 10 minutes
Total Time: 10 minutes

1 cup fruit, such as sliced bananas, apple, pear, peach, or your favorites
1 cup fresh berries
¼ cup Coconut Yogurt (page 262)
1½ tablespoons tahini
2 teaspoons blackstrap molasses (optional)
1 tablespoon hemp and/or chia seeds
1 tablespoon cacao nibs

1. Place the fruit and berries in bowls. Top with the coconut yogurt. Drizzle with the tahini and molasses.
2. Top with the hemp seeds and cacao nibs before serving.

VARIATIONS

- Double up on the hemp, chia, and cacao.
- Add 1 tablespoon of seeds, such as pumpkin or sunflower, or chopped nuts, such as walnuts or pecans.
- Replace the tahini with almond butter or peanut butter.

Berry Chia Bowl with Pomegranate

Berries are back again, this time paired with potent chia seeds and pomegranate. Chia seeds, as you saw on page 76, are a powerful antiaging food. When soaked, chia forms a delicious and satisfying pudding, complemented by sweet strawberries, dates, and cardamom, for a low-glycemic and high-fiber dessertlike breakfast. Prep your toppings while the chia seeds are soaking. You can prepare the chia mixture the night before as well.

TOTAL YIELD: 12 OUNCES
> Serving Size: 6 ounces
> Number of Servings: 2
> Prep Time: 5 minutes
> Soak Time: 20 minutes
> Total Time: 25 minutes

1 cup water

¾ cup chopped strawberries

3 to 4 Medjool dates, pitted

⅛ teaspoon ground cardamom

¼ cup chia seeds

¼ cup Coconut Yogurt (page 262, or store-bought)

2 tablespoons pomegranate arils

2 tablespoons cacao nibs

1. Place the water, strawberries, dates, and cardamom in a blender and blend well. Transfer to a bowl along with the chia seeds and mix well. Allow to sit until the liquid is absorbed, 15 to 20 minutes, stirring occasionally.
2. Transfer to individual bowls. Top with the coconut yogurt, pomegranate arils, and cacao nibs.

VARIATIONS

- Replace the strawberries with other fruit, such as blueberries, mango, or peach.
- Add 1 teaspoon of pure vanilla extract along with the water.
- Add ¼ teaspoon of ground cinnamon along with the cardamom.

Chlorella Smoothie Bowl

Hold off on drinking that smoothie! Pour it into a bowl and load it up with extras, such as fresh chopped fruit, seeds, nuts, and antiaging superfoods. Chlorella is a dried version of a blue-green algae that is rich in protein, vitamins, minerals, carotenoids, and antioxidants that can help protect cells from damage. It is highly nutrient dense, containing B complex vitamins, beta-carotene, vitamin E, manganese, zinc, copper, iron, selenium, and essential fatty acids. Enjoy this smoothie bowl with a slice of Banana Pineapple Bread (page 133).

TOTAL YIELD: 32 OUNCES

Serving Size: 16 ounces
Number of Servings: 2
Prep Time: 10 minutes
Total Time: 10 minutes

BASE

10 ounces frozen mixed berries, or 2 cups fresh
1 fresh or frozen large banana
1 to 2 cups almond, soy, hemp, or rice milk, depending on desired consistency and strength of blender
2 tablespoons almond or peanut butter
1 tablespoon chlorella powder
2 tablespoons chia seeds

TOPPINGS

Colorful fresh fruit, such as kiwi, strawberries, raspberries, blueberries, mango; dried nuts or seeds; coconut flakes; goji berries; and/or cacao nibs. You get the idea!

1. Combine all the base ingredients in a blender and blend until smooth.
2. Transfer to a bowl and top with your toppings of choice.

VARIATIONS

- Experiment with different fruit instead of the berries.
- Try different plant-based milks or even coconut water. Yum!

Superfood Buckwheat Pancakes

What's light, fluffy, oil-free, and loaded with nutrients? If you guessed these buckwheat pancakes . . . you win a prize. What's the prize? You get to have them for breakfast one day! We made ours with gluten-free flour and they totally delivered. Buckwheat provides sustained energy and lots of minerals and fiber for protecting against heart disease and diabetes. Top with the usual pancake suspects, such as pure maple syrup or date syrup, fresh fruit, additional superfoods, such as cacao nibs or goji berries, or perhaps a schmear of almond butter, and dig in!

TOTAL YIELD: 24 OUNCES
> Serving Size: 4 ounces
> Number of Servings: 6
> Prep Time: 10 minutes
> Cook Time: 20 minutes
> Total Time: 30 minutes

DRY

1 cup buckwheat flour

1 cup flour, such as a gluten-free flour blend (for homemade, see page 254), spelt, whole wheat pastry, or unbleached all-purpose

¼ cup hemp seeds (optional)

1½ tablespoons baking powder

2 tablespoons vegan granulated sugar (optional)

½ teaspoon sea salt

WET

1¾ cups plant-based milk, such as almond or soy

¼ cup applesauce

1 teaspoon pure vanilla extract (optional)

Oil for cooking, unless using a nonstick pan

1. Place the dry ingredients in a bowl and mix well. Place the wet ingredients in another bowl and mix well. Add the wet to the dry and mix well.
2. Preheat a griddle to high, or place a sauté pan over medium-high heat. Add a splash of oil. Spoon out ½ cup of batter per pancake and cook until the sides start to brown and the center begins to bubble, about 3 minutes, depending on the heat of the pan. Flip and cook for 3 more minutes, or until the other side is brown and the pancakes are cooked through. Flip again if necessary to ensure even cooking. Enjoy warm.

VARIATIONS

- Replace the buckwheat flour with spelt flour, whole wheat pastry, or unbleached all-purpose flour.
- Add ½ cup of blueberries, sliced strawberries, or sliced banana, placing the fruit directly on the pancakes while the first side is cooking.
- Add ¼ cup of vegan chocolate chips or cacao nibs to the batter along with the hemp seeds.

Banana Pineapple Bread

Wondering what to do with overripe bananas? Try this healthy breakfast treat for a sweet way to take in those morning vitamins. Pineapples provide tons of skin-smoothing vitamin C plus natural anti-inflammatory bromelain. Bananas have B vitamins and tryptophan that help start the morning with a balanced mood. Serve warm with a schmear of tahini and Roasted Squash Butter (page 264) or your vegan butter of choice.

TOTAL YIELD: 1 (9-INCH) LOAF
    Serving Size: 1 slice
    Number of Servings: 12
    Prep Time: 15 minutes
    Cook Time: 50 minutes
    Total Time: 1 hour 5 minutes

DRY

2 cups flour, such as a gluten-free flour blend (for homemade, see page 254), or spelt, whole wheat pastry, or unbleached all-purpose
1 teaspoon baking powder
½ teaspoon ground cinnamon (optional)
¼ teaspoon ground allspice (optional)
¼ teaspoon sea salt

WET

1½ cups mashed banana (3 to 4 bananas)
½ cup small-diced pineapple
¼ cup tightly packed pitted and chopped dates
2 tablespoons pure maple syrup, coconut nectar, or date syrup (for homemade, see page 109) (optional)
1 teaspoon pure vanilla extract (optional)
½ cup soy, almond, or coconut milk
¼ cup safflower oil or applesauce (for oil-free)

Oil for pan

1. Preheat the oven to 350°F. Place the dry ingredients in a bowl and mix well. Place the wet ingredients in another bowl and mix well. Add the wet to the dry and mix well.
2. Transfer to a well-oiled loaf pan and bake for 50 minutes, or until a toothpick inserted into the center comes out dry.

VARIATIONS

- Add ½ cup of chopped crystallized ginger to the wet ingredients.
- Add ½ cup of vegan dark chocolate chips to the wet ingredients.
- Replace the pineapple with mango, peach, or papaya.

Savory Grits

For those down-home kind of days when you are looking for a grounding breakfast, you can rely on this simple recipe to deliver. Easily digestible grits provide a healthy dose of carbohydrate and fiber, along with some iron, and vitamins A and C for immunity. The tahini and nutritional yeast combo creates a cheesy flavor and helps provide prolonged energy and mood balancing B vitamins and magnesium. Serve on its own garnished with smoked paprika, or top with Smoky Mushrooms (page 254), Braised Kale with Shallots and Slivered Almonds (page 185), or Magical Mushroom Medley (page 184).

TOTAL YIELD: 28 OUNCES
  Serving Size: 7 ounces
  Number of Servings: 4
  Prep Time: 5 minutes
  Cook Time: 15 minutes
  Total Time: 20 minutes

3½ cups water
¾ cup corn grits
¼ teaspoon sea salt
1 to 2 cloves garlic, pressed or minced
½ teaspoon dried onion flakes
Pinch of crushed red pepper flakes (optional)
1 cup chopped spinach
2 tablespoons tahini
1½ tablespoons nutritional yeast

1. Place the water in a medium-size pot and bring to a boil. Lower the heat to low, add the grits, salt, garlic, onion flakes, and red pepper flakes, if using, and cook for 10 minutes, stirring frequently at first, then occasionally.
2. Add the spinach and cook until wilted, about 2 minutes. Add the tahini and nutritional yeast, mix well, serve, and enjoy!

VARIATIONS

- Add ½ cup of shredded vegan cheese.
- Add 2 tablespoons of vegan butter.
- Consider using smoked salt instead of sea salt.
- Replace the spinach with other greens, such as arugula, kale, dandelion greens, or mustard greens.

Ancient Sunrise

These ancient grains—millet, quinoa, and amaranth—have just as much potency today as they did centuries ago. Gluten-free, the grains provide a refreshing blend both flavor- and nutrient-wise, providing ample amounts of protein, fiber, iron, and magnesium, to start off the day right. Top with your favorite fresh or dried fruit, nuts, seeds, and superfoods. We love ours with a dollop of vegan yogurt, a spoonful of tahini or other nut butter, and a splash of plant-based milk.

TOTAL YIELD: 26 OUNCES
    Serving Size: 13 ounces
    Number of Servings: 2
    Prep Time: 5 minutes
    Cook Time: 20 minutes
    Total Time: 25 minutes

3¾ cups water
½ cup uncooked quinoa
¼ cup uncooked amaranth
½ cup uncooked millet
¾ teaspoon ground cinnamon
¼ teaspoon ground cardamom
Pinch of sea salt

Place all the ingredients in a medium-size pot over medium heat. Cook until all the grains are cooked, about 20 minutes, stirring frequently.

VARIATIONS

- Top with your favorite superfoods, such as chia seeds, hemp seeds, ground flaxseeds, or chlorella.

- Replace the millet and amaranth with grits.

- Add desired sweetener to taste.

Superseed Baked French Toast

It is highly unlikely you will encounter this superfood version of *pain perdu* while strolling the Champs-Élysées. Seeds add both a satisfying crunch and a boost of protein for sustained energy from a traditionally carb-heavy dish. For the full Parisian effect, use a thick-sliced bread, serve with pure maple syrup, and garnish with powdered sugar and fresh berries.

TOTAL YIELD: 6 SLICES
Serving Size: 2 slices
Number of Servings: 3
Prep Time: 10 minutes
Cook Time: 30 minutes
Total Time: 40 minutes

6 to 8 slices bread

DIPPING MIXTURE

1 cup almond, soy, or coconut milk
3 tablespoons almond butter
1 tablespoon pure maple syrup (optional)
½ teaspoon ground cinnamon

SUPERSEED CRUST

½ cup pumpkin seeds, raw or toasted
¼ cup sunflower seeds, raw or toasted
¼ cup hemp seeds
¼ teaspoon ground cinnamon or cardamom

1. Preheat the oven to 400°F.
2. Place the dipping mixture ingredients in a bowl and whisk well. Place the superseed crust ingredients in a food processor and process until well ground. Transfer to a shallow dish.
3. Dip each piece of bread in the dipping mixture until soaked through. Place on the plate with the superseed crust and coat both sides of the bread with the crust. Transfer to a parchment paper–lined baking sheet.
4. Place in the oven and bake for 15 minutes. Carefully flip and bake for an additional 15 minutes before serving. Enjoy!

VARIATIONS

- Experiment with different types of bread.
- Replace the sunflower and pumpkin seeds with almonds and walnuts.
- Add 2 tablespoons of desiccated coconut to the seed mixture.

Tofu Rancheros

Welcome to the official tofu scramble of Mexico, delicious and satisfying, complete with all the flavors of the region. For special mornings, or days when you need a more hearty, grounding meal, this high-protein dish with a flavorful herb and spice combo will get you going without weighing you down. We recommended adding the extra ingredients listed in the variations, for the full fiesta. Serve with a side of tortillas or Herb-Roasted Potatoes (page 199), sliced avocados, and dollop of Vegan Sour Cream (page 274).

TOTAL YIELD: 24 OUNCES

Serving Size: 8 ounces
Number of Servings: 3
Prep Time: 10 minutes
Cook Time: 15 minutes
Total Time: 25 minutes

1 teaspoon olive oil, or 2 tablespoons water
½ cup thinly sliced yellow onion
14 ounce extra-firm tofu, drained well and crumbled
1½ teaspoons chili powder
⅓ cup salsa, fire-roasted tomatoes, or chopped fresh tomato (½-inch pieces)
½ cup cooked black beans (see page 102)
2 tablespoons nutritional yeast
½ teaspoon sea salt, or to taste depending on the saltiness of the salsa
⅛ teaspoon ground black pepper
2 to 3 tablespoons finely chopped fresh cilantro

1. Place a medium-size sauté pan over medium-high heat. Heat the oil. Add the onion and cook for 3 minutes, stirring frequently and adding a small amount of water if necessary to prevent sticking.
2. Add the tofu and chili powder and cook for 3 minutes, stirring frequently. Add the salsa and black beans and cook for 5 minutes, stirring frequently.
3. Add the nutritional yeast, salt, and black pepper and mix well. Add the cilantro and mix well before serving.

VARIATIONS

- Add two pressed or minced garlic cloves and ½ teaspoon of ground turmeric along with the onion.

- Add ½ teaspoon of ground cumin and ¼ teaspoon of chipotle powder along with the chili powder.

- Add ½ cup of grated vegan cheese along with the nutritional yeast.

- Add ½ cup of chopped mushrooms along with the onion.

- Omit the beans and salsa and add diced bell pepper, spinach, or your favorite veggies.

- Omit the Mexican seasonings and add ½ cup of Pepita Pesto with Avocado (page 265).

TWELVE

SUSTAINING SOUPS AND STEWS

Soup's on! With these amazing veggie-based soups and stews, your journey into liquid nutrition takes a quantum leap forward. In many culinary traditions from around the world, soups and stews play an important role in health and longevity. Kundalini Kitchari (page 154) is a shining example of healing stew made with super antiaging copper-rich mung beans and inflammation-reducing, heart-healthy curry spices. You can also branch out from tradition with the cooling Raw Chilled Strawberry Soup (page 141) with ginger, cilantro, and cucumber, to rehydrate while supporting both digestion and detoxification.

It doesn't get easier than our selection of one-pot soups, where you are cutting up veggies and putting them in the pot, as simple as it gets. You can bulk up these one-pot soups by adding legumes, beans, and/or pasta. Create creamy vegan soups by adding nuts, such as cashews, as with the Creamy Corn Chowder with Fire-Roasted Tomatoes and Dill (page 146), or plant-based milks, such as coconut, as in the Coco-Lemongrass Soup

TIMELESS TIPS: SOUP HACKS

- Stock up on vegetable stock! Save your veggie clippings as you prep the rest of your meals—then check out the soup stock method on page 248. Out of homemade stock? Keep backup stock in your pantry—a bouillon cube, packaged stock, or powdered broth. Remember to reduce the salt listed in the recipe if using a store-bought stock that already has sodium in it.
- Curry up! Keep a couple of jars of curry paste—red and green—on hand for your Thai soups.
- Use leftover rice or quinoa either directly in your soup, or place in a bowl and top with soup.
- Double up your soups and freeze some for later use.
- Consider purchasing a slow cooker or Instant Pot to make your soup-making experience that much easier and more efficient. Follow the manufacturers' instructions for use.

(page 143). You can also blend in white beans; starchy veggies, such as potatoes; and even silken tofu to create creaminess in your soups.

Here you'll find soups of all kinds, from lighter, raw soups, such as Raw Chilled Strawberry mentioned above, to the heartier Adzuki Bean Tempeh Chili (page 152), which is a full meal in itself.

Note that all of the soups in this chapter can be made without processed oil, which is a huge plus for those with cardio issues who are looking to eliminate oil from their diet. But if you wish, you can add 1 to 1½ tablespoons of oil to a hot pot and sauté the initial vegetables (typically onion) before following the rest of the recipe.

Raw Chilled Strawberry Soup

Chill out with this refreshing raw soup that is the perfect antidote to a hot summer day. Get your vitamin C in an innovative way with this unique blend of flavors and a refreshing and rejuvenating nutrient profile. Serve with a dollop of Smoky Cashew Cream (page 266) and black sesame seeds or Black Sesame Gomasio (page 253).

TOTAL YIELD: 24 OUNCES
Serving Size: 12 ounces
Number of Servings: 2
Prep Time: 15 minutes
Total Time: 15 minutes

1 cup water
3 cups strawberries
2 tablespoons freshly squeezed lime juice
1 tablespoon peeled and minced fresh ginger
1 tablespoon finely chopped fresh cilantro
¾ cup seeded and diced cucumber
2 tablespoons balsamic vinegar
¼ teaspoon chipotle powder
Pinch of sea salt
Pinch of ground black pepper

1. Place the water, strawberries, lime juice, and ginger in a blender and blend until smooth. Transfer to a bowl. Add the cilantro and mix well.
2. Place the cucumber, balsamic vinegar, chipotle powder, salt, and black pepper in another bowl and mix well. To serve, pour the soup into bowls and top with the cucumber mixture.

VARIATIONS

Add 1 tablespoon of pure maple syrup, coconut nectar, or date syrup (for homemade, see page 109) or to taste, along with the strawberries.

Replace the strawberries with blueberries or peaches.

Miso Roots Soup

One of Japan's secrets of longevity? Miso paste! Miso is a nutrient-rich, cultured soybean paste that has been part of the human diet for thousands of years. Root vegetables provide ample grounding minerals and protective antioxidants, while mushrooms and ginger together exude their powerful immunity-boosting properties. This soup is pure medicine in a delicious and comforting broth. Enjoy at the beginning of a meal that may include Domo Arigato Arame Salad (page 159) and Black Rice Sushi with Wasabi Mayo (page 222).

TOTAL YIELD: 48 OUNCES

    Serving Size: 12 ounces
    Number of Servings: 4
    Prep Time: 10 minutes
    Cook Time: 20 minutes
    Total Time: 30 minutes

5 cups water or vegetable stock (for homemade, see page 248)
2 cups diced root vegetables (try carrot, parsnip, turnip, and/or celeriac)
1 cup sliced yellow onion
1 cup thinly sliced shiitake mushrooms
1 tablespoon peeled and minced fresh ginger
¼ cup dried arame
1½ tablespoons store-bought miso paste
1 tablespoon finely chopped fresh cilantro
2 teaspoons wheat-free tamari or other soy sauce, or to taste
Sea salt and ground black pepper
Pinch of crushed red pepper flakes

1. Place the water in a 3-quart pot over medium-high heat. Add the root vegetables, onion, shiitake mushrooms, and ginger and cook until the vegetables are just tender, about 15 minutes, stirring occasionally. Add the arame and cook for 5 minutes.
2. Remove a small amount of liquid from the pot and place in a small bowl or measuring cup along with the miso paste. Stir well until the miso is dissolved and return the liquid to the pot. Add the cilantro.
3. Season with the tamari, salt and pepper to taste, and the red pepper flakes before serving.

VARIATIONS

- Add 1 cup spinach or arugula along with the arame.
- Add ¼ cup of thinly sliced green onion with the cilantro.
- Add ¼ teaspoon of ground turmeric, or 2 teaspoons peeled and chopped fresh turmeric, along with the ginger.
- Add two to three pressed or minced garlic cloves in addition to or instead of the ginger.
- Add 1 cup of cubed extra-firm tofu, optionally roasted (see pages 104–105).

Coco-Lemongrass Soup

Dream of pristine beaches in Thailand with this soul-satisfying combo of coconut and lemongrass. Meanwhile, enjoy the excellent protective benefits of mineral- and antioxidant-rich cruciferous bok choy. If you can find kaffir lime leaves, do yourself a favor and toss in a few along with the lemongrass for the full effect. Serve with Black Gomasio Crusted Tofu (page 215) and Pilau Rice (page 198).

TOTAL YIELD: 48 OUNCES
Serving Size: 12 ounces
Number of Servings: 4
Prep Time: 15 minutes
Cook Time: 25 minutes
Total Time: 40 minutes

3 cups water or vegetable stock (for homemade, see page 248)
1 (13.5-ounce) can coconut milk (1¾ cups)
¾ cup diced shallot
3 to 4 cloves garlic, pressed or minced
2 to 3 stalks lemongrass, crushed
1½ cups chopped tomato
2 cups chopped bok choy or baby bok choy
2 tablespoons finely chopped fresh cilantro
1¼ teaspoons sea salt, or to taste
¼ teaspoon ground black pepper
¼ teaspoon crushed red pepper flakes (optional)

1. Place the water in a 3-quart pot over medium-high heat. Add the coconut milk, shallot, garlic, and lemongrass and cook for 10 minutes, stirring occasionally. Add the tomato and cook for 10 minutes, stirring occasionally. Add the bok choy and cook for 5 minutes, stirring occasionally.
2. Add the cilantro, salt, black pepper, and red pepper flakes, if using, and stir well before serving.

VARIATIONS

- Add 1 cup of small firm, extra-firm, or super-firm tofu cubes, optionally roasted (see pages 104–105).

- Add ½ cup of sliced mushrooms along with the bok choy.

- Add ⅓ cup of uncooked basmati rice along with the coconut milk. Cook until the rice is just tender.

- Add 1 tablespoon of store-bought curry paste along with the coconut milk. Amazing!

- Add three kaffir lime leaves along with the lemongrass. Remove before serving.

- Replace the coconut milk with soy, rice, or almond milk.

Roasted Red Pepper Soup with Fennel

Light your fire with this heart-healthy soup featuring lycopene-rich red bell peppers. The onion, celery, and garlic trio itself has major heart health benefits due to blood pressure-balancing and circulation-enhancing qualities. Plenty of potassium here! Also, fennel can improve digestion, lower cholesterol, and even help treat anemia.

We recommend adding the balsamic vinegar to round out the goodness and flavor. Top with a dollop of Smoky Cashew Cream (page 266) or Vegan Sour Cream (page 274) and serve with Skillet Corn Bread (page 204) and a side salad.

TOTAL YIELD: 52 OUNCES
  Serving Size: 8 ounces
  Number of Servings: 6+
  Prep Time: 10 minutes
  Cook Time: 30–50 minutes, depending on method of roasting peppers
  Total Time: 40–60 minutes, depending on method of roasting peppers

4 cups water or vegetable stock (for homemade, see page 248)
1 cup diced yellow onion
½ cup thinly sliced celery
3 to 4 cloves garlic, pressed or minced (optional)
1½ teaspoons Italian Spice Mix (page 251, or store-bought)
4 to 5 medium-size red bell peppers
Olive oil
¾ cup chopped cashews, raw or roasted unsalted
¼ teaspoon crushed red pepper flakes (optional)
1½ teaspoons sea salt, or to taste
⅛ teaspoon ground black pepper
1 cup chopped fennel bulb
2 teaspoons balsamic vinegar (optional)
2 tablespoons chiffonaded fresh basil

1. Preheat the oven to 400°F or HIGH broil. Place the water in a 3-quart pot over medium-high heat. Add the onion, celery, garlic, and Italian Spice Mix and cook for 20 minutes, stirring occasionally. Lower the heat to low.

2. Meanwhile, place the peppers on a well-oiled or non-stick baking sheet and lightly oil the peppers. If roasting at 400°F, cook until the skin of the peppers is bubbly and charred, about 45 minutes, using tongs to flip once or twice. If using the HIGH broil setting, broil until the skin becomes black and charred, flipping frequently with the tongs to ensure even cooking, about 10 minutes, depending on the heat of the oven. Place the peppers in a bowl and cover with a lid or plate to steam. Allow to sit for 15 minutes, or until cool enough to handle. Carefully remove all or most of the skin, and all the seeds. Roughly measure out 2¼ cups for this recipe. Set aside 2 tablespoons of the liquid as well. Place in the soup pot, then add the cashews, red pepper flakes, if using, salt, and black pepper, and stir well.

3. Carefully transfer the soup to a blender and blend until very creamy. Be careful not to overfill the blender. You will probably need to blend in two batches, using another pot or bowl to transfer the first blended batch.

4. Return the soup to the pot, increase the temperature to medium-high, add the fennel, and cook until just tender, about 10 minutes, stirring occasionally. Add the balsamic vinegar, if using, and stir well. Garnish with the basil before serving.

VARIATIONS

- Add 1 teaspoon of wheat-free tamari along with the balsamic vinegar.

- If you have a gas stove, you can roast the peppers by placing them directly over the flame and using your handy tongs to flip them until charred on all sides.

- Once blended, add one 15-ounce can of drained cannellini or navy beans.

- Add 1 cup of fresh or fire-roasted corn after blending.

- You can also roast the fennel, by combining 1 cup of chopped fennel bulb, 1 teaspoon olive oil, and a pinch each of salt and pepper in a bowl and mixing well. Roast at 375°F until just tender, about 20 minutes. Add to the soup after blending. Highly recommended by our recipe tester!

Creamy Corn Chowder with Fire-Roasted Tomatoes and Dill

Creamy and satisfying, a simple soup to celebrate the bounty of summer's harvest. Unprocessed, organic, whole corn is an amazing food in that it delivers plenty of vitamin C, B vitamins, beta-carotene, fiber, potassium, magnesium, and even protein, all in a low-calorie package. It also contains the skin- and eye-specific antioxidants lutein and zeaxanthin. Use fire-roasted corn for a double fire-roasted effect. Top with chopped avocado and enjoy with Papas, Bean, and Greens Burritos (page 237).

TOTAL YIELD: 70 OUNCES

Serving Size: 14 ounces
Number of Servings: 5
Prep Time: 15 minutes
Cook Time: 20 minutes
Total Time: 35 minutes

4½ cups water or vegetable stock (for homemade, see page 248)

1 cup diced yellow onion

½ cup thinly sliced celery

4 to 5 cloves garlic

3 cups fresh or frozen corn, divided

½ cup cashews, raw, roasted unsalted, or toasted (see page 106)

1 (14.5-ounce) can diced fire-roasted tomatoes, or 1½ cups chopped fresh tomato

1 tablespoon minced fresh dill

1½ teaspoons sea salt, or to taste

¼ teaspoon ground black pepper, or to taste

1. Place the water in a 2-quart pot over medium-high heat. Add the onion, celery, garlic, and 2 cups of the corn and cook for 15 minutes, stirring occasionally. Add the cashews and stir well.

2. Transfer to a blender and blend until creamy. Return the mixture to the pot. Add the remaining ingredients, including the remaining cup of corn, and cook for 5 minutes, stirring occasionally. Stir well before serving.

VARIATIONS

- Add ¼ teaspoon of crushed red pepper flakes or chipotle powder, or ½ teaspoon smoked paprika, along with the garlic.

- If you're using fresh corn, try grilling the corn cobs before using in this recipe.

- Replace the tomatoes with chopped potatoes and cook until just tender.

- Replace the corn with other vegetables, such as asparagus, zucchini, broccoli, or cauliflower.

- Replace the cashews with macadamia nuts, blanched almonds, or pine nuts.

- Replace the cashews and 1 cup of water with 1½ cups of soy, rice, coconut, or almond milk.

- Add 1 tablespoon of a Global Spice Blend, such as Italian, Moroccan, or Indian (pages 249–252), along with the onion.

Grecian Braised Cauliflower Soup

Witnessing the beauty of Aphrodite pales in comparison to the euphoria you will experience while enjoying this soup. Cauliflower is a huge source of vitamin K; vitamins B_5, B_6, and B_9, potassium, manganese, fiber, and lots of vitamin C. The lovely florets also contain numerous phytonutrients, such as indole-3-carbinol and sulforaphane, which may help protect against certain cancers. Garnish with a liberal amount of finely chopped flat-leaf parsley. Serve with Roasted Butternut Squash Penne with Sage (page 242) and get ready to smash some plates!

TOTAL YIELD: 60 OUNCES

    Serving Size: 12 ounces
    Number of Servings: 5
    Prep Time: 10 minutes
    Cook Time: 30 minutes
    Total Time: 40 minutes

1½ tablespoons olive oil, or ¼ cup water
1 cup diced yellow onion
3 to 4 cloves garlic, pressed or minced
5 cups small cauliflower florets
1 teaspoon sea salt, or to taste
⅛ teaspoon ground black pepper
2 teaspoons dried oregano
1 teaspoon ground cinnamon
3 cups water or vegetable stock (for homemade, see page 248)
1 (14.5-ounce) can fire-roasted tomatoes, or 1½ cups diced fresh tomato
1 (15-ounce) can fava or cannellini beans, or 1½ cups cooked
1 tablespoon balsamic vinegar (optional)
Pinch of crushed red pepper flakes (optional)

1. Place a 3-quart pot over medium-high heat. Heat the oil. Add the onion, garlic, cauliflower, salt, black pepper, and oregano and cook for 5 minutes, stirring frequently and adding a small amount of water or veggie stock if necessary to prevent sticking. Add the cinnamon, water, and fire-roasted tomatoes and cook for 20 minutes, stirring occasionally.
2. Add the fava beans and cook for 5 minutes, stirring occasionally.
3. Add the balsamic vinegar and red pepper flakes, if using, and stir well. Season with salt and pepper before serving.

VARIATIONS

- Replace the cauliflower with broccoli, cabbage, or assorted mixed vegetables.

- Replace the fava beans with cannellini, kidney, navy, or pinto.

- Add 1 tablespoon Italian Spice Mix (page 251) along with the oregano.

Three Sisters Soup

The Native American trinity consists of squash, beans, and corn—three ancient ingredients that have sustained a huge population with the foundational nutrients of a healthy diet. This is a truly superpowered antiaging soup. Top with toasted sunflower seeds or pumpkin seeds and a dollop of Vegan Sour Cream (page 274). Enjoy along with Kale Millet Tabbouleh (page 164) for a soup and salad combo that delivers!

TOTAL YIELD: 64 OUNCES
  Serving Size: 13 ounces
  Number of Servings: 5
  Prep Time: 10 minutes
  Cook Time: 25 minutes
  Total Time: 35 minutes

6 cups water or vegetable stock (for homemade, see page 248)
¾ cup diced yellow onion
½ cup thinly sliced celery
1 tablespoon adobo seasoning or Italian Spice Mix (page 251, or store-bought)
1½ cups chopped butternut squash (1-inch pieces)
1 (15-ounce) can kidney or navy beans, or 1½ cups cooked (see page 102)
¾ cup fresh or frozen corn
1 tablespoon minced fresh dill, or 2 tablespoons finely chopped fresh flat-leaf parsley
Sea salt and ground black pepper
Pinch of crushed red pepper flakes (optional)

1. Place the water in a 3-quart pot over medium-high heat. Add the onion, celery, adobo seasoning, and butternut squash and cook for 15 minutes, stirring occasionally.
2. Add the kidney beans and corn and cook for 10 minutes, stirring occasionally.
3. Add the dill and season with salt and black pepper to taste and the red pepper flakes, if using, before serving.

VARIATIONS

🔥 Add three to four pressed or minced garlic cloves along with the onion.

🔥 Replace the butternut squash with other squash, such as delicata, kabocha, buttercup, or acorn.

🔥 Replace the butternut squash with sweet potatoes, such as garnet, jewel, or purple.

🔥 Replace the beans with black, pinto, or fava beans.

🔥 Replace the dill with 2 tablespoons of minced fresh cilantro or basil.

Shiitake Hot Pot Noodle Soup

Now is your chance to break out your decorative hot pot! Shiitake mushrooms are king of the natural flavor enhancers as well as a highly anti-inflammatory food. They are a great source of vitamin B$_7$ and copper, and are well known for beta-glucan, an antioxidant said to protect against diabetes. Garnish with thinly sliced green onion. Serve in a hot pot for a "wow" presentation, along with Marvelous Macro Meal (page 226) and finish off with Mango Rice Pudding with Salted Caramel (page 293).

TOTAL YIELD: 48 OUNCES
Serving Size: 8 ounces
Number of Servings: 6
Prep Time: 10 minutes
Cook Time: 20 minutes
Total Time: 30 minutes

5 cups water or vegetable stock (for homemade, see page 248)
¾ cup thinly sliced white or yellow onion
1 cup shiitake mushrooms, stems removed
1 cup veggies (try chopped bok choy, sliced carrots, spinach, broccoli flowerets, or snow peas)
½ teaspoon Chinese five-spice powder or garam masala
1 tablespoon wheat-free tamari or other soy sauce
3 ounces thin rice noodles
2 tablespoons loosely chopped fresh cilantro
¼ teaspoon cayenne pepper or crushed red pepper flakes (optional)
Sea salt and ground black pepper

1. Place the water in a 3-quart pot over medium-high heat. Add the onion and shiitake mushrooms and cook for 3 minutes, stirring occasionally.
2. Add the assorted veggies and Chinese five-spice and cook until the hardest vegetable is just tender, about 10 minutes, stirring occasionally.
3. Add the tamari and rice noodles and cook until just tender, about 5 minutes. Add the cilantro, cayenne, if using, and salt and black pepper to taste, and mix well before serving.

VARIATIONS

- Add 2 teaspoons of curry powder instead of the Chinese five-spice powder.
- Add 1 tablespoon of peeled and minced fresh ginger and/or two minced garlic cloves along with the onion.
- Experiment with different veggies.
- Add 1 cup of diced extra-firm tofu along with the shiitake mushrooms.

Purple Potato Soup

You know you are heading in the right culinary direction when your soup is purple! The deeper the color, the higher the antioxidant benefit. Purple potatoes have four times as much anthocyanin as a russet potato, making them excellent for brain and heart health. Enjoy with Asian Couscous (page 208) and Brazenly Braised Tempeh (page 219) for a complete meal.

TOTAL YIELD: 64 OUNCES

> Serving Size: 8 ounces
> Number of Servings: 8
> Prep Time: 15 minutes
> Cook Time: 25 minutes
> Total Time: 40 minutes

4 cups water or vegetable stock (for homemade, see page 248)

1 (13.5-ounce) can coconut milk (1¾ cups)

1 cup diced yellow onion

¾ cup thinly sliced celery

3 to 4 cloves garlic, pressed or minced

3 cups chopped purple sweet potato, unpeeled (½-inch pieces)

1 cinnamon stick

1 teaspoon sea salt, or to taste

¼ teaspoon crushed red pepper flakes (optional)

2 tablespoons finely chopped fresh cilantro

1. Place the water in a 3-quart pot over medium-high heat. Add the coconut milk, onion, celery, garlic, sweet potato, and cinnamon stick. Cook for 20 minutes, stirring occasionally.
2. Add the salt and red pepper flakes, if using, and cook for 5 minutes.
3. Remove the cinnamon stick, add the cilantro, and stir well before serving.

VARIATIONS

- Add ½ teaspoon of wheat-free tamari or other soy sauce along with the salt.
- Replace the purple sweet potato with other potato, such as jewel or garnet, red bliss potato, or Peruvian purple potato.
- Replace the coconut milk with soy, rice, or almond milk.

Parsnip Leek Soup

Parsnips are the new carrot! The white version of the beloved carrot provides a generous amount of potassium and fiber as well as vitamins C and E, making it a heart-healthy and pancreas-loving (potentially antidiabetes) food. Leeks, in the Allium family like their cousin garlic, add the benefits of sulfur, as well as folate and polyphenols, which help lower chronic inflammation. The synergy of the parsnip and fennel highly benefits the digestive system, as well as the body's absorption of all these nutrients. Top with a dollop of Vegan Sour Cream (page 274) and toasted pumpkin seeds and enjoy this creamy goodness along with Club Med Pasta Salad (page 168) and Roasted Tofu with Almond Sauce (page 221).

TOTAL YIELD: 64 OUNCES
Serving Size: 8 ounces
Number of Servings: 8
Prep Time: 15 minutes
Cook Time: 25 minutes
Total Time: 40 minutes

3 cups water or vegetable stock (for homemade, see page 248)
3 cups unsweetened soy or almond milk
1¼ cups thinly sliced leek, rinsed and drained well
4 to 5 cloves garlic, pressed or minced
3 cups chopped parsnip (½-inch pieces)
½ cup chopped fennel bulb
1 cup garden or sweet peas
½ cup halved cherry tomatoes
1½ teaspoons sea salt, or to taste
⅛ teaspoon ground black pepper
Pinch of cayenne pepper (optional)

1. Place a 3-quart pot over medium-high heat. Add the water, soy milk, leek, garlic, parsnip, and fennel and cook for 20 minutes, stirring occasionally.
2. Carefully transfer to a blender in two or three batches and blend until creamy. Return the mixture to the pot.
3. Add the peas and tomatoes and cook for 5 minutes. Season with salt and black pepper, and cayenne, if using, before serving.

VARIATIONS

- Add 1 tablespoon of Italian Spice Mix (page 251) along with the onion.

- Replace the leeks with onion.

- Replace the parsnip with potato.

- Add 1 tablespoon of chopped fresh dill or 2 tablespoons of finely chopped fresh parsley before serving.

Adzuki Bean Tempeh Chili

A certified heartburn-free chili coming at
you! Adzuki beans originate in East Asia
and the Himalayas and are a nutrient-
packed source of fiber and protein. They
are said to have a warming effect on the
body—perfect for the autumn and winter months. Cultured tempeh adds a nice
earthy quality and digestive benefit. Adding beta-carotene–rich pumpkin will increase calcium and magnesium, as well as
vitamins C and E and some B vitamins, all
to enhance not only your immunity but also
glowing skin health. Enjoy with a dollop of
Vegan Sour Cream (page 274) and a sprinkle of toasted pumpkin seeds, and garnish
with a sprig of cilantro.

TOTAL YIELD: 48 OUNCES
    Serving Size: 12 ounces
    Number of Servings: 4
    Prep Time: 10 minutes
    Cook Time: 25 minutes
    Total Time: 35 minutes

1 tablespoon olive oil, or 3 tablespoons
    water
1 cup diced yellow onion
8 ounces finely chopped soy tempeh
1 (15-ounce) can adzuki beans, or 1½ cups
    cooked (see page 102)
1 (14.5-ounce) can fire-roasted tomatoes,
    or 1½ cups diced fresh tomato
2 teaspoons chili powder
¼ teaspoon chipotle powder (optional)
1 to 1½ cups water or vegetable stock (for
    homemade, see page 248)
2 tablespoons freshly squeezed lime juice
½ teaspoon sea salt, or to taste
1 tablespoon wheat-free tamari or other
    soy sauce (optional)
2 tablespoons minced fresh cilantro

1. Place a 3-quart pot over medium-high heat. Heat the oil. Add the onion and cook for 3 minutes, stirring frequently and adding small amounts of water if necessary to prevent sticking. Add the tempeh and cook for 3 minutes, stirring frequently. Lower the heat to medium.
2. Add the adzuki beans, fire-roasted tomatoes, chili powder, and chipotle powder, if using, and cook for 15 minutes, stirring occasionally. Add the water to your desired consistency, lime juice, salt, and tamari, if using, and gently stir well. Cook for 5 minutes.
3. Add the cilantro and stir well before serving.

VARIATIONS

- Add four to five pressed or minced garlic cloves and ½ teaspoon of ground cumin along with the onion.

- For a **Pumpkin Chili**, add ½ cup of pure pumpkin puree or 1½ cups of roasted and cubed pumpkin along with the tomatoes. To roast the pumpkin, preheat an oven to 400°F. Carefully slice the pumpkin into halves or quarters and remove the seeds. Place on a baking sheet along with about ½ inch of water. Roast until just tender, about 35 minutes, depending on the size of the pumpkin. Do not overcook. Allow to cool and scoop out the flesh. Cut into ½-inch pieces for use in this recipe. You can also replace the pumpkin with squash, such as butternut, buttercup, or kabocha.

- Alternative method: Instead of roasting the pumpkin, you can peel and chop the pumpkin into 1-inch cubes. Add along with the tempeh and cook for an additional 20 minutes.

Kundalini Kitchari

You can feel your chakras open with every spoonful of this traditional Ayurvedic recipe. *Kitchari* translates as "mixture," though it commonly includes two grains or a grain and legume. Here we are using mung beans and rice. Mung beans are known to be easily digestible, and contain impressive amounts of magnesium, potassium, and B vitamins, including folate. Curry powder has considerable health benefits, such as lowering inflammation, supporting heart health, and even improving liver function, making this dish a powerfully medicinal food. Plan ahead and soak the mung beans the night before for optimal digestion. Serve with Arugula Walnut Salad with Cashew Dill Dressing (page 161) or Sunny Kale Salad (page 162).

TOTAL YIELD: 60 OUNCES
    Serving Size: 12 ounces
    Number of Servings: 5
    Prep Time: 10 minutes
    Soak Time: 12 hours
    Cook Time: 40 minutes
    Total Time: 50 minutes plus soak time

¾ cup dried mung beans
6 cups water or vegetable stock (for homemade, see page 248)
½ cup uncooked short-grain brown rice
1 cup diced yellow onion
1 tablespoon curry powder
1 teaspoon cumin seeds
2½ cups assorted vegetables, such as diced carrot, small broccoli or cauliflower florets, chopped zucchini, chopped cabbage, chopped fennel, and shredded kale or collards
2 tablespoons finely chopped fresh cilantro
Sea salt and ground black pepper

1. Place the mung beans in a bowl or jar with ample water to cover. Allow to sit overnight or for up to 12 hours. Rinse and drain well. You should have about 1¾ cups of beans once they are soaked.
2. Place the fresh water in a 3-quart pot over medium-high heat. Add the rice, onion, curry powder, and cumin seeds and cook for 30 minutes, stirring occasionally.
3. Add the assorted veggies and cook until the mung beans are soft and chewy and the vegetables are just tender, about 10 minutes, stirring occasionally.
4. Add the cilantro, and season with salt and pepper to taste before serving.

VARIATIONS

⚘ There are as many variations of this recipe as verses of the Upanishads. Experiment with different veggies.

⚘ Add 1 tablespoon of peeled and minced fresh ginger or three to four pressed or minced garlic cloves along with the onion.

⚘ Add 2 teaspoons of brown mustard, fenugreek, coriander, and/or fennel seeds along with the onion.

⚘ Replace the mung beans with split peas (see pages 102–103).

⚘ Replace the rice with other grains.

THIRTEEN

SUPERFOOD SALADS AND DRESSINGS

Wherein lies one of the biggest secrets to creating a younger you? The humble salad. It's an accessible entry point to a plant-based diet; most people can wrap their mind around a salad. Just get a little more creative! Start adding new ingredients and you will find yourself addicted to them in no time. Enjoy a colorful salad as many days of the week as you can to kick your longevity program into high gear.

Salads are a wonderful way to load up on varieties of protective antioxidants from the extensive array of greens and other colorful veggies we can choose from. Try the Sunny Kale Salad (page 162) for a recipe with the poster child for superfoods, kale. Salads can also be where we can enjoy a daily serving of cultured foods, such as sauerkraut (Ruby Kraut, page 259) or kimchi.

A celebration of garden-fresh goodness, salads can range from light (Tomato Cucumber with Pine Nuts, page 158) to more substantial meals in themselves, such as Cool Bean Salad with Fava, Farro, and Fennel page (169), which includes a grain, a bean, as well as your greens.

Wondering what to include in your salad? It's limited only by your imagination. Salads can include cooked veggies, such as with the Wilted Collard Salad (page 166), sea vegetables (Domo Arigato Arame Salad, page 159), or pasta (Club Med Pasta Salad, page 168). Or how are these for a starting point? (Don't feel that you need to include all of them!)

- **Different types of greens,** such as buttercup, romaine lettuce, or mixed salad greens. Try arugula, baby spinach, and baby kale.

- **Sprouts**, such as alfalfa, clover, broccoli, sunflower, buckwheat, pea, mung bean, lentil, and crunchy mixed sprouts.
- **Raw vegetables**, such as carrots, beets, daikon, avocados, celery, bell peppers, zucchini, broccoli, cauliflower, cabbage, tomatoes, cucumbers, kohlrabi, corn, onion (red, white, or green), or your favorites.
- Rotate through **different cuts**: slice, dice, chop, and grate. Break out the spiralizer and go to town!
- Add **cooked vegetables** that can be steamed, grilled, roasted, or sautéed.
- **Seeds and nuts** that are raw or toasted, such as sunflower seeds, pumpkin seeds, hazelnuts, almonds, pecans, walnuts, hemp seeds, sesame seeds, and more.
- Bulk it up with **legumes**: add cooked chickpeas, pinto beans, black beans, fava beans, kidney, green lentils, black lentils, edamame, or roasted tofu or tempeh cubes.
- Don't forget **grains**, such as quinoa, rice, millet, or buckwheat.

Of course, dressings make all the difference in how your salad experience unfolds. Try our luscious oil-free dressing made with chia seeds, Oil-Free Roasted Red Pepper Dressing (page 170), or a Zesty Lemon Sriracha Dressing (page 171), to put a sparkle on your salad.

Did we forget anything? We would love to hear about your creative salad ideas! E-mail info@doctorandchef.com.

> ## TIMELESS TIPS: SALAD HACKS
>
> - **Add flair to your salads:** Consider investing in a spiralizer, to create thick or thin noodles (see page 307), or a handheld mandoline for perfect veggie slices.
> - **Dress it up.** Prepare dressing recipes from this book, or purchase a few of your favorite store-bought varieties to have on hand to enhance your salads.
> - **On the go?** Keep some mason jars on hand to create Salad in a Jar (page 157). Prepare one or two salads in advance.
> - **Use leftovers as a salad base.** What did you have for dinner that can be repurposed as a salad by mixing in some organic lettuce or greens? Pineapple Fried Rice (page 203), Quintessential Quinoa Pilaf (page 186), Braised Kale with Shallots and Slivered Almonds (page 185), and many of the other recipes in this book can be magically transformed into salad the following day.

Salad in a Jar

Colorful, convenient, and portable. Fill your mason jar with veggies of choice and you are good to go when travel plans hit and you don't want to miss on your daily plant-based health boost. Serve along with your favorite salad dressing, such as Oil-Free Roasted Red Pepper (page 170), Turmeric Tahini (page 172), Avo Goddess (page 160), or Zesty Lemon Sriracha (page 171). Looking to take a single portion of dressing with you? Fill a 2-ounce glass or plastic to-go container and fit it right in the jar!

TOTAL YIELD: 32 OUNCES
Serving Size: 16 ounces
Number of Servings: 2
Prep Time: 10 minutes
Total Time: 10 minutes

2 cups arugula
1 cup halved cherry tomatoes
½ cup seeded and chopped cucumber
¼ cup peeled and spiralized carrot
¼ cup seeded and julienned yellow bell pepper
¼ cup shredded purple cabbage
2 tablespoons sunflower or pumpkin seeds

1. Place the arugula in the bottom of a 1-quart mason jar. If you want two individual servings, use two pint-size mason jars instead of a 1-quart jar.
2. Top with the cherry tomatoes, cucumber, carrot, bell pepper, purple cabbage, and sunflower seeds.
3. Seal with a lid and you're ready to travel with your salad!

VARIATIONS

- Go to town with creating your ultimate salad jar by experimenting with different greens as well as different chopped veggies, such as zucchini, gold bar squash, broccoli, jicama, green onion, and fennel bulb.

- Add peeled and grated vegetables, such as beets, kohlrabi, daikon, or parsnip.

- Add your favorite nuts and seeds, such as pecan, hazelnut, walnut, or sesame.

- Add sprouts, such as sunflower, buckwheat, or pea.

- Add a crunch with vegan croutons (for homemade, see page 189).

- We feel obligated to mention that instead of using a mason jar, you can also place all the ingredients in a bowl and enjoy your salad!

Tomato Cucumber with Pine Nuts

Hello, ultraeasy! Whip up this simple and invigorating salad in no time as a side dish for your El Tortilla Pizza (page 224), Mushroom Risotto (page 233), or Marvelous Macro Meal (page 226) and receive potassium, vitamin C, and healthy fats for a balanced and detoxifying nosh. Check out the variations and include as many as you can to increase the joy of your palate.

TOTAL YIELD: 24 OUNCES

    Serving Size: 6 ounces
    Number of Servings: 4
    Prep Time: 15 minutes
    Total Time: 15 minutes

1¼ cups seeded and chopped cucumber
   (½-inch pieces)
1 cup chopped tomato (½-inch pieces)
½ cup peeled, pitted, and diced avocado
3 tablespoon diced red onion
2 tablespoons pine nuts
3 tablespoons freshly squeezed lemon juice
¼ cup fresh or frozen corn
2 teaspoons balsamic vinegar (optional)
Sea salt and ground black pepper
Pinch of crushed red pepper flakes
   (optional)

Combine all the ingredients in a bowl and mix well.

VARIATIONS

- Add ¼ cup of diced fennel bulb, one pressed or minced garlic clove, and 1 tablespoon of finely chopped fresh flat-leaf parsley and/or basil.
- Add 2 tablespoons of nutritional yeast.
- Add 2 tablespoons of finely chopped olives.
- Replace the cucumber and tomato with other chopped veggies, such as zucchini, cabbage, red onion, jicama, or daikon radish.
- Add 1 tablespoon olive oil.

Domo Arigato Arame Salad

Give thanks for this satisfying salad that has the flavor of the sea, imparted from the sea vegetable arame. A great source of iodine to support the thyroid and help boost detoxification. Serve along with Marvelous Macro Meal (page 226) or Black Gomasio Crusted Tofu (page 215) and Miso Roots Soup (page 142).

TOTAL YIELD: 12 OUNCES SALAD, 3 OUNCES DRESSING

    Serving Size: 4 ounces salad, 1 ounce dressing
    Number of Servings: 3
    Prep Time: 5 minutes
    Soak Time: 30 minutes
    Total Time: 35 minutes

1 cup arame
½ cup fresh or frozen corn
¼ cup seeded and diced red bell pepper
¼ cup thinly sliced green onion

ARAME DRESSING

¼ cup arame soak water or water
2 teaspoons toasted sesame oil
2 teaspoons rice vinegar
2 teaspoons wheat-free tamari or
    other soy sauce
Pinch of cayenne pepper (optional)
Sea salt and ground black pepper

1. Place the arame in a bowl with ample hot water to cover. Allow to sit until the arame becomes soft, about 20 minutes. Drain the arame well, reserving ¼ cup of the water for the dressing. Place the arame in a bowl with the corn, bell pepper, and green onion and mix well.
2. Make the dressing: Combine the dressing ingredients in a separate bowl and mix well.
3. Add the dressing to the arame mixture and mix well.

VARIATIONS

- Add 2 tablespoons of tahini to the dressing.
- Add 1 tablespoon of minced fresh cilantro.
- Add 1 cup of sautéed mushrooms or Magical Mushroom Medley (page 184).
- Add ½ cup of grated carrot, beet, daikon, or parsnip.
- Add 2 teaspoons of peeled and minced fresh ginger, one pressed and minced garlic clove, and/or ½ teaspoon of Chinese five-spice powder.
- Omit the oil for an oil-free salad.

Daikon with Avo Goddess Dressing

In the town of Glastonbury, in the shadow of the ancient hill Tor, sits one of England's only temples to the Goddess. Ancient manuscripts reveal that the recipe for this oil-free dressing has stood the test of time. (We're kidding, of course, but we **do** think this salad is perfect nourishment for your inner god or goddess!) Daikon, a highly detoxifying, skin-clearing, and immunity- and bone-strengthening radish, is the perfect choice of root to accompany this burst of supernutritious plant flavors. Top with cherry tomatoes and toasted pine nuts, and serve along with Pilau Rice (page 198), or Quintessential Quinoa Pilaf (page 186) and Herb-Roasted Tofu (page 220).

TOTAL YIELD: 24 OUNCES SALAD, 8 OUNCES DRESSING

    Serving Size: 4 ounces salad, 1⅓ ounces dressing
    Number of Servings: 6
    Prep Time: 15 minutes
    Total Time: 15 minutes

3 cups peeled and thinly sliced or chopped daikon radish
½ cup thinly sliced white or red onion
1 tablespoon finely chopped fresh cilantro

AVO GODDESS DRESSING

1 cup water
½ cup peeled, pitted, and mashed avocado
¼ cup chopped fresh cilantro
3 tablespoons freshly squeezed lime juice
1 clove garlic (optional)
2 teaspoons raw apple cider vinegar or coconut vinegar
½ teaspoon sea salt, or to taste
¼ teaspoon chili powder or chipotle powder
⅛ teaspoon ground black pepper

1. Place the daikon and white onion in a bowl and mix well.
2. Prepare the dressing: Place all the dressing ingredients in a blender and blend well.
3. Pour the dressing over daikon mixture and mix well. Top with the cilantro before serving.

VARIATIONS

- Add 2 tablespoons of your favorite chopped olive along with the daikon.
- Replace the daikon with jicama or chopped vegetables of your choosing, such as broccoli, carrots, radishes, corn, tomatoes, or cucumbers.
- Add ¼ teaspoon of wheat-free tamari or other soy sauce to the dressing.
- Add 1 teaspoon of curry powder to the dressing.
- Replace the cilantro with fresh basil, and the lime juice with lemon juice. Add 2 teaspoons of Italian Spice Mix (page 251).

Arugula Walnut Salad with Cashew Dill Dressing

You may not have noticed the waiver at the beginning of the book that releases us from liability if you become addicted to this creamy oil-free dressing. The dill adds a nice kick as well as myriad benefits for digestion, allergies, and even arthritis. Serve with Jackfruit Tacos (see page 216), Marvelous Macro Meal (page 226), or Quinoa Quiche (page 235).

TOTAL YIELD: 32 OUNCES SALAD, 6 OUNCES DRESSING

> Serving Size: 8 ounces salad, 1½ ounces dressing
> Number of Servings: 4
> Prep Time: 10 minutes
> Soak Time: 20 minutes
> Total Time: 30 minutes

CREAMY CASHEW DILL DRESSING

½ cup raw cashew pieces
½ cup water
2 tablespoons nutritional yeast
1 tablespoon minced fresh dill
1 clove garlic
1 tablespoon raw apple cider vinegar
½ teaspoon sea salt, or to taste
Pinch of crushed red pepper flakes
  (optional)

SALAD

4 cups arugula
½ cup chopped walnuts
¼ cup dried currants or cranberries
  (optional)

1. Prepare the dressing: Place the cashews in a bowl with ample water to cover. Allow to sit for 20 minutes for up to a few hours. Rinse and drain well. Transfer to a blender with all the remaining dressing ingredients, including the ½ cup of fresh water, and blend until creamy.
2. Arrange the arugula on plates. Drizzle with the dressing. Top with the walnuts, and the currants, if using. Enjoy!

VARIATIONS

- Replace the arugula with spinach, mixed organic greens, or chopped veggies of your choosing.
- Add the usual salad suspects, such as grated carrots or chopped cucumbers.
- Replace the walnuts with other nuts and seeds.

Sunny Kale Salad

Brighten up your day with the epitome of nutrient-dense foods. Kale has an optimal omega-3 to omega-6 ratio, as well as vitamins A, C, E, and K; the minerals calcium and iron; and its list of antiaging benefits is seemingly endless. The kale is mixed with a creamy sunflower seed sauce to enhance absorption of all the healing nutrients. Garnish with Black Sesame Gomasio (page 253) and serve as a power boost along with Mac n Cheez (page 230).

TOTAL YIELD: 48 OUNCES SALAD, 8 OUNCES SAUCE

> Serving Size: 8 ounces salad, 1⅓ ounces sauce
> Number of Servings: 6
> Prep Time: 15 minutes
> Soak Time: 20 minutes
> Total Time: 25 minutes

6 cups shredded kale

1 cup halved cherry tomatoes

¼ cup raw sunflower seeds

SUNSEED SAUCE

½ cup raw sunflower seeds

½ cup water

3 to 4 tablespoons freshly squeezed lemon juice

2 tablespoons finely chopped fresh cilantro

1 clove garlic

2 tablespoon nutritional yeast

¾ teaspoon sea salt, or to taste

⅛ teaspoon ground black pepper

¼ teaspoon crushed red pepper flakes (optional)

1. Place the kale in a large bowl.
2. Prepare the sauce: Place the ½ cup of sunflower seeds in a bowl with ample water to cover. Allow to sit for 20 minutes up to a few hours. Rinse and drain well. Transfer to a blender with the ½ cup of fresh water, lemon juice, cilantro, garlic, nutritional yeast, salt, black pepper, and red pepper flakes, if using, and blend until creamy.
3. Transfer to the kale and mix well. Top with the cherry tomatoes and remaining ¼ cup of sunflower seeds before serving.

VARIATIONS

- Replace the kale with other greens, such as arugula, chard, or mixed salad greens.

- Replace the sunflower seed sauce with Turmeric Tahini Dressing (page 172) or Zesty Lemon Sriracha Dressing (page 171).

- Add any or all of the following to the kale: ½ cup of shredded carrot or beet, ¼ cup of corn, or ¼ cup of shredded purple cabbage.

Raw Fettuccine Alfreda

It's true . . . raw pasta is a thing. Your spiralizer is your friend when it comes to creating gluten-free pasta on demand. This pasta is made from B vitamin–rich zucchini, and the heart-healthy creamy sauce is cashew based. Don't forget basil's additional anti-aging and anti-inflammatory benefits. Serve as part of a raw feast that may include Raw Choco-Cherry Bombs (page 281) for dessert.

TOTAL YIELD: 32 OUNCES
 Serving Size: 16 ounces
 Number of Servings: 2
 Prep Time: 15 minutes
 Total Time: 15 minutes

4 cups spiralized zucchini (see note)
½ cup cashew cheese (for homemade, see
  page 179)
2 tablespoons chiffonaded fresh basil
2 tablespoons diced sun-dried tomato,
  pimiento, or roasted red pepper (see page
  170)
1 tablespoon diced kalamata olives,
  or 2 teaspoons capers
1 tablespoon finely chopped fresh flat-leaf
  parsley
2 tablespoons pine nuts, optionally toasted

Place the spiralized zucchini, cashew cheese, basil, sun-dried tomato, olives, and parsley in a bowl and mix well. Top with the pine nuts before serving.

VARIATIONS

- Replace the zucchini with gold bar squash, carrots, beets, or strips of medium-soft coconut meat sliced into noodle size.

- Add ½ teaspoon of minced fresh rosemary.

- Replace the cashew cheese with Artful Almond Sauce (page 270).

- Replace the cashew cheese with Chunky Tomato Sauce (page 267) and serve warm. (Don't tell the raw police.)

NOTE:

To spiralize zucchini, follow manufacturers' instructions based on the model you are using. Be sure to chop the spiralized zucchini into 6-inch or smaller pieces for ease of eating!

Kale Millet Tabbouleh

Africa meets the Middle East in this light yet filling salad. Traditionally made with bulgur wheat, this gluten-free version of the Middle Eastern staple includes millet. With origins in Africa, millet is a good source of trace minerals, B vitamins, and fiber, with specific antioxidants that may help prevent heart disease, diabetes, and even asthma. Serve along with Chimichurri Grilled Cauliflower Steaks (page 201) and Herb-Roasted Tofu (page 220).

TOTAL YIELD: 40 OUNCES
   Serving Size: 10 ounces
   Number of Servings: 4
   Prep Time: 10 minutes
   Cook Time: 25 minutes
   Cooling Time: 15 minutes
   Total Time: 50 minutes, unless served with
      warm millet

1¼ cups water or vegetable stock (for
   homemade, see page 248)
½ cup uncooked millet
¾ teaspoon sea salt, or to taste, divided
2 cups shredded kale
1 cup chopped tomato (½-inch pieces)
¼ cup diced red onion
¼ cup finely chopped fresh flat-leaf parsley
3 tablespoon freshly squeezed lemon juice
2 tablespoons olive or hemp seed oil
   (optional)
⅛ teaspoon ground black pepper
¼ teaspoon crushed red pepper flakes
   (optional)

1. Place the water, millet, and ½ teaspoon of the sea salt in a 2-quart pot over high heat. Bring to a boil. Cover, lower the heat to low, and cook until all the liquid is absorbed, about 25 minutes. Fluff with a fork.
2. Meanwhile, place the remaining ingredients, including the remaining ¼ teaspoon of salt, in a large bowl and mix well.
3. Add the cooked millet and mix well. Serve warm or cold.

VARIATIONS

※ Replace the millet with quinoa, rice, couscous, or bulgur wheat (see pages 100–101).

※ Add ½ cup of cooked chickpeas, 2 tablespoons of your favorite chopped olives, and/or ¼ cup of chopped artichoke hearts or hearts of palm.

※ Add 1 cup of sautéed mushrooms or mushrooms from the Magical Mushroom Medley (page 184).

Sally's Super Simple Slaw

Say that five times fast and see what happens! Zesty and nutritious, cabbage contains reputed anticancer and digestion-healing glucosinolates, vitamins C and K, manganese, and more. While vegan mayonnaise may not be the ultimate health food, we consider it a valuable transition food for those that love the flavor of mayo and wish to eliminate the cholesterol-laden egg-based version. Serve Sally's Super Simple Slaw with something special, such as our scrumptious Sweet Potato Black Bean Sliders (page 228).

TOTAL YIELD: 32 OUNCES
Serving Size: 8 ounces
Number of Servings: 4
Prep Time: 15 minutes
Total Time: 15 minutes

4 cups shredded cabbage (try a mixture of red and green cabbage)
½ cup finely chopped fennel
½ cup thinly sliced green onion
1 teaspoon minced fresh dill
¼ cup plus 2 tablespoons vegan mayonnaise (for homemade, see page 273)
1 tablespoon apple cider vinegar or coconut vinegar
1 tablespoon stone-ground or Dijon mustard
¾ teaspoon sea salt, or to taste
⅛ teaspoon ground black pepper
⅛ teaspoon crushed red pepper flakes (optional)

1. Place the cabbage, fennel, green onion, and dill in a large bowl and mix well.
2. Place the mayonnaise, vinegar, mustard, salt, black pepper, and crushed red pepper flakes, if using, in a small bowl and mix well.
3. Transfer to the cabbage mixture and mix well before serving.

VARIATIONS

- Add 1 teaspoon of celery seeds, 1½ teaspoons of wheat-free tamari or other soy sauce, and one pressed or minced garlic clove along with the mustard.

- Add ¼ teaspoon of chipotle powder along with the salt and black pepper.

- Add ½ cup of pumpkin or sunflower seeds along with cabbage.

- Replace the dill with 1 tablespoon of minced fresh cilantro or 2 tablespoons of chiffonaded fresh basil.

- Not into mayo? Feel free to omit it and add an extra 1½ teaspoons of vinegar and mustard. You can also replace the mayo with an equivalent amount of pureed cashews. To puree cashews, place the cashews in a strong blender and add just enough water to puree when blending.

Wilted Collard Salad

After a late night jazz concert on Bourbon Street in New Orleans, you are probably craving some wilted collards. Come home to find some leftover rice or quinoa? Score! High in vitamins A and K as well as calcium, manganese, B vitamins, and some vitamin C, yummy collards will put that pep back in your step. Enjoy with the simple dressing in the recipe or use your favorite. Top with a sprinkle of Black Sesame Gomasio (page 253) and serve along with Herb-Roasted Tofu (page 220) and Creamy Corn Chowder with Fire-Roasted Tomatoes and Dill (page 146).

TOTAL YIELD: 24 OUNCES
> Serving Size: 12 ounces
> Number of Servings: 2
> Prep Time: 10 minutes
> Cook Time: 15 minutes
> Total Time: 25 minutes

1 bunch collard greens, rinsed well
Sea salt
1½ teaspoons olive oil, or 2 tablespoons water
1 teaspoon Cajun Spice Mix (page 249, or store-bought) or curry powder
2 cups mixed organic salad greens
1 cup cooked and cooled quinoa or rice (see note)
Juice of 1 lemon
1½ tablespoons hemp, flax, or olive oil (optional)
2 tablespoons nutritional yeast
Ground black pepper

1. Stem the collards by removing the thickest part of the stem with a sharp knife or tearing it away from the leaf with your hands. Leaving some of the top portion of the stem is okay. Slice the collard leaves into 1-inch strips.
2. Place a small sauté pan over high heat. Heat the olive oil. Add the collards, Cajun Spice Mix, and an optional pinch of sea salt. Cook until the collards are just wilted and are still a vibrant dark green, stirring constantly.
3. Place the salad greens in a large bowl. Add the quinoa and collards and gently toss well. Top with the lemon juice, a drizzle of hemp oil, and the nutritional yeast. Season with salt and pepper to taste.

VARIATIONS

- Replace the collards with kale, spinach, chard, or arugula.
- Add other raw and chopped vegetables, such as radishes, bell peppers, cabbage, or red onion.
- Too impatient to wait for your quinoa to cool? Go ahead and use warm and even hot cooked quinoa or rice in the recipe.

NOTE:

To cook the quinoa, place 1 cup of water, ½ cup of uncooked quinoa, optionally rinsed and drained, and ¼ teaspoon of sea salt in a small pot over high heat. Bring to a boil. Cover, lower the heat to low, and cook until all the liquid is absorbed, about 10 minutes. Turn off the heat, keep covered, and allow to sit for 5 minutes. Fluff with a fork. Allow to cool for this recipe.

THE ULTIMATE AGE-DEFYING PLAN

Butter Bean Salad

Lima bean to some, butter bean to others, this protein-rich creamy salad has Persian origins. Along with all of the other mineral, protein, and fiber benefits, the lima is an excellent source of molybdenum, important for blood sugar balance and essential enzyme actions. Garnish with smoked paprika and serve with Braised Kale with Shallots and Slivered Almonds (page 185), Lemony Herbed Cauliflower Roast (page 211), and Pilau Rice (page 198).

TOTAL YIELD: 28 OUNCES
 Serving Size: 7 ounces
 Number of Servings: 4
 Prep Time: 15 minutes
 Total Time: 15 minutes

2 (15-ounce) cans butter beans, or 3 cups cooked (see page 102)
¼ cup thinly sliced celery
¼ cup diced red onion
3 tablespoons vegan mayonnaise (for homemade, see page 273)
1 tablespoon minced fresh dill
2 teaspoons raw apple cider vinegar
1¼ teaspoons Dijon or stone-ground mustard
½ teaspoon sea salt, or to taste
¼ teaspoon wheat-free tamari or other soy sauce (optional)
Pinch of crushed red pepper flakes (optional)

Place all the ingredients in a bowl and mix well.

VARIATIONS

- Add one pressed or minced garlic clove along with the mustard.

- Replace the mayonnaise with unsweetened Coconut Yogurt (page 262).

- Replace the butter beans with cannellini, navy, or fava beans.

Club Med Pasta Salad

Oh, the joys of the Mediterranean! Sun-kissed produce, olives dripping from the trees, and endless miles of beaches. Can you feel it? We hope you do when you experience this dish—so simple to prepare. Not to mention brain-boosting and overall tissue-rejuvenating from high amounts of antioxidants and healthy fats. Serve along with Cool Bean Salad with Farro, Fava, and Fennel (page 169) and Roasted Red Pepper Soup with Fennel (page 144).

TOTAL YIELD: 64 OUNCES

> Serving Size: 8 ounces
> Number of Servings: 8
> Prep Time: 15 minutes
> Cook Time: 10 minutes
> Total Time: 25 minutes

12 ounces elbow rice pasta

¼ cup chopped kalamata olives or your favorite

3 cups finely chopped spinach

1 (15-ounce) can diced fire-roasted tomatoes, or 1½ cups diced tomato

1 tablespoon olive oil (optional)

½ cup thinly sliced red onion

½ cup chopped artichoke hearts

2 tablespoons finely chopped fresh flat-leaf parsley

1 tablespoon balsamic vinegar (optional)

Sea salt and ground black pepper

Pinch of crushed red pepper flakes (optional)

1. Cook the pasta according to the package instructions. Drain well.
2. Meanwhile, combine all the remaining ingredients in a bowl and mix well.
3. Add the cooked pasta while it is still hot, and mix well. Serve warm or at room temperature.

VARIATIONS

- Add 2 tablespoons of nutritional yeast.

- Add 7 ounces of sliced vegan sausage that has been sautéed for 5 minutes.

- Add ½ cup of grated vegan cheese.

- Add ¼ cup of Zesty Lemon Sriracha Dressing (page 171) or add a **Simple Balsamic Dressing**. For this, combine 2 tablespoons of olive oil, 2 teaspoons of balsamic vinegar, 1 teaspoon of pure maple syrup, ¾ teaspoon of Dijon mustard, a pinch of sea salt, a pinch of ground black pepper, and a pinch of red pepper flakes in a bowl and whisk well.

Cool Bean Salad with Farro, Fava, and Fennel

Farro is an ancient form of wheat, popular in ancient Rome as the gladiators' energy food of choice for the big games. Protein-rich and a good source of iron, B vitamins, and zinc, farro pairs well with equally nutritionally dense fava beans, which alone served historically as a sustaining food during famine in Sicily. Fennel, a familiar ingredient in Mediterranean cuisine, is high in phytonutrients, including a unique volatile oil compound called anethole, which is showing promise in preventing cancer growth.

Garnish with thinly sliced green onion, top with a dollop of Vegan Sour Cream (page 274) and serve along with Sunny Kale Salad (page 162) or Wilted Collard Salad (page 166).

TOTAL YIELD: 32 OUNCES
Serving Size: 8 ounces
Number of Servings: 4
Prep Time: 10 minutes
Cook Time: 30 minutes
Total Time: 40 minutes

½ cup uncooked farro (1 cup cooked)
1¾ cups water or vegetable stock (for homemade, see page 248)
½ teaspoon sea salt, or to taste
1 (15-ounce) can fava beans, or 1½ cups cooked
½ cup chopped fresh fennel bulb
1 tablespoon minced fresh dill
3 tablespoons pitted and chopped kalamata olives or your favorite
2 tablespoons freshly squeezed lemon juice
2 teaspoons balsamic vinegar
2 teaspoons olive oil (optional)

1. Place the farro, water, and salt in a 2-quart pot over medium-high heat. Cook for 30 minutes, or until the farro is tender. Drain any excess liquid. Rinse in a colander with cold water until the farro is at room temperature.
2. Transfer to a bowl, add the remaining ingredients, and mix well before serving.

VARIATIONS

- Add hot sauce to taste. Or add a pinch of cayenne pepper or crushed red pepper flakes.

- Replace the farro with quinoa, millet, or rice (see pages 100–101).

- Replace the fava beans with cannellini, pinto, or navy beans.

- Replace the dill with 2 tablespoons minced fresh cilantro, basil, or flat-leaf parsley.

- Add 1 tablespoon of a Global Spice Blend, such as Italian, Ethiopian, or Cajun (pages 249–252).

- Replace the fennel with cucumber, artichoke hearts, or hearts of palm.

- It would be radical . . . this can be a hot bean salad. Simply heat the fava beans over low heat while the farro is cooking. Do not rinse the farro under cold water and mix while hot with the fava beans and remaining ingredients.

Oil-Free Roasted Red Pepper Dressing

You will never miss the oil in this flavorful and robust dressing. Cooking the bell peppers actually enhances absorption of their antioxidant lycopene, found in the inner skin. Try tossed with Grilled Vegetables Extraordinaire (page 178), drizzled over Polenta Croutons (page 189), or on your salad of choice. Go rogue and serve as a dipping sauce for Curried Cauliflower Pakora (page 200) or Coco Jackfruit Nuggets (page 183).

TOTAL YIELD: 12 OUNCES

> Serving Size: 2 ounces
> Number of Servings: 6
> Prep Time: 15 minutes
> Cook Time: 10 minutes if broiling or roasting peppers over fire, 45 minutes if roasting in oven
> Cooling Time: 15 minutes
> Total Time: 40 to 1 hour, 15 minutes depending on roasting method

Oil for pan
1 large red bell pepper
¾ cup water
1½ tablespoons chia seeds
1½ tablespoons raw apple cider vinegar
2½ teaspoons pure maple syrup, coconut nectar, date syrup (for homemade, see page 109), or 2 pitted dates
2 teaspoons Dijon mustard
¾ teaspoon sea salt, or to taste
½ teaspoon onion flakes
1 teaspoon garlic flakes
Pinch of cayenne pepper (optional)

1. Preheat the oven to 400°F or HIGH broil. Place the pepper on a well-oiled or non-stick baking sheet and lightly oil the pepper. If roasting at 400°F, cook until the skin on the peppers is bubbly and charred, about 45 minutes, using tongs to flip once or twice. If using the HIGH broil setting, broil until the skin becomes black and charred, flipping frequently with tongs to ensure even cooking, about 10 minutes, depending on the heat of the oven. Place the pepper in a bowl, then cover with a lid or plate. Allow to sit for 15 minutes, or until cool enough to handle.

2. Carefully remove all or most of the skin, and all the seeds. Measure out ½ cup for this recipe, along with 1 teaspoon of the roasting liquid. Transfer to a blender with the remaining ingredients and blend well.

VARIATIONS

- Add 2 teaspoons of balsamic vinegar and ¼ teaspoon of wheat-free tamari or other soy sauce.

- Add 2 tablespoons of toasted coconut (see page 106). You can also use the toasted coconut as a garnish on the dressing when served with salad or grilled vegetables.

Zesty Lemon Sriracha Dressing

Bring a zing and a zap to your salads . . . turning an ordinary dish into an extraordinary flavor sensation. Lemon is the ultimate detoxifier, refresher, and alkinizer. Serve with your salad of choice, or use as a dipping sauce for Smoky Truffled Baked Broccoli Fries (page 180).

TOTAL YIELD: 4 OUNCES
    Serving Size: 1 ounce
    Number of Servings: 4
    Prep Time: 10 minutes
    Total Time: 10 minutes

¼ cup olive oil
3 tablespoons freshly squeezed lemon juice
1½ teaspoons Dijon mustard
1½ teaspoons sriracha
1½ teaspoons pure maple syrup, coconut nectar, or date syrup (for homemade, see page 109) (optional)
½ teaspoon minced fresh dill
⅛ teaspoon sea salt, or to taste (try with smoked salt)
Pinch of ground black pepper

Place all the ingredients in a bowl and whisk well.

VARIATIONS

- For an oil-free version, omit the oil. Place 3 tablespoons of water and 1 tablespoon of chia seeds in a small bowl for 10 minutes, stirring occasionally. Transfer to a blender with the remaining ingredients and blend.

- Replace the dill with 1 teaspoon of minced fresh chervil, summer savory, parsley, or cilantro.

- Add 1 tablespoon of prepared horseradish.

Turmeric Tahini Dressing

An ancient hippie recipe passed down from generation to generation in the natural food world, this oil-free dressing is so rich and creamy thanks to tahini, which is a great source of calcium and magnesium for the heart, muscles, and brain. Turmeric adds its antioxidant, heart-protective, pain-reducing, and brain-boosting touches. Serve with your Salad in a Jar (page 157) or use as a sauce for your Marvelous Macro Meal (page 226).

TOTAL YIELD: 8 OUNCES
Serving Size: 1 ounce
Number of Servings: 8
Prep Time: 10 minutes
Total Time: 10 minutes

1 tablespoon store-bought miso paste
¾ cup water
½ cup tahini
1 teaspoon Dijon or stone-ground mustard
1 tablespoon nutritional yeast
1½ teaspoons wheat-free tamari or other soy sauce
1 tablespoon freshly squeezed lemon juice
½ teaspoon ground turmeric
2 tablespoons thinly sliced green onion (optional)
1 clove garlic, pressed or minced (optional)
Sea salt and ground black pepper

1. Place the miso paste in a bowl. Add the water slowly, whisking well.
2. Add the remaining ingredients and mix well.

VARIATIONS

🖉 Add ½ teaspoon of minced fresh dill or 1 tablespoon of finely chopped fresh cilantro or flat-leaf parsley.

🖉 Replace the tahini with almond butter.

Berry Peach Smoothie, Maca Pepita Elixir, Hydration Station, and Kale Kiwi Avocado Juice (credit: Elizabeth Arraj) [pages 121, 118, 115, 117]

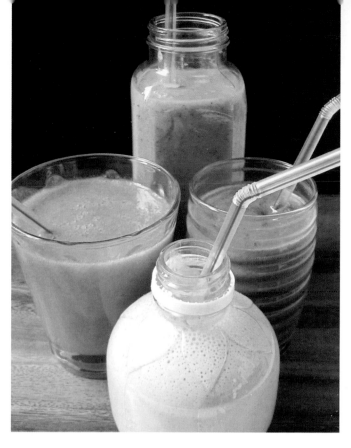

Chlorella Smoothie Bowl (credit: Elizabeth Arraj) [page 131]

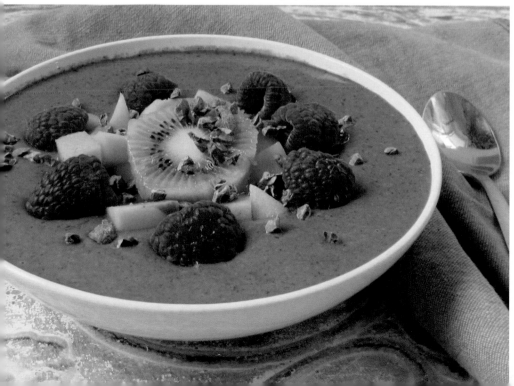

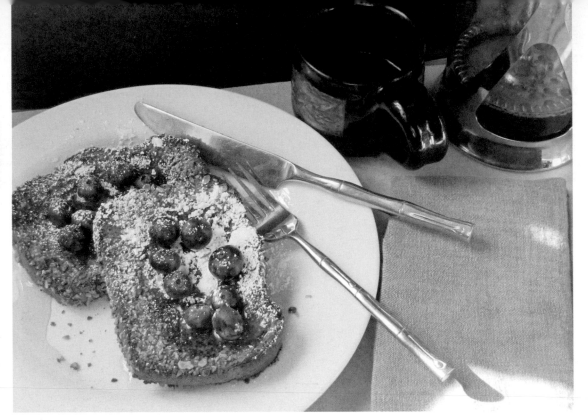

Superseed Baked French Toast (credit: Elizabeth Arraj) [page 136]

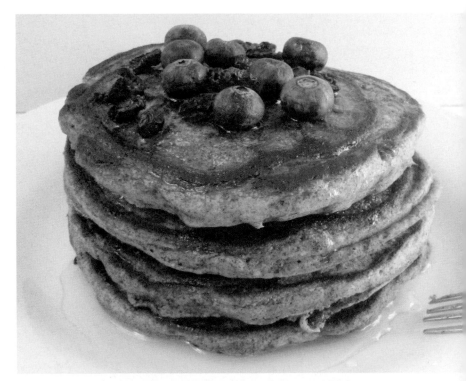

Superfood Buckwheat Pancakes (credit: Elizabeth Arraj) [page 132]

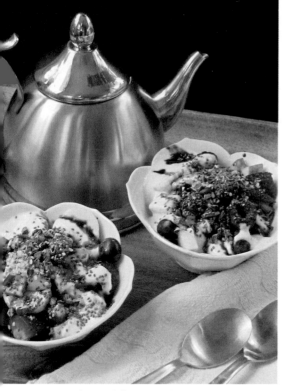

Berry Good Breakfast Bowl
(credit: Elizabeth Arraj) [page 129]

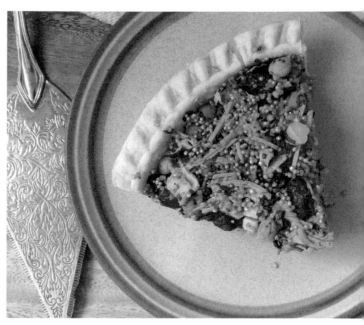

Quinoa Quiche (credit: Elizabeth Arraj) [page 235]

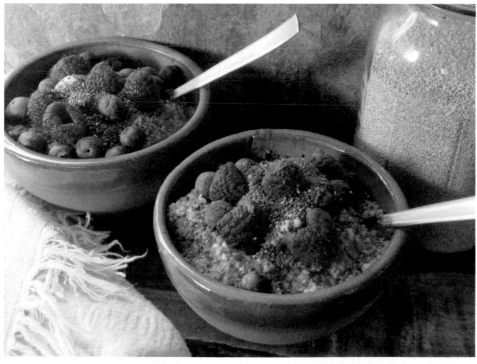

Ancient Sunrise (credit: Elizabeth Arraj) [page 135]

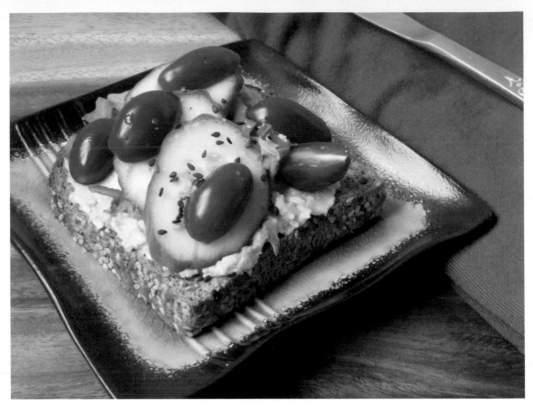

Smashed Avocado Toast Supreme (credit: Elizabeth Arraj) [page 127]

Sweet Potato Black Bean Sliders (credit: Olivia Wallace) [page 228]

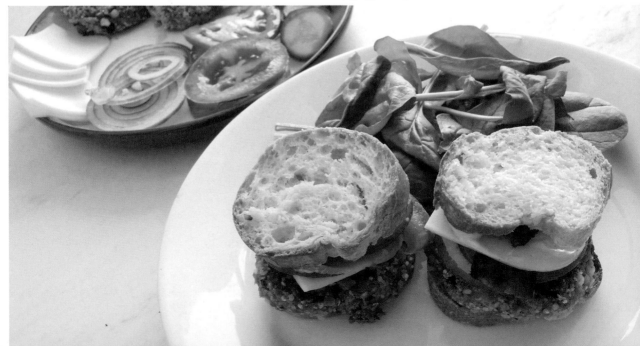

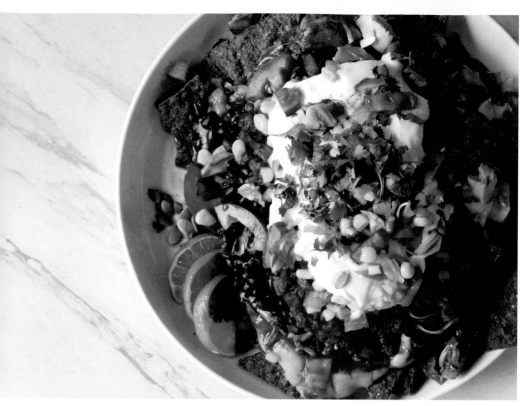

Loaded Nachos (credit: Olivia Wallace) [page 206]

Stacked Avocados (credit: Elizabeth Arraj) [page 195]

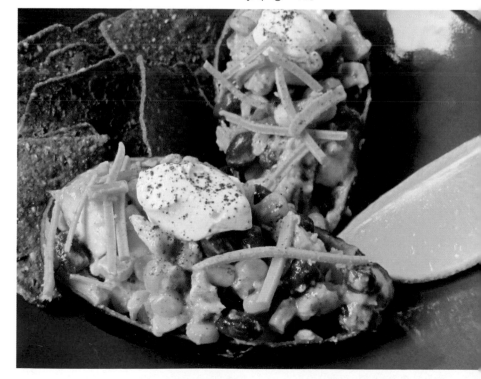

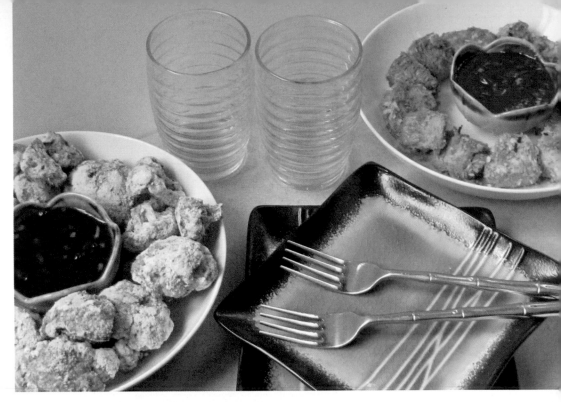

Curried Cauliflower Pakora and Coco Jackfruit Nuggets
(credit: Elizabeth Arraj) [pages 200, 183]

Cashew Cheese–Stuffed Sweet Peppers, Raw Fettuccine Alfreda, and Smoky
Roasted Beets (credit: Elizabeth Arraj) [pages 179, 163, 182]

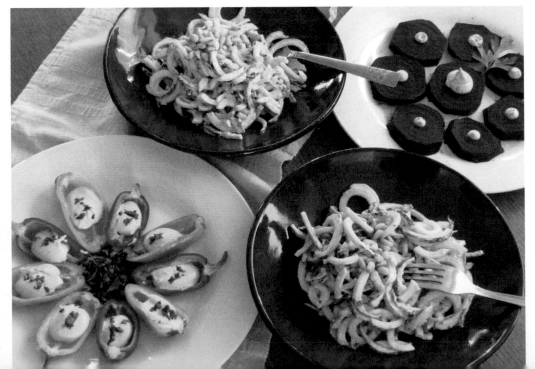

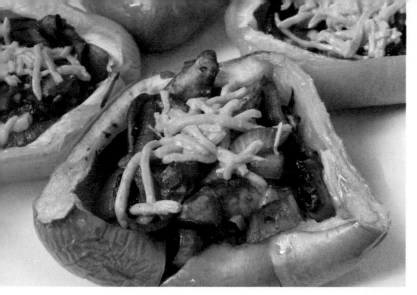

Portobello Cheez Steak Stuffed Peppers
(credit: Elizabeth Arraj) [page 232]

Baked Sesame Zucchini Fries
(credit: Mark Reinfeld) [page 193]

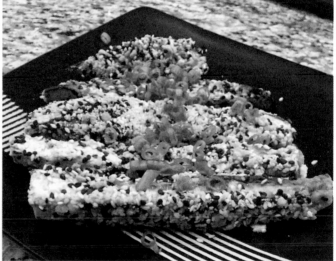

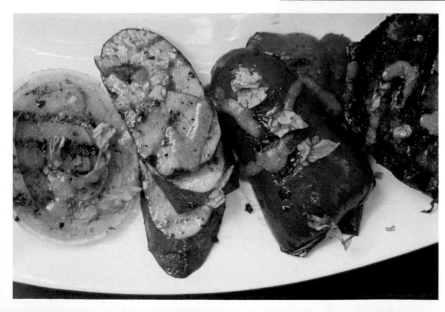

Grilled Vegetables Extraordinaire
(credit: Elizabeth Arraj)
[page 178]

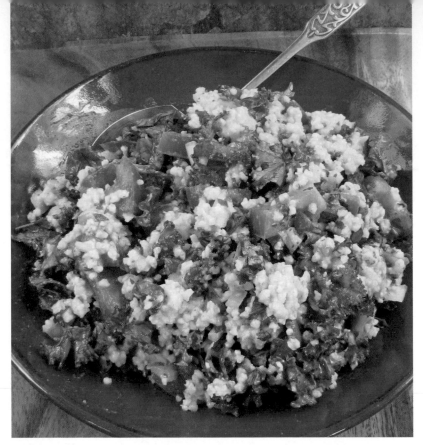

Kale Millet Tabbouleh
(credit: Elizabeth Arraj)
[page 164]

Quintessential Quinoa Pilaf (credit: Elizabeth Arraj) [page 186]

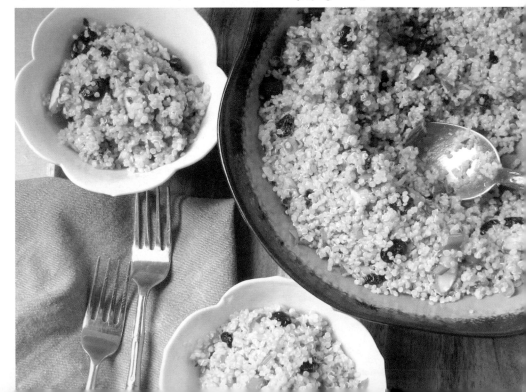

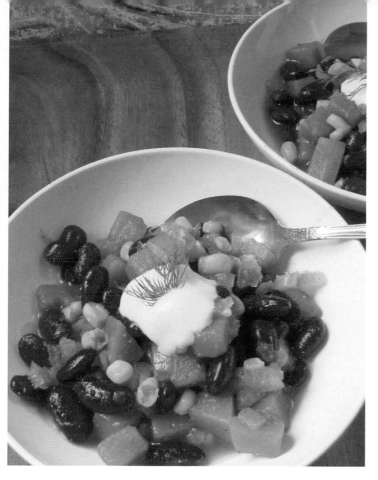

Three Sisters Soup
(credit: Elizabeth Arraj) [page 148]

BBQ Jackfruit with Quintessential Quinoa Pilaf, Pilau Rice, Vegan Sour Cream, and Black Sesame Gomasio (credit: Mark Reinfeld) [pages 217, 186, 198, 274, 253]

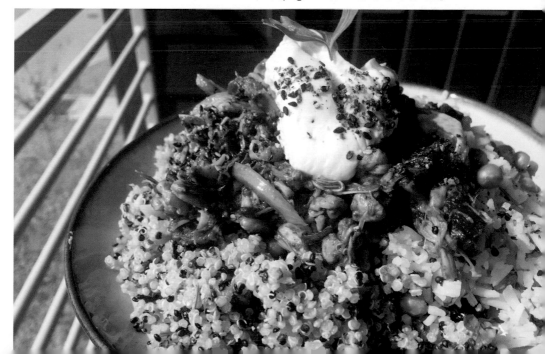

Roasted Butternut Squash
Penne with Sage
(credit: Elizabeth Arraj)
[page 242]

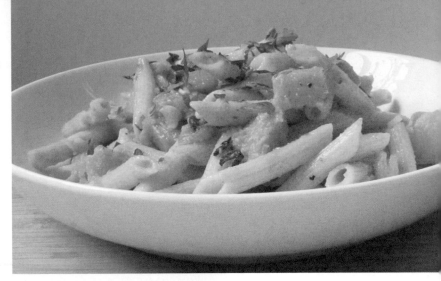

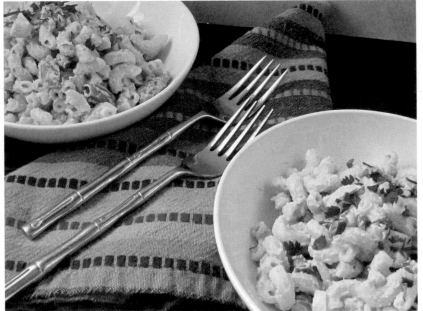

Mac n Cheez
(credit: Elizabeth Arraj) [page 230]

Garlicky Whipped Parsnips
(credit: Elizabeth Arraj)
[page 192]

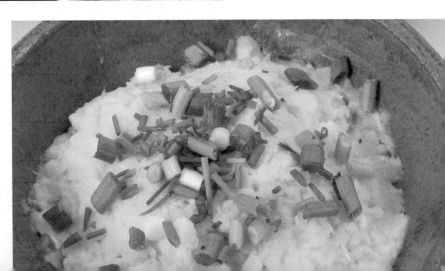

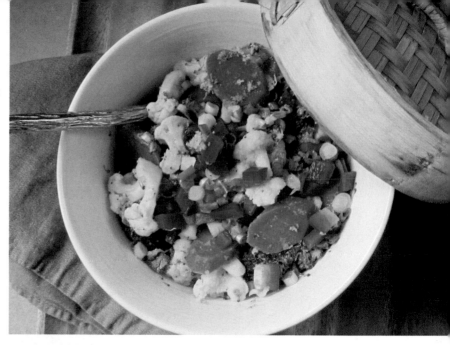

Steamed Supreme
(credit: Elizabeth Arraj)
[page 176]

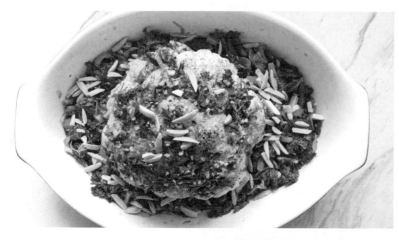

Lemony Herbed Cauliflower Roast
with Braised Kale with Shallots
and Slivered Almonds
(credit: Olivia Wallace)
[pages 211, 185]

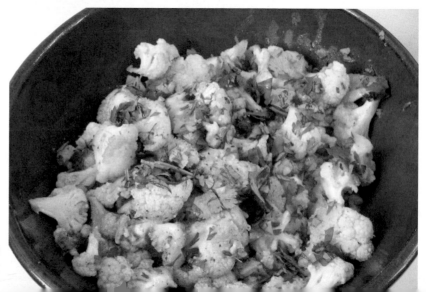

Coco Cauliflower
(credit: Elizabeth Arraj)
[page 197]

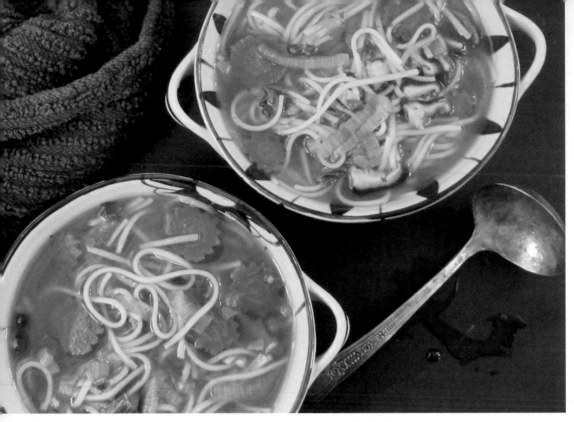

Shiitake Hot Pot Noodle Soup (credit: Elizabeth Arraj) [page 149]

Creamy Corn Chowder with Fire-Roasted Tomatoes and Dill
(credit: Olivia Wallace) [page 146]

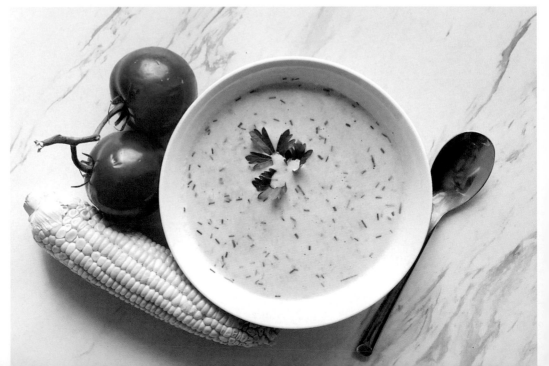

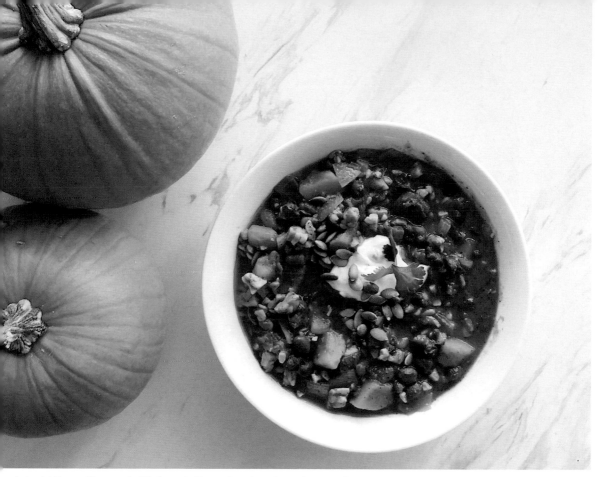

Adzuki Bean Tempeh Chili with Pumpkin (credit: Olivia Wallace) [page 152]

Roasted Red Pepper Soup with Fennel (credit: Mark Reinfeld) [page 144]

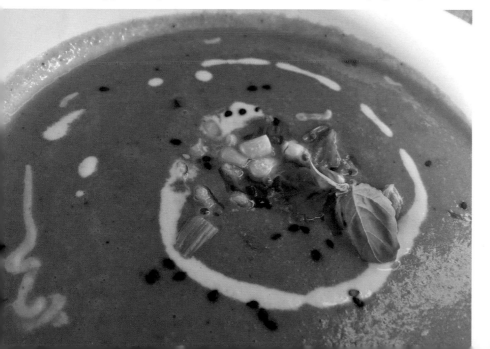

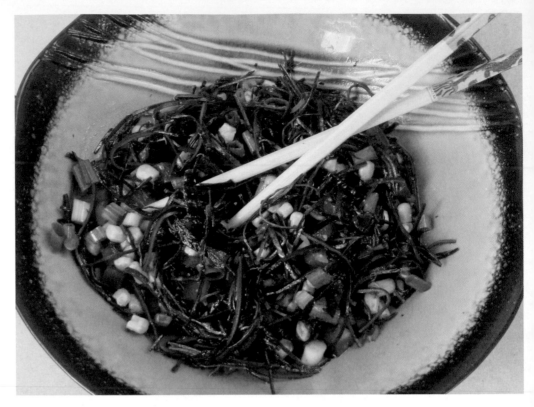

Domo Arigato Arame Salad (credit: Elizabeth Arraj) [page 159]

Brats and Kraut (credit: Elizabeth Arraj) [page 243]

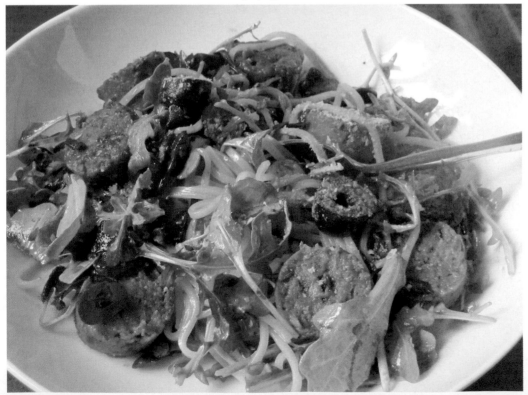

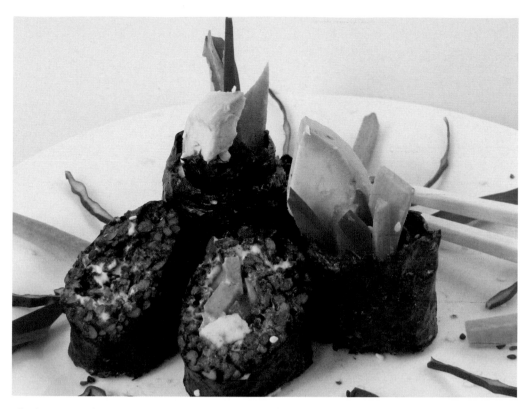

Black Rice Sushi with Wasabi Mayo (credit: Elizabeth Arraj) [page 222]

Black Gomasio Crusted Tofu (credit: Elizabeth Arraj) [page 215]

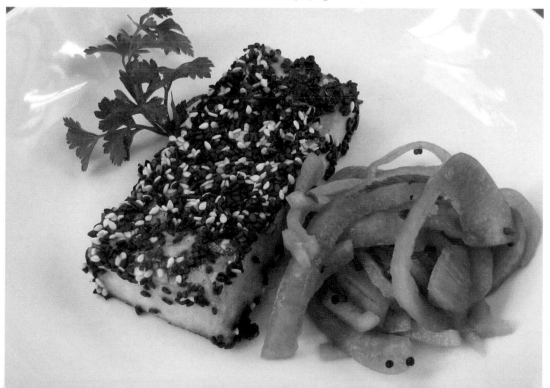

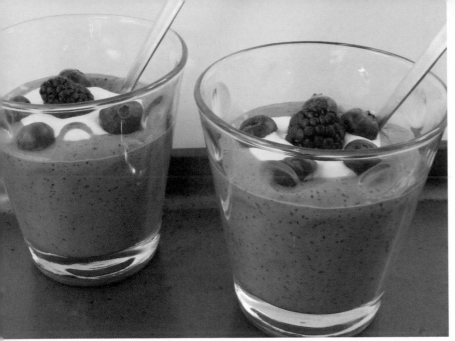

Berry Mousse
(credit: Elizabeth Arraj)
[page 290]

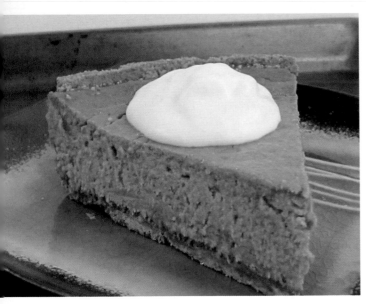

The Great Pumpkin Cheezcake
(credit: Elizabeth Arraj) [page 294]

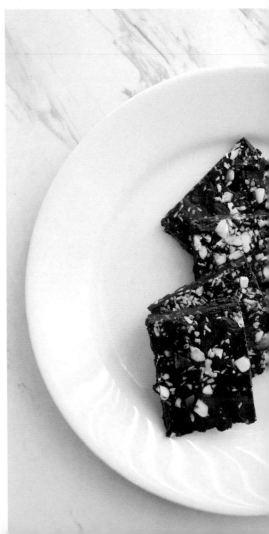

Superfood Chocolate Bark
(credit: Olivia Wallace)
[page 284]

FOURTEEN

AGELESS APPETIZERS AND SIDE DISHES

Welcome to largest chapter in the book! Why so big? Because these recipes are so yummy and versatile! They can be appetizers, snacks, side dishes, or even the main course if you combine a few of them and serve your meal tapas style. Let's load up on the good stuff for lifelong health!

If you're new to cooking or a plant-based diet, or just want supersimple preparation, check out Steamed Supreme (page 176), Rainbow Roasted Roots (page 196), and Grilled Vegetables Extraordinaire (page 178) to get up to speed on steaming, roasting, and grilling basics. Want to enjoy the ultimate age-defying side dish? Steam up a bunch of greens until just tender—rotate through kale, chard, collards, spinach, dandelion greens, and others as available. Drizzle with some lemon juice or lime juice and add a pinch of a Global Spice Blend (pages 249–252) and you are good to go!

Turn here when the savory snack attack hits: Enter the world of spreads, with Garlicky Hummus (page 194) and Cheezy Artichoke Dip (page 205). Curry Cauliflower Pakora (page 200), Baked Sesame Zucchini Fries (page 193), and Coco Jackfruit Nuggets (page 183) are all crowd-pleasers when served with a dipping sauce from Chapter 16. The Loaded Nachos (page 206) are perfect for Super Bowl Sunday. We would also love to introduce you to the debut of Smoky Truffled Baked Broccoli Fries (page 180): your new favorite way to enjoy broccoli!

Sides, such as Pineapple Fried Rice (page 203), Pilau Rice (page 198), and Quintessential Quinoa Pilaf (page 186) pair well with many of the main dishes in Chapter 15. Enjoy your Skillet Corn Bread (page 204) with a soup or stew from Chapter 12 when you are looking for some down-home goodness.

One of the keys to maintaining a healthy diet is to be able to snack on healthy foods. The best way to ensure that is to keep a vegan snack arsenal within easy reach. Chop up carrot and celery sticks, cucumber boats, radishes, sticks of broccoli stalks, and/or jicama sticks. Apple slices are good, too, though they won't stay fresh as long as the other foods. Chopped red cabbage is great, too, but be warned: your fingertips stay purple for days afterward if you eat it with your fingers (been there, done [and still do] that!). Nut butters and spreads, such as hummus, guacamole, and vegan cheese, are excellent to have on hand as well.

A little lime or lemon juice can go a long way. Squeeze it on cucumber, jicama, and papaya spears. Top with a pinch of chili or curry powder, or any of the Global Spice Blends (pages 249–252).

Prepare grains, such as rice or quinoa, in advance and in larger batches. They have a longer shelf life than many dishes and can be there when you need them to round out your main meal.

You can also prep veggies in advance. Chop up some broccoli and cauliflower, carrots, and other veggies that can then be steamed or roasted at a later time. Use within three to four days, or until they lose their firmness.

And for an over-the-top tapas experience, combine some of your favorite recipes in this chapter and serve them on small plates. Consider Coco Cauliflower (page 197), Miso Ginger Glazed Eggplant (page 202), Rosemary Polenta Croutons (page 189) with Pepita Pesto with Avocado (page 265), Braised Kale with Shallots and Slivered Almonds (page 185), Cumin Chickpeas (page 188), and whatever else strikes your fancy. Take a photo of your best tapas feast and share it with us at info@doctorandchef.com.

Lemon Dill Asparagus Spears

Revered since ancient Greek and Roman times, tender asparagus shoots herald the arrival of spring. And you, too, can celebrate its tantalizing nutritional excellence. Perhaps our ancestors sensed that asparagus contains many essential antioxidants, including rutin, which supports blood circulation and eye health, and is one of the highest sources of glutathione, an antioxidant necessary in the liver's detoxification pathways?

For best results with this dish, place in a dehydrator set to 118°F for 2 hours. If you have not yet geared up with a dehydrator, you can use the lowest setting on your regular oven for about 20 minutes, or until the asparagus turns a darker green and is just tender. Serve along with your Hummus Panini with Balsamic Massaged Kale (page 239) and Arugula Walnut Salad with Cashew Dill Dressing (page 161).

TOTAL YIELD: 24 OUNCES
> Serving Size: 6 ounces
> Number of Servings: 4
> Prep Time: 10 minutes
> Marinate Time: 20 minutes
> Total Time: 30 minutes

1 bunch thin asparagus, very bottoms trimmed, sliced thinly on diagonal (about 3 cups)
2 teaspoons olive oil (optional)
2 tablespoons freshly squeezed lemon juice
1 teaspoon minced fresh dill
1 teaspoon red wine vinegar
¼ teaspoon sea salt, or to taste
Pinch of crushed red pepper flakes (optional)
½ teaspoon truffle oil (optional)
¼ cup seeded and diced red bell pepper

1. Place all the ingredients, except the bell pepper, in a bowl and mix well.
2. Allow to sit for 20 to 30 minutes before serving for the flavors to absorb. Garnish with the bell pepper before serving.

VARIATIONS

- Add ¼ cup of diced orange and yellow bell pepper along with the red bell pepper.

- Add one pressed or minced garlic clove along with the asparagus.

- Go Mexican by replacing the dill with 1 tablespoon of fresh cilantro and adding 1 teaspoon of chili powder.

- Go Indian by replacing the dill with 1 tablespoon of cilantro and adding 1 teaspoon of curry powder.

- Although it's a code one raw food violation, you can roast the asparagus until just tender, about 10 minutes in a 300°F oven. Alternatively, you can grill the asparagus until just tender. For either of these methods, brush the asparagus with olive oil before cooking. Combine the remaining ingredients in a bowl and mix well. When the asparagus is done cooking, add to the bowl and toss well before serving.

Steamed Supreme

Simplicity is the mother of beauty. That is no more evident than when you sit down to a big bowl of colorful and perfectly steamed veggies. Also, your life expectancy expands with each bite! Enjoy as part of your Monk Bowls (see page 209), and prepare for nirvana! You can also top with Turmeric Tahini Dressing (page 172) or a double batch of Chimichurri Topping (page 201), and serve as a side to Portobello Cheez Steak Stuffed Peppers (page 232) or Brats and Kraut (page 243).

TOTAL YIELD: 24 OUNCES

Serving Size: 8 ounces
Number of Servings: 3
Prep Time: 10 minutes
Cook Time: 10 minutes
Total Time: 20 minutes

2 cups small broccoli florets
2 cups small cauliflower florets
1 cup diagonally sliced carrots (½-inch slices)
3 tablespoons hemp or flax oil
2 tablespoons nutritional yeast
Sea salt and ground black pepper
½ cup seeded and diced red bell pepper
½ cup thinly sliced green onion

1. Place a steamer basket in a 2-quart pot and fill with water until it reaches the bottom of the steamer basket. Cover, place over high heat, and bring to a boil.
2. Lower the heat to medium. Place the broccoli, cauliflower, and carrots in the steamer basket and cook until the veggies are just tender, about 10 minutes.
3. Transfer to a bowl. Top with the hemp oil and nutritional yeast. Season with salt and black pepper to taste. Garnish with the bell pepper and green onion before serving.

VARIATIONS

- You probably guessed that you can rotate through steaming your favorite veggies, including zucchini, cabbage, onion, celery, garlic, bok choy, kale, collards, and more!

- Feel free to add 1 cup of cubed extra-firm tofu or tempeh along with the vegetables while steaming.

- For an oil-free variation, replace the oil with 2 tablespoons freshly squeezed lemon or lime juice.

Santorini Okra Tomato

Traveling through Greece as a vegan is easier than you think . . . so, don't pass up that trip of a lifetime. But there's no need to travel farther than your own kitchen to experience fantastic Greek cuisine, vegan style. Using tomatoes as a base for veggies is a popular method of cooking on the islands, as with this okra-based dish. Okra is well known for its digestive tissue–healing and blood sugar–regulating properties.

Top with a sprinkle of pine nuts and serve with Lemony Herbed Cauliflower Roast (page 211), Cool Bean Salad with Farro, Fava, and Fennel (page 169), Pilau Rice (page 198), or Club Med Pasta Salad (page 168).

TOTAL YIELD: 32 OUNCES
Serving Size: 8 ounces
Number of Servings: 4
Prep Time: 10 minutes
Cook Time: 20 minutes
Total Time: 30 minutes

1 tablespoon olive oil, or 3 tablespoons water

¾ cup sliced thinly sliced yellow onion

3 to 4 cloves garlic, pressed or minced

1 tablespoon Italian Spice Mix (page 251, or store-bought)

4 cups chopped fresh or frozen (1 pound bag) okra (½-inch pieces)

1 (14.5-ounce) can diced fire-roasted tomatoes, or 1½ cups chopped fresh tomato

2 tablespoons finely chopped fresh flat-leaf parsley

1 tablespoon balsamic vinegar

Sea salt and ground black pepper

Pinch of crushed red pepper flakes (optional)

1. Place a medium-size sauté pan over medium-high heat. Heat the oil. Add the onion and cook for 3 minutes, stirring frequently, adding small amounts of water or vegetable stock if necessary to prevent sticking. Add the garlic and Italian Spice Mix and cook for 2 minutes, stirring frequently.
2. Lower the heat to medium. Add the okra and fire-roasted tomatoes and cook until the okra is just tender, about 15 minutes, stirring frequently.
3. Add the remaining ingredients and stir well before serving.

VARIATIONS

- Add 1 teaspoon of wheat-free tamari or other soy sauce.
- Add 1 tablespoon of chiffonaded fresh basil.
- Add 1 cup of cooked and drained black-eyed peas or fava beans.
- For an Indian flair, replace the Italian Spice Mix with Indian Spice Mix (page 251) and replace the parsley with fresh cilantro.
- For a taste of the South, replace the Italian Spice Mix with Cajun Spice Mix (page 249).

Grilled Vegetables Extraordinaire

Even vegans like to break out the grill! When grilling season hits, gird yourself with your apron and tongs and harvest some veggies. Marinade adds to the nutrient benefits, and gentle grilling locks in moisture and can even enhance absorption of certain antioxidants. Try drizzling with roasted Oil-Free Roasted Red Pepper Dressing (page 170) or Simple Balsamic Dressing (page 168) and serve with Brazenly Braised Tempeh (page 219) and Herb-Roasted Potatoes (page 199) or rice.

TOTAL YIELD: 24 OUNCES WHEN CHOPPED

Serving Size: 6 ounces
Number of Servings: 4
Prep Time: 10 minutes
Cook Time: 20 minutes
Total Time: 30 minutes

VEGGIE BASTING SAUCE

2 tablespoons olive oil
1 tablespoon Italian Spice Mix (page 251, or store-bought)
1 tablespoon balsamic vinegar
½ teaspoon sea salt, or to taste
¼ teaspoon crushed red pepper flakes (optional)
⅛ teaspoon ground black pepper, or to taste

1 large portobello mushroom, gills removed
1 large red bell pepper, quartered and seeded
1 large zucchini, cut into ½-inch slices
1 medium-size yellow onion, cut into ½-inch rings
2 tablespoons chiffonaded fresh basil for garnish

1. Preheat a grill to high. Prepare the basting sauce by placing all the sauce ingredients in a bowl and mixing well.
2. Place the mushroom, bell pepper, zucchini, and onion on the grill and grill until just tender and char marks appear, about 10 minutes, basting frequently with a pastry brush and flipping occasionally to ensure even cooking.
3. Serve the veggies whole or chopped. Top with any remaining basting sauce and basil before serving.

VARIATIONS

- Experiment with different veggies, such as baby bok choy, broccoli, cauliflower, carrots, or parsnips. Grill until just tender.

- Add 2 teaspoons of wheat-free tamari or other soy sauce to the basting sauce.

- Replace the Italian Spice Mix with Cajun Spice Mix (page 249), Ethiopian Spice Mix (page 250), or Mexican Spice Mix (page 252).

Cashew Cheese–Stuffed Sweet Peppers

Cashews are changing the world! Cashews, the tropical nut that provides ample protein, minerals, and healthy fats, is being used extensively as the base for vegan cheese. Soon, no cheese will remain unconquered by plant-based chefs, as pretty much every cheese can now be veganized. Enjoy this quick version as a creamy and cheesy filling in the colorful and crunchy petite sweet peppers or other veggies, such as celery sticks, cherry tomatoes, or cucumber slices. Please also remember to enjoy the cashew cheese whenever a non-dairy-based cheese is called for, such as a topping for El Tortilla Pizza (page 224) or instead of the store-bought vegan cream cheese in Cheezy Artichoke Dip (page 205).

TOTAL YIELD: 8 OUNCES CHEESE; 8 PEPPERS

> Serving Size: 2 ounces cheese; 2 peppers
> Number of Servings: 4
> Prep Time: 5 minutes
> Soak Time: 20 minutes
> Total Time: 25 minutes

QUICK CASHEW CHEESE
1 cup raw cashew pieces
½ cup water
3 tablespoons freshly squeezed lemon juice
2 tablespoons nutritional yeast
½ teaspoon sea salt, or to taste
½ teaspoon minced fresh rosemary
1 teaspoon onion flakes
1 clove garlic, pressed or minced

½ cup Quick Cashew Cheese
8 small (petite) sweet peppers
1 tablespoon finely chopped fresh flat-leaf parsley

1. Prepare the cashew cheese: Soak the cashews in a bowl of water with ample room to cover. Allow to sit for 20 minutes up to a few hours. Rinse and drain well. Transfer to a blender with the remaining cheese ingredients, including the ½ cup of fresh water, and blend until creamy.
2. Slice the peppers in half lengthwise. Fill with a dollop of cashew cheese. Leftover cheese can last for a few days in a glass jar in the fridge.
3. Garnish with the parsley before serving.

VARIATIONS
- Add 1 teaspoon of miso along with the rosemary.
- Add 1 cup of seeded and chopped red bell pepper to the cheese.
- Add 1 tablespoon of a Global Spice Blend, such as Cajun, Moroccan, Indian, or Italian (pages 249–252), to the cheese before blending.
- You can grill the peppers before using in this recipe (see page 105).

Smoky Truffled Baked Broccoli Fries

Not so fast with tossing those leftover broccoli stalks! They can actually be transformed into a gorgeous appetizer. For years we have been trimming the stalks and mixing them in with our stir-fries. It wasn't until we cut them into a French fry shape that we realized this hidden treasure. And then discovered that they have the same nutritional benefits as the florets; even slightly more calcium, iron, and vitamin C. Save your stalks. (And use the florets in such recipes as Thai Red Coconut Curry [page 231] or Roasted Cauliflower and Broccoli [page 181].) Serve on its own or as a side for Sweet Potato Black Bean Sliders (page 228).

TOTAL YIELD: 12 FRIES
    Serving Size: 4 fries
    Number of Servings: 3
    Prep Time: 10 minutes
    Cook Time: 15 minutes
    Total Time: 25 minutes

1 tablespoon olive oil, or ¼ cup water
⅛ teaspoon sea salt, or to taste
Pinch of ground black pepper
⅛ teaspoon smoked paprika
    or chipotle powder
3 medium-size broccoli stalks,
    peeled and cut into 12 strips
    about ¼ by 4 inches each
1 teaspoon freshly squeezed lemon juice
⅛ teaspoon truffle oil
1 tablespoon nutritional yeast

1. Preheat the oven to 375°F. Place the olive oil, salt, pepper, and paprika on a small baking sheet and mix well. Add the broccoli strips and coat well.
2. Bake for 15 minutes, or until just tender.
3. Drizzle with the lemon juice and truffle oil and top with the nutritional yeast before serving.

VARIATION

- Replace the broccoli stalks with carrots or . . . dare we say . . . potatoes.

Roasted Cauliflower and Broccoli

Cruciferous is king! Take full advantage of the benefits of these superfood cousins with this simple yet flavorful roasted dish. The phytochemicals in this category of veggies are well known in both cancer prevention and in boosting liver detoxification pathways. Top with chopped hazelnuts and serve with Roasted Butternut Squash Penne with Sage (page 242) or Quinoa Quiche (page 235) and a large side salad.

TOTAL YIELD: 16 OUNCES
Serving Size: 8 ounces
Number of Servings: 2
Prep Time: 10 minutes
Cook Time: 30 minutes
Total Time: 40 minutes

2 cups broccoli florets
2 cups cauliflower florets
1 cup diagonally cut carrot
½ cup water or vegetable stock (for homemade, see page 248)
1 tablespoon olive oil (optional), plus more for pan
¼ teaspoon sea salt, or to taste
¼ teaspoon ground black pepper
Pinch of crushed red pepper flakes (optional)
2 tablespoons freshly squeezed lemon juice
2 tablespoons chiffonaded fresh basil
1 tablespoon nutritional yeast
½ teaspoon balsamic vinegar

1. Preheat the oven to 425°F. Place the broccoli, cauliflower, carrot, water, oil, if using, salt, black pepper, and crushed red pepper flakes, if using, in a large bowl and toss well.
2. Transfer to a lightly oiled baking sheet. Cook for 25 minutes, stirring once or twice to ensure even cooking.
3. Change the oven temperature to HIGH broil and cook for 5 minutes. Add the lemon juice, basil, nutritional yeast, and balsamic vinegar, and mix well before serving.

VARIATIONS

- Replace the veggies with others of your choosing and roast until just tender.

- Toss the roasted veggies in Simple Balsamic Dressing (page 168), Zesty Lemon Sriracha Dressing (page 171), or Oil-Free Roasted Red Pepper Dressing (page 170) before serving.

- Add 1 tablespoon of Global Spice Blend, such as Italian, Mexican, or Indian (pages 249–252) before serving.

Smoky Roasted Beets

According to the venerable Tom Robbins, author of *Jitterbug Perfume* (a reliable nutritional resource if there ever was one), beets contain one of the secrets to immortality. He may be on to something as beets contain a variety of nutrients that may help prevent heart disease and certain types of cancer. Beets are known to purify the blood, and also aid in forestalling macular degeneration, improve circulation, prevent cataracts, and mediate respiratory problems. Serve as an elegant appetizer or part of a tapas feast with a dollop of vegan cheese (for homemade, see page 179) between each slice of beet.

TOTAL YIELD: 2 BEETS, 10 SLICES
    Serving Size: 5 slices
    Number of Servings: 2
    Prep Time: 5 minutes
    Cook Time: 45 minutes
    Total Time: 50 minutes

2 large red beets
Drizzle of olive oil
¼ teaspoon sea salt, or to taste
¼ teaspoon ground black pepper (try smoked)
Juice of 1 lemon
½ teaspoon smoked paprika
Parsley sprigs

1. Preheat the oven to 400°F. Cut off the very bottom of the beets so they can lie flat. Clean the beets well and place on a parchment paper–lined baking sheet. Drizzle with the olive oil and top with the salt and pepper.
2. Roast until a knife can easily pass through a beet, 45 to 50 minutes depending on the size of the beet.
3. Carefully peel off the skin. Slice into ¼-inch slices. Drizzle with the lemon juice and top with the smoked paprika. Garnish with parsley sprigs before serving.

VARIATIONS

- Replace the red beets with gold beets, Chiogga beets, turnips, rutabagas, even carrots or parsnips, and roast until just tender.

- Drizzle with Zesty Lemon Sriracha Dressing (page 171), Oil-Free Roasted Red Pepper Dressing (page 170), or Simple Balsamic Dressing (page 168).

Coco Jackfruit Nuggets

Hard hat warning! Beware of walking under a jackfruit tree, as the whole fruit, hanging from a small stem, can weigh as much as 80 pounds! Jackfruit is a rising star in the culinary world. The seeds are a wonderful source of protein and the flesh of the young fruit can be used to create a vegan "pulled pork." Or used to replace chicken in your nuggets . . . providing minerals, fiber, and sustained energy, without any cholesterol or saturated fat. (PS: The ripe flesh is awesome in smoothies!) Serve these nuggets with Apricot BBQ Sauce (page 269) or Smoky Sweet Chili Garlic Sauce (page 263).

TOTAL YIELD: ABOUT 15 NUGGETS
Serving Size: 5 nuggets
Number of Servings: 3
Prep Time: 10 minutes
Cook Time: 20 minutes
Total Time: 30 minutes

1 (14-ounce can) (1½ cups) young jackfruit, drained well (7.9 ounces dry weight)
1 tablespoon olive oil (optional)

JACKFRUIT NUGGET COATING
¼ cup nutritional yeast
3 tablespoons shredded unsweetened coconut
½ teaspoon onion flakes
½ teaspoon garlic flakes
¼ teaspoon sea salt, or to taste
⅛ teaspoon crushed red pepper flakes
⅛ teaspoon ground black pepper

1. Preheat the oven to 375°F. Place the jackfruit and olive oil, if using, in a bowl and toss well.
2. Prepare the coating: Place the coating ingredients in a small bowl and mix well.
3. Place the jackfruit, one piece at a time, in the bowl of coating. Cover each piece completely with the coating and place on a well-oiled or parchment paper–lined baking sheet.
4. Bake for 10 minutes. Flip with tongs. Bake for an additional 5 to 10 minutes, or until the coating is golden brown. Serve warm.

VARIATIONS

⚘ Replace the jackfruit with artichoke hearts or 1-inch cubes of tofu.

⚘ Add ¼ cup of bread crumbs to the coating.

⚘ Add 1 teaspoon of a Global Spice Blend, such as Italian, Ethiopian, or Cajun (pages 249–252).

Magical Mushroom Medley

One bite and you will know that you are in for an amazing culinary journey with the superfood of superfoods. The fungi kingdom has so much to offer, including unique compounds found in all 'shrooms that can inhibit the growth of cancer cells, regulate blood pressure, improve immune response, reduce oxidative stress, help the liver work better, and more. Garnish with a pinch of smoked paprika, and serve as a side with Savory Baked Seitan (page 225), Brazenly Braised Tempeh (page 219), or as part of an English breakfast (see page 126).

TOTAL YIELD: 10 OUNCES

Serving Size: 5 ounces
Number of Servings: 2
Prep Time: 5 minutes
Cook Time: 15 minutes
Total Time: 20 minutes

1 teaspoon olive oil, or 3 tablespoons water
¼ cup diced shallot
3 to 4 cloves garlic, pressed or minced
2¾ cups halved or quartered cremini mushrooms
½ teaspoon sea salt, or to taste
Pinch of ground black pepper
⅛ teaspoon ground nutmeg
¼ cup seeded and diced red bell pepper
1 teaspoon minced fresh dill, plus a few sprigs for garnish
¼ teaspoon wheat-free tamari or other soy sauce, or to taste (optional), or additional salt

1. Place a medium-size sauté pan over medium-high heat. Heat the oil. Add the shallot and cook for 1 minute. Add the garlic and cook for 1 minute, stirring constantly and adding small amounts of water or vegetable stock if necessary to prevent sticking. Add the mushrooms, salt, black pepper, and nutmeg and cook for 5 minutes, stirring frequently.

2. Add the bell pepper and cook for 5 minutes, stirring frequently. Add the dill and tamari, if using, and stir well. Garnish with dill sprigs before serving.

VARIATIONS

- Add 1 tablespoon of mirin along with the dill, or to taste.

- Add crushed red pepper flakes or cayenne pepper to taste.

- Add a drizzle of truffle oil before serving.

- Replace the dill with 1 tablespoon of minced fresh cilantro or flat-leaf parsley.

- Add 2 teaspoons of a Global Spice Blend, such as Italian, Moroccan, or Ethiopian (pages 249–252).

Braised Kale with Shallots and Slivered Almonds

Get your greens on! This glorious and nutritious dish is a wonderful way to balance some of the heavier foods you may occasionally indulge in, especially during the holiday season. Give yourself a yummy boost of energy and nutrition, courtesy of the superfood kale. Serve with Brazenly Braised Tempeh (page 219), Mushroom Leek Gravy (page 276), and Quintessential Quinoa Pilaf (page 186).

TOTAL YIELD: 12 OUNCES
Serving Size: 6 ounces
Number of Servings: 2
Prep Time: 10 minutes
Cook Time: 15 minutes
Total Time: 25 minutes

1 tablespoon olive oil, or 3 tablespoons water
¼ cup diced shallot
4 to 5 cloves garlic, pressed or minced
1 large bunch kale, chopped into ½-inch pieces (about 6 cups)
¼ cup vegetable stock (for homemade, see page 248) or water, plus more if needed
1 tablespoon freshly squeezed lemon juice
1 teaspoon soy sauce or wheat-free tamari or other soy sauce
1½ teaspoons mirin (optional)
¼ teaspoon crushed red pepper flakes (optional)
¼ cup slivered almonds, optionally toasted in a 350°F oven for 10 minutes

1. Place a large sauté pan over medium-high heat. Heat the oil. Add the shallots and cook for 3 minutes, stirring frequently. Add the garlic and cook for 2 minutes, stirring frequently and adding small amounts of water or vegetable stock if necessary to prevent sticking.
2. Add the kale and cook for 5 minutes, or until all the kale is just tender and still a vibrant green, using tongs to stir and evenly cook.
3. Add the vegetable stock, lower the heat to low, and cook for 3 minutes, stirring frequently with the tongs. If you have a cover for the sauté pan, feel free to use it.
4. Add the lemon juice, soy sauce, mirin, if using, and red pepper flakes, if using, and stir well. Place on a serving platter and top with the almonds before serving.

VARIATIONS

- Replace the kale with other dark leafy greens, such as collards or chard.
- You can sauté the almonds in coconut oil or vegan butter until just toasted, instead of toasting in the oven.
- Replace the almonds with hazelnuts or pecans.
- Add 1 tablespoon of peeled and minced fresh ginger along with or instead of the garlic.

Quintessential Quinoa Pilaf

From the Andes with love, protein-rich quinoa forms the base of this versatile pilaf. Cranberries add vibrancy and tang as well as loads of antioxidant and anti-inflammatory benefits. Serve with Black-Eye Cabbage (page 212) or Himalayan Lentils and Greens (page 214) and as part of your Monk Bowls (see page 209).

TOTAL YIELD: 32 OUNCES
>   Serving Size: 8 ounces
>   Number of Servings: 4
>   Prep Time: 10 minutes
>   Cook Time: 15 minutes
>   Total Time: 25 minutes

1¾ cups water or vegetable stock
   (for homemade, see page 248)
1 cup uncooked quinoa
½ teaspoon sea salt, or to taste
¼ cup dried cranberries
¼ cup slivered almonds
2 tablespoons finely chopped fresh
   flat-leaf parsley
¼ cup thinly sliced green onion
Ground black pepper
Pinch of crushed red pepper flakes

1. Place the water, quinoa, and salt in a 2-quart pot over high heat. Bring to a boil. Cover, lower the heat to low, and cook until all the liquid is absorbed, about 15 minutes. Turn off the heat, keep covered, and allow to sit for 5 minutes. Fluff with a fork.
2. Transfer to a bowl along with the remaining ingredients and mix well. Serve warm or cold.

VARIATIONS

- Add 2 tablespoons of chopped kalamata olives or olive of your choice and 1 cup of frozen peas and carrots.

- Add 1 cup of chopped grilled or roasted veggies (see pages 105 and 178).

- Replace the quinoa with rice, millet, or buckwheat (see pages 100–101).

- Replace the parsley with fresh cilantro or basil and add 2 teaspoons of Indian Spice Mix (page 251), Italian Spice Mix (page 251), or Mexican Spice Mix (page 252).

- Replace the almonds with walnuts, pistachio nuts, or pumpkin seeds and replace the cranberries with currants or chopped dried apricots.

- Add 1 cup of rinsed and drained cooked chickpeas, kidney beans, or French lentils.

Baked Cajun Veggie Fritters

All of the bayou is talkin' about these plant-based fritters. Garbanzo (chickpea) flour is a wonderful whole food gluten-free option for creating a perfect fritter texture, plus it adds protein, fiber, and iron to the already dense nutrition of your favorite veggies. Serve with Sriracha Aioli (page 275) before enjoying your Black-Eye Cabbage (page 212) and BBQ Jackfruit (page 217).

TOTAL YIELD: 16 OUNCES/12 FRITTERS
  Serving Size: 3 fritters
  Number of Servings: 4
  Prep Time: 10 minutes
  Cook Time: 35 minutes
  Total Time: 45 minutes

½ cup water
1 tablespoon chia seeds
1 cup grated zucchini
½ cup garbanzo flour
½ cup peeled and grated potato
½ cup minced yellow onion
2 to 3 cloves garlic, pressed or minced (optional)
¼ cup grated carrots
1 tablespoon Cajun Spice Mix (page 249, or store-bought)
1 teaspoon sea salt, or to taste
⅛ teaspoon ground black pepper
Pinch of cayenne pepper (optional)

1. Preheat the oven to 400°F. Combine the water and chia seeds in a small bowl and stir well. Allow to sit for 10 minutes, or until a gel forms, stirring once or twice to make sure all the seeds are submerged in water.
2. Meanwhile, place all the remaining ingredients in a bowl and mix well. Add the chia seed mixture and mix well. Allow to sit for 10 minutes.
3. Form into twelve patties, about ⅛ cup each, and place on a well-oiled or parchment paper–lined baking sheet. Bake for 18 minutes, then flip and cook for an additional 18 minutes. Serve warm.

VARIATIONS

↝ Add ½ teaspoon of wheat-free tamari or other soy sauce.

↝ Add 2 tablespoons of minced fresh parsley or cilantro, or 2 teaspoons of minced fresh dill.

↝ Add 1 tablespoon of coconut flakes.

↝ Replace the chia seeds and water with an equal amount of aquafaba (see page 272).

Cumin Chickpeas

One of the earliest cultivated legumes, chickpeas have been gracing our tables for over 7,500 years. Talk about longevity! Chickpeas are an excellent source of molybdenum and manganese, both important in energy production, tissue healing, and bone strength. They also provide folate, copper, healthy fiber, phosphorus, protein, iron, and zinc, and are really just fun to eat. This is a beyond simple way to add the protein component to your Monk Bowls (see page 209) or Marvelous Macro Meal (page 226). Enjoy with Quintessential Quinoa Pilaf (page 186) or Pilau Rice (page 198), and a veggie dish, such as Braised Kale with Shallots and Slivered Almonds (page 185) or Roasted Cauliflower and Broccoli (page 181).

TOTAL YIELD: 12 OUNCES
>Serving Size: 6 ounces
>Number of Servings: 2
>Prep Time: 5 minutes
>Cook Time: 10 minutes
>Total Time: 15 minutes

1 (15-ounce) can chickpeas, drained, or 1½ cups cooked chickpeas (see page 102) plus a small amount of water
3 to 4 cloves garlic, pressed or minced
¼ cup diced yellow onion (optional)
¾ teaspoon ground cumin, optionally toasted (see page 106)
2 tablespoons freshly squeezed lemon juice
1 tablespoon minced fresh cilantro
Sea salt and ground black pepper
Pinch of chipotle powder, cayenne pepper, or crushed red pepper flakes (optional)

1. Place the chickpeas in a small pot over medium heat. Add the garlic, onion, if using, and cumin and cook for 10 minutes, stirring occasionally and lowering the heat to low, if necessary, to prevent boiling over.
2. Add the lemon juice, cilantro, and seasonings to taste. Mix well before serving.

VARIATIONS

Replace the garlic with peeled and minced fresh ginger.

Since you are a master of the Template Recipe by now, you probably realize you can replace the chickpeas with other beans, such as kidney, navy, cannellini, pinto, fava, or black beans. Or replace them with pulses, such as green or black lentils.

Replace the cumin with 1 tablespoon of a Global Spice Blend. such as Mexican, Italian, Cajun, Moroccan, or Indian (pages 249–252).

Replace the cilantro with fresh basil or parsley, or 2 teaspoons of minced fresh dill.

Rosemary Polenta Croutons

Calling all gluten-free eaters: behold your crouton! It uses polenta, a corn-based grain used extensively in northern Italian cuisine, which retains all the benefits of low-calorie whole corn, such as trace B vitamins, beta-carotene, protein, and iron, after it is ground into meal. (The stone-ground process keeps more of the grain intact, so the most nutrients are retained.)

Serve as a tapas dish with a dollop of Pepita Pesto with Avocado (page 265) or on top of Arugula Walnut Salad with Cashew Dill Dressing (page 161) or Raw Fettuccine Alfreda (page 163).

TOTAL YIELD: 12 OUNCES
  Serving Size: 3 ounces
  Number of Servings: 4
  Prep Time: 5 minutes
  Cook Time: 25 minutes
  Total Time: 30 minutes plus 20 minutes for
    cooling time if served cold

1¾ cups water, vegetable stock (for
  homemade, see page 248), or
  unsweetened soy or almond milk
½ cup polenta
½ teaspoon sea salt, or to taste
⅛ teaspoon ground black pepper
¾ teaspoon minced fresh rosemary
½ teaspoon dried oregano
⅛ teaspoon crushed red pepper flakes
2 tablespoons nutritional yeast

1. Place the water in a medium-size pot over high heat. Bring to a boil. Lower the heat to low. Add the polenta, salt, pepper, rosemary, oregano, and red pepper flakes and cook for 10 minutes, stirring constantly. Cover and cook for 20 minutes, or until the polenta is completely cooked through, stirring occasionally. Add the nutritional yeast and mix well.

2. Transfer to a well-oiled small baking sheet (about 5 by 8 inches, the kind that fits into a toaster oven) so that the polenta is about ¾ inch high. Allow to cool until firm enough to cut, either at room temperature or by placing in the refrigerator.

3. Cut into ¾-inch cubes and gently separate the cubes on the pan so they are not sticking together.

4. Heat the oven to HIGH broil. Place the pan in the oven and bake until the cubes are just crispy on the outside, about 5 minutes. Enjoy warm or cold.

VARIATIONS

⌇ Looking for an hors d'oeuvres dish? Break out the cookie cutter or cut the polenta into larger rectangles and serve with a dollop of Pepita Pesto with Avocado (page 265) or Chimichurri Topping (page 201).

⌇ Add 1 tablespoon of olive oil along with the polenta.

⌇ Add ¼ cup of shredded vegan mozzarella-style cheese along with the nutritional yeast.

⌇ Add 2 teaspoons of Italian Spice Mix (page 251) along with the polenta.

⌇ For Mexican flair, replace the rosemary and oregano with 1½ teaspoons of chili powder, ⅛ teaspoon of chipotle powder, and 1 tablespoon of minced fresh cilantro.

Sweet Chili Brussels Sprouts

Your grandmother always told you to eat your Brussels sprouts, but she would be amazed to know they can taste so good. Brussels are a member of the cruciferous veggie group, and an excellent source of vitamins C and K as well as vitamins B_1, B_6, and B_9 (folate), manganese, choline, copper, potassium, phosphorus, dietary fiber, and omega-3 fatty acids. Short on time? You can omit the chili sauce for cilantro lime Brussels sprouts that would still make your grandma proud. Serve as a tapas-style appetizer or as a side dish along with Pecan Sage Holiday Loaf (page 244), Garlicky Whipped Parsnips (page 192), and Mushroom Leek Gravy (page 276).

TOTAL YIELD: 24 OUNCES
    Serving Size: 6 ounces
    Number of Servings: 4
    Prep Time: 5 minutes
    Cook Time: 25 minutes
    Total Time: 30 minutes

4 cups bottom-trimmed and halved Brussels sprouts
1 tablespoon olive oil (optional), plus more for pan
½ cup water or vegetable stock (for homemade, see page 248)
½ teaspoon sea salt, or to taste
⅛ teaspoon ground black pepper
¼ teaspoon chipotle powder (optional)
¼ to ½ cup Smoky Sweet Chili Garlic Sauce (page 263, or store-bought sweet chili sauce)
1 tablespoon freshly squeezed lime juice
1½ tablespoons finely chopped fresh cilantro

1. Preheat the oven to 425°F. Place the Brussels sprouts, oil, if using, water, salt, pepper, and chipotle powder, if using, in a bowl and toss well. Transfer to a lightly oiled baking sheet and bake for 15 minutes.
2. Remove from the oven, add the chili sauce and lime juice, and stir well. Return the pan to the oven and bake until the Brussels sprouts are just tender, about 10 minutes.
3. Add the cilantro and stir well before serving.

VARIATIONS

- Replace the Brussels sprouts with cauliflower or broccoli florets.
- Replace the sweet chili sauce with Apricot BBQ Sauce (page 269), and serve along with Mac n Cheez (page 230).

Sweet and Spicy Plantains

The powerhouse cousin of the banana, plantains are a true superfood and survival food for their high vitamin, mineral, and fiber content as well as strong tissue-healing properties. Make sure your plantains' peel is black in color, with some speckles of yellow. The riper they are, the sweeter they are, and the happier you will be with this recipe. Serve with a drizzle of pure maple syrup or a jerk sauce as a start to a meal that may include Thai Red Coconut Curry (page 231) and Mango Rice Pudding with Salted Caramel (page 293).

TOTAL YIELD: 16 OUNCES
Serving Size: 4 ounces
Number of Servings: 4
Prep Time: 10 minutes
Cook Time: 30 minutes
Total Time: 40 minutes

½ cup coconut, soy, or almond milk
1 tablespoon freshly squeezed lime juice
1 tablespoon minced fresh cilantro
¼ teaspoon chipotle powder
⅛ teaspoon ground allspice
⅛ teaspoon ground cinnamon
Pinch of sea salt
2 ripe plantains, diagonally sliced ½ inch thick (2½ cups)
Oil for pan (optional)

1. Preheat the oven to 400°F. Place the coconut milk, lime juice, cilantro, chipotle powder, allspice, cinnamon, and salt in a bowl and mix well. Add the plantains and mix well.
2. Transfer the plantains to a parchment paper–lined or well-oiled baking sheet, reserving the excess liquid. Bake for 20 minutes.
3. Flip the plantains and coat them with the excess liquid. Bake for more 10 minutes. The plantains should be nice and tender.

VARIATIONS

- No luck finding plantains? Try with just ripe, not-too-soft bananas.
- Instead of baking, you can sauté the plantains in oil until golden brown and tender.

Garlicky Whipped Parsnips

Worshipped by garlic lovers, reviled by vampires, this creamy and garlicky dish features parsnips, a sweet carrotlike tuber with a ton of immunity-boosting micronutrients and lots of heart-healthy, blood sugar-balancing fiber. Top with Mushroom Leek Gravy (page 276) and serve along with Black Gomasio Crusted Tofu (page 215), Brazenly Braised Tempeh (page 219), or Pecan Sage Holiday Loaf (page 244).

TOTAL YIELD: 16 OUNCES
Serving Size: 8 ounces
Number of Servings: 2
Prep Time: 10 minutes
Cook Time: 15 minutes
Total Time: 25 minutes

3 cups peeled and chopped parsnips
   (½-inch pieces)
2 tablespoons olive oil, or ¼ cup water
1 tablespoon minced garlic
½ cup unsweetened soy, almond,
   or coconut milk
¼ teaspoon sea salt, or to taste
⅛ teaspoon ground black pepper
Pinch of cayenne pepper (optional)
¼ teaspoon paprika or smoked paprika
1 tablespoon finely chopped fresh chives
1 tablespoon thinly sliced green onion

1. Place a steamer basket in a medium-size pot and fill with water until it reaches the bottom of the steamer basket. Cover, place over high heat, and bring to a boil.
2. Lower the heat to medium. Add the parsnips to the steamer basket, cover, and steam until very tender, about 15 minutes. Transfer the parsnips to a mixing bowl.
3. Meanwhile, place a small sauté pan over low heat. Heat the oil and add the garlic, and cook until the garlic is golden brown, about 5 minutes, stirring frequently and being careful not to burn. Add to the cooked parsnips. Add the soy milk, salt, black pepper, and cayenne, if using, and whisk until creamy. (Alternatively, you can transfer the mixture to a stand mixer and whisk with the whisk attachment.) Garnish with the paprika, chives, and green onion before serving.

VARIATIONS

- Replace the parsnips with peeled potatoes.
- Replace half of the parsnips with cauliflower florets.
- Add 1 teaspoon of minced fresh dill or 1 tablespoon of minced fresh cilantro or parsley.
- Add ½ teaspoon of minced fresh rosemary, 1 teaspoon of fresh oregano, and 2 teaspoons of fresh marjoram.
- Add 1 tablespoon of a Global Spice Blend, such as Ethiopian, Cajun, or Mexican (pages 249–252).

Baked Sesame Zucchini Fries

Move over, French fries! These black and white fries are crispy on the outside and creamy on the inside. Pure deliciousness in every bite. Sesame seeds are little power-packed gems that add protein and essential minerals to a dish, the black containing more fiber and a slightly different mineral profile with both copper and zinc. Zucchini is a known cleansing food, light on digestion, and with manganese and vitamin C that offer both protection and healing to the body. Serve as an appetizer with Smoky Sweet Chili Garlic Sauce (page 263) or a store-bought sweet-and-sour sauce. You can also serve as a side dish to Sweet Potato Black Bean Sliders (page 228) or Black Rice Sushi with Wasabi Mayo (page 222).

TOTAL YIELD: 24 STICKS
  Serving Size: 6 sticks
  Number of Servings: 4
  Prep Time: 20 minutes
  Cook Time: 15 minutes
  Total Time: 35 minutes

⅓ cup flour, such as a gluten-free flour blend (for homemade, see page 254), spelt, whole wheat pastry, or unbleached all-purpose

1½ large zucchini, peeled, cut in half, sliced lengthwise, and then sliced into 1 by 1 by 6-inch strips

Oil for pan (optional)

DIPPING INGREDIENTS

1 cup almond, soy, or coconut milk

1½ teaspoons toasted sesame oil (optional)

¼ teaspoon Chinese five-spice powder

COATING

¼ cup plus 2 tablespoons bread crumbs (try panko or gluten-free)

¼ cup white sesame seeds

2 tablespoons black sesame seeds

¼ teaspoon sea salt

¼ teaspoon Chinese five-spice powder

1. Preheat the oven to 400°F. Place the flour on a small plate. Place the dipping ingredients in a bowl and whisk well. Place the coating ingredients in another bowl and mix well.
2. To form sticks, place zucchini strips in the flour and coat well. Using one hand, place the zucchini in the dipping liquid and transfer to the bowl of coating. Using your other hand, coat the zucchini strips well and place on a well-oiled or parchment paper–lined baking sheet.
3. Bake for 10 minutes, flip, and cook for another 5 minutes, or until slightly golden and crispy.

VARIATIONS

- Replace the zucchini with eggplant or parsnip.
- Add 1 tablespoon of shredded coconut to the coating.
- Replace the sesame seeds with finely chopped nuts or seeds, such as pecans, walnuts, pistachios, or macadamia nuts.

Garlicky Hummus

A wise vegan sage once said, "When all else fails, turn to hummus." Enjoyed for millennia in the Middle East, the core ingredients of hummus—chickpeas and tahini—are chock-full of protein, iron, calcium, magnesium, zinc, and B vitamins, including folate. It certainly earns its status as a go-to source for strength and endurance. This is a garlicky twist to the ultimate vegan survival food. Serve with crudités and chips for a protein-rich snack, or as the spread of choice for the Hummus Panini with Balsamic Massaged Kale (page 239)

TOTAL YIELD: 16 OUNCES

> Serving Size: 4 ounces
> Number of Servings: 4
> Prep Time: 15 minutes
> Cook Time: 10 minutes
> Total Time: 25 minutes

3 tablespoons olive oil, or ¼ cup water
1½ tablespoons minced garlic
1 (15-ounce) can chickpeas, drained and rinsed, or 1½ cups cooked (see page 102)
¼ cup tahini
¼ cup water
¼ cup freshly squeezed lemon juice
¾ teaspoon sea salt, or to taste
½ teaspoon ground cumin
¼ teaspoon chipotle powder
⅛ teaspoon ground black pepper

1. Heat the olive oil in a small pot over low heat. Add the garlic and cook until just golden brown in color, being careful not to burn, about 7 minutes, stirring frequently.
2. Transfer to a food processor with the remaining ingredients and process until smooth.

VARIATIONS

🌿 You can omit the cooked garlic and add 2 teaspoons of raw minced or pressed garlic.

🌿 Add 1 teaspoon of minced fresh rosemary and 2 tablespoons of minced kalamata olives.

🌿 Add 1 tablespoon of a Global Spice Blend, such as Moroccan or Ethiopian (pages 249–252).

🌿 Add 2 tablespoons of minced fresh cilantro and 1 tablespoon of Mexican Spice Mix (page 252) or Indian Spice Mix (page 251).

🌿 Reserve the liquid from the can of chickpeas (aquafaba) (see page 272). Use in this recipe if extra liquid is needed to reach desired consistency, or use in Vegan Fluff (page 283) or Aqua Mayo (page 272).

Stacked Avocados

All the flavor and nothing but nutrition in this energy-balancing whole food snack. For a superstacked avocado, add a dollop of Vegan Sour Cream (page 274) and salsa. Serve as an appetizer or snack with chips and a couple of lime wedges and prepare to be wowed!

TOTAL YIELD: 4 HALVES AVOCADO, 16 OUNCES FILLING

Serving Size: ½ avocado, 4 ounces filling
Number of Servings: 4
Prep Time: 15 minutes
Total Time: 15 minutes

2 medium to large avocados
½ cup cooked black beans (see page 102)
**½ cup fresh or frozen corn
    (try fire-roasted)**
3 tablespoons minced red onion
1 tablespoon finely chopped fresh cilantro
1½ tablespoons freshly squeezed lime juice
¼ teaspoon chipotle powder
¼ teaspoon sea salt, or to taste
**¼ teaspoon ground black pepper, or to
    taste**

1. Slice the avocados in half lengthwise and remove the pit. Carefully score the avocado, to form ½-inch cubes, and scoop out with a spoon (you should have 1½ cups of avocado flesh). Save the skins.
2. Place the black beans, corn, red onion, cilantro, lime juice, chipotle powder, salt, and pepper in a bowl and mix well. Add the avocado and gently mix well. Mound the mixture in the avocado skins for the ultimate presentation.

VARIATIONS

- Add one minced garlic clove and 1 teaspoon of seeded and diced jalapeño pepper along with the red onion.

- Go Indian by adding 1½ teaspoons of curry powder and ½ teaspoon of ground cumin along with the red onion.

- Add 1 tablespoon olive oil along with the black beans.

Rainbow Roasted Roots

Roots go deep and can bring healing to your body and soul! Some of the original vegetarians were actually called "diggers" because of the value placed on root veggies, which bring us vital disease-fighting minerals and vitamins straight from the goodness of the earth. Enjoy with your Sweet Potato Black Bean Sliders (page 228), Pecan Sage Holiday Loaf (page 244), and Mushroom Leek Gravy (page 276).

TOTAL YIELD: 32 OUNCES
    Serving Size: 8 ounces
    Number of Servings: 4
    Prep Time: 15 minutes
    Cook Time: 45 minutes
    Total Time: 60 minutes

5 cups chopped colorful root vegetables (1-inch pieces) (try gold and red beet, carrot, parsnip, rutabaga, purple and/or garnet sweet potato)

¾ cup thickly sliced onion

3 to 5 whole garlic cloves, or 2 to 3 cloves, pressed or minced

1½ tablespoons olive oil, or ¼ cup vegetable stock (for homemade, see page 248) or water

½ cup water or vegetable stock

½ teaspoon sea salt, or to taste (try smoked)

⅛ teaspoon ground black pepper

½ teaspoon minced fresh rosemary

Pinch of crushed red pepper flakes (optional)

1 tablespoon chopped fresh sage

1. Preheat the oven to 400°F. Place all the ingredients, except the sage, in a bowl and mix well. Transfer to a baking sheet and roast until the firmest veggie is just tender, about 45 minutes depending on the vegetables. Check after 30 minutes for tenderness in case the veggies are ready by then.
2. Add the sage and mix well before serving.

VARIATIONS

- Replace the sage with fresh dill or 2 tablespoons of finely chopped fresh parsley, cilantro, or basil.

- Add 1 tablespoon of Italian Spice Mix (page 251), Mexican Spice Mix (page 252), or Moroccan Spice Mix (page 252) along with the veggies.

- Toss with salad dressings, such as Zesty Lemon Sriracha (page 171) or Simple Balsamic Dressing (page 168), after roasting.

- Change the size of the veggies and cook until just tender. The smaller the chop, the quicker the cook time.

Coco Cauliflower

Word on the street is that cauliflower is the new kale. We'd believe it, considering its huge nutrient profile, which can improve health in just one serving! Its mild flavor and texture are perfect with the aromatic Eastern spice flavors and sweet coconut. Try this simple and rich dish and decide for yourself. Serve with BBQ Jackfruit (page 217) and Pilau Rice (page 198).

TOTAL YIELD: 16 OUNCES
   Serving Size: 8 ounces
   Number of Servings: 2
   Prep Time: 10 minutes
   Cook Time: 25 minutes
   Total Time: 35 minutes

4 cups cauliflower florets
2 tablespoons water
1½ tablespoons olive oil
½ teaspoon sea salt, or to taste
⅛ teaspoon ground black pepper
Pinch of cayenne pepper
½ cup coconut milk
1½ teaspoons curry powder
½ teaspoon cumin seeds
2 tablespoons finely chopped fresh cilantro

1. Preheat the oven to 400°F. Place the cauliflower, water, olive oil, salt, black pepper, and cayenne on a baking sheet and mix well. Roast the cauliflower until just tender, about 25 minutes, stirring once or twice to ensure even cooking. Transfer to a bowl.
2. Meanwhile, place the coconut milk, curry powder, and cumin seeds in a small bowl and whisk well. Add to the cooked cauliflower and mix well. Garnish with the cilantro before serving.

VARIATIONS

- Replace the coconut milk with soy milk, rice milk, or Pumpkin Seed Milk (page 116).

- Add 2 teaspoons of store-bought red or green curry paste to spice it up!

- For a taste of Mexico, replace the curry powder with chili powder.

Pilau Rice

Billed as the official rice pilaf of the Taj Mahal, pilau rice can take many forms. Green peas have many impressive benefits, such as protein, iron, fiber, and B vitamins; eating them is said to help protect against osteoporosis and limit neuronal damage in the brain that can cause such diseases as Alzheimer's. The herbs used here have a nourishing and healing effect on digestion and immunity.

Top with 1 teaspoon of Black Sesame Gomasio (page 253) and serve along with Himalayan Lentils and Greens (page 214) or Spinach Chickpeas (page 213). Finish with a glass of Cacao Turmeric Elixir (page 120).

TOTAL YIELD: 32 OUNCES

Serving Size: 8 ounces
Number of Servings: 4
Prep Time: 5 minutes
Cook Time: 25 minutes
Total Time: 30 minutes

1 teaspoon cumin seeds
½ teaspoon mustard seeds
1 cup uncooked white basmati rice
1½ cups water or vegetable stock (for homemade, see page 248)
1 teaspoon cardamom pods
½ teaspoon sea salt, or to taste
¼ teaspoon saffron threads (optional)
½ cup fresh or frozen garden or sweet peas
1 tablespoon finely chopped fresh cilantro

1. Place a dry 2-quart pot over high heat. Add the cumin and mustard seeds. Cook for 2 minutes, or until the seeds start popping, stirring constantly.
2. Add the rice, water, cardamom pods, salt, and saffron threads, if using, and bring to a boil.
3. Cover, lower the heat to low, and cook until all the liquid is absorbed, about 15 minutes. Turn off the heat, keep covered, and allow to sit for 5 minutes. Fluff with a fork.
4. Add the peas and cilantro and gently mix well before serving.

VARIATIONS

- Add 1 tablespoon of sesame oil or vegan butter, along with the rice.
- Add ½ teaspoon of ground turmeric along with the salt and pepper.
- Add one cinnamon stick and two bay leaves along with the rice; remove before serving.

Herb-Roasted Potatoes

Rosemary adds more to dishes than just its aromatic flavor. Its oil improves memory and concentration, and increases the anti-oxidant capacities of other plants. Serve as part of an epic brunch along with Tofu Rancheros (page 137) and Smashed Avocado Toast Supreme (page 127). End with a glass of Citrus Cleanse (page 117).

TOTAL YIELD: 20 OUNCES
Serving Size: 10 ounces
Number of Servings: 2
Prep Time: 5 minutes
Cook Time: 50 minutes
Total Time: 55 minutes

4 cups chopped potatoes (½-inch pieces) (try russet, Yukon gold, or your favorites)
1 to 1½ tablespoons olive oil, or ¼ cup water or vegetable stock (for homemade, see page 248)
2 tablespoons water or vegetable stock
½ teaspoon sea salt, or to taste
⅛ teaspoon ground black pepper (try smoked)
1¼ teaspoons minced fresh rosemary
¼ teaspoon smoked paprika

1. Preheat the oven to 400°F. Place the potatoes, olive oil, water, salt, and pepper on a baking sheet and toss well.
2. Roast for 30 minutes. Remove from the oven and stir well. Return the pan to the oven and roast for 15 to 20 minutes, or until golden brown and cooked through.
3. Add the rosemary and smoked paprika and toss well before serving.

VARIATIONS

- Add ½ teaspoon of wheat-free tamari or other soy sauce along with rosemary.
- Replace the rosemary with fresh dill.
- Add 2 tablespoons of nutritional yeast along with the rosemary.
- Drizzle with truffle oil before serving.
- Replace the potatoes with a mixture of chopped parsnips and carrots.

Curried Cauliflower Pakora

From Rishikesh with love, these crunchy nuggets, coated with protein-rich garbanzo flour, can transport you to the banks of the Ganges. A delicious way to receive plenty of vitamins B$_5$, B$_6$, B$_9$ (folate), C, K, and choline from one of the healthiest foods on earth. Serve with Smoky Sweet Chili Garlic Sauce (page 263) or Apricot BBQ Sauce (page 269).

TOTAL YIELD: ABOUT 16 PIECES

Serving Size: 4 pieces
Number of Servings: 4
Prep Time: 10 minutes
Cook Time: 40 minutes
Total Time: 50 minutes

1 cup garbanzo flour
2 teaspoons minced fresh cilantro
1½ teaspoons curry powder
1 teaspoon ground cumin
¼ teaspoon sea salt
⅛ teaspoon ground black pepper
Pinch of cayenne pepper (optional)
¾ cup unsweetened almond or soy milk
1 medium-size cauliflower, divided into small florets (about 16 florets)

1. Preheat the oven to 375°F. Combine the garbanzo flour, cilantro, curry powder, cumin, salt, black pepper, and cayenne, if using, in a bowl and mix well.
2. Pour the almond milk into a separate bowl.
3. Dip each cauliflower floret into the almond milk with one hand. Use your other hand to place the floret in the bowl in the flour mixture and coat well.
4. Place on a parchment paper–lined baking sheet. Bake for 20 minutes. Carefully flip and cook until golden brown and just tender, about 20 minutes, depending on the size of the florets. Serve warm.

VARIATIONS

- Replace the cauliflower with broccoli florets, chopped zucchini, or 1-inch cubes of tofu.

- For a taste of Mexico, replace the curry powder with chili powder and add ½ teaspoon of ground cumin and ⅛ teaspoon of chipotle powder.

- Replace the garbanzo flour with other flours, such as a gluten-free flour blend (for homemade, see page 254), whole wheat pastry, or unbleached all-purpose flour.

Chimichurri Grilled Cauliflower Steaks

Certified cow-free steaks that are guaranteed to satisfy the cowboy or cowgirl in your life, offering brain-boosting B vitamins and choline, plenty of heart-healthy fiber and antioxidants, and no destructive saturated fat or cholesterol. Nutritional powerhouse cauliflower is paired with a zesty herb chimichurri topping, which adds even more antioxidant vitalizing properties. Top with toasted pumpkin seeds or sunflower seeds and serve with Brazenly Braised Tempeh (page 219) or Herb-Roasted Tofu (page 220) and Quintessential Quinoa Pilaf (page 186). PS: Feel free to use the chimichurri topping over your steamed and grilled vegetables.

TOTAL YIELD: 1 CAULIFLOWER, 8 OUNCES TOPPING

> Serving Size: 1 slice
> Number of Servings: 4
> Prep Time: 15 minutes
> Cook Time: 15 minutes
> Total Time: 30 minutes

1 medium-size cauliflower, cut vertically into ½-inch slices (4 to 5 slices)
12 to 15 cherry tomatoes

BASTING SAUCE

2 tablespoons olive oil, or ¼ cup water
⅛ teaspoon sea salt
⅛ teaspoon ground black pepper

CHIMICHURRI TOPPING

2 tablespoons water
1½ tablespoons olive oil (optional)
½ teaspoon sea salt, or to taste

⅛ teaspoon ground black pepper
¼ cup finely chopped fresh parsley
2 tablespoons finely chopped fresh cilantro
3 tablespoons freshly squeezed lime juice
½ teaspoon chili powder
1 garlic clove, pressed or minced

1. Preheat a grill. Place the basting sauce ingredients in a small bowl and mix well. Place the cauliflower steak on the grill and, basting periodically with the basting sauce, using a pastry brush, grill for 5 minutes. Flip and grill for an additional 5 minutes, or until the cauliflower is just tender, depending on the heat of the grill.
2. Place the cherry tomatoes on a skewer and grill until just tender, flipping a few times to ensure even cooking, about 5 minutes, depending on the heat of the grill.
3. Meanwhile, place the chimichurri topping ingredients in a bowl and whisk well. Pour over the cauliflower steaks and top with the cherry tomatoes before serving.

VARIATIONS

- Add ½ teaspoon Italian Spice Mix (page 251) to the basting sauce.
- Add 1 tablespoon of nutritional yeast to the chimichurri topping.
- Not ready to break out the grill? You can roast the cauliflower instead. To do so, preheat the oven to 400°F. Place the cauliflower on a baking sheet. Top with the basting sauce and flip to ensure even coating. Cook until cauliflower is just tender, about 25 minutes, depending on the size of the slices.
- Replace the cauliflower with portobello mushroom, tofu, or tempeh cutlets. Grill until char marks appear on both sides and the food is thoroughly heated through.

Miso Ginger Glazed Eggplant

Sweet, savory, and succulent. What more can you ask for from a vegetable dish? Eggplant is a good source of fiber, B vitamins, and vitamin K, and is known for helping with weight loss and lowering cholesterol. Serve along with Black Rice Sushi with Wasabi Mayo (page 222) and Domo Arigato Arame Salad (page 159).

TOTAL YIELD: 24 OUNCES
    Serving Size: 6 ounces
    Number of Servings: 4
    Prep Time: 10 minutes
    Cook Time: 30 minutes
    Total Time: 40 minutes

3 to 4 small Chinese or purple eggplants, sliced into 1-inch slices (about 4 cups)
¼ cup water
1 tablespoon sesame oil, or 2 tablespoons additional water
¼ teaspoon sea salt, or to taste
⅛ teaspoon ground black pepper
Oil for pan (optional)
¼ cup thinly sliced green onion

MISO GLAZE

¼ cup water
1 tablespoon store-bought miso paste
1 tablespoon pure maple syrup (optional)
1 teaspoon wheat-free tamari or other soy sauce
1½ teaspoons rice vinegar
2 teaspoons peeled and minced fresh ginger

1. Preheat the oven to 400°F. Place the eggplant, ¼ cup of water, and the sesame oil, salt, and pepper in a bowl and toss well. Transfer to a well-oiled or nonstick baking sheet, place in the oven, and roast for 20 minutes. Flip or stir the eggplant and cook until soft, about 10 more minutes.

2. Meanwhile, prepare the glaze: Place the water and miso paste in a small pot over medium heat. Whisk well. Add the maple syrup, if using, and the tamari, rice vinegar, and ginger, and cook for 10 minutes, stirring occasionally and being careful not to boil.

3. To serve, drizzle the glaze over the eggplant and top with the green onion.

VARIATIONS

- Add 2 teaspoons of toasted sesame oil to the miso glaze.

- Add ¼ cup orange juice to the miso glaze.

- Replace the eggplant with 14 ounces of extra-firm tofu, cut into 1-inch cubes.

- For a thicker sauce, place 1 teaspoon of arrowroot powder in a small dish with 2 tablespoons of water and whisk well. Add to the pot at the end of step 2 and stir constantly until the glaze thickens, about 2 minutes. Lower the heat to low and drizzle over the eggplant.

Pineapple Fried Rice

Aloha, people! Pineapple, with its high vitamin C content and natural enzymes, brings a nutritive and sweet vibe to this dish, which is Hawaii's answer to leftover rice. If you have rice already cooked, use 3 cups for this recipe. Feel free to use pineapple juice for the liquid instead of blending fresh pineapple as the recipe suggests. Garnish with thinly sliced green onion and black and white sesame seeds. Serve with Sunny Kale Salad (page 162) and Brazenly Braised Tempeh (page 219) or Roasted Tofu with Almond Sauce (page 221).

TOTAL YIELD: 26 OUNCES
  Serving Size: 6.5 ounces
  Number of Servings: 4
  Prep Time: 10 minutes
  Cook Time: 60 minutes if rice is not cooked, 15
    if using leftover rice
  Total Time: 25 to 1 hour 10 minutes

1 cup uncooked long-grain brown rice

2¼ cups water or vegetable stock (for homemade, see page 248), divided

½ teaspoon sea salt, or to taste

1 cup cubed pineapple (¼-inch cubes), divided

½ teaspoon tamari (optional)

Pinch of crushed red pepper flakes (optional)

1 tablespoon toasted sesame oil, or ¼ cup water or vegetable stock

1 cup thinly sliced yellow onion

¾ cup frozen peas and carrots

¼ cup seeded and diced red bell pepper

1 tablespoon finely chopped fresh cilantro

1. Place the rice, 2 cups of the water, and the salt in a 2-quart pot over medium-high heat. Bring to a boil. Cover, lower the heat to low, and cook until all the liquid is absorbed, about 40 minutes.

2. Meanwhile, place ½ cup of the pineapple cubes in a blender along with the remaining ¼ cup of water, the tamari, if using, and the red pepper flakes, if using, and blend well. Set aside. (Alternatively, you can use ½ cup of pineapple juice instead of the cubes; simply add the tamari and red pepper flakes, if using, into the juice.)

3. Place a large sauté pan over medium-high heat. Heat the oil. Add the onion and cook for 3 minutes, stirring frequently.

4. When the rice is done cooking, add to sauté pan and cook for 5 minutes, stirring frequently. Add the pineapple mixture and cook for 3 minutes, or until all the liquid is absorbed, stirring frequently.

5. Lower the heat to medium, add the peas and carrots and bell pepper, and cook for 3 minutes, stirring frequently. Add the remaining ½ cup of chopped pineapple and cook for 5 minutes, stirring frequently. Add the cilantro and stir well before serving.

VARIATIONS

* For **Cauliflower Pineapple Rice**, replace the cooked rice with very finely chopped cauliflower.

* Add three to four pressed or minced garlic cloves along with the onion.

* Add ½ teaspoon of Chinese five-spice powder along with the onion.

* Add ½ cup of thinly sliced shiitake mushrooms along with the onion.

* Add ¼ cup of fresh or frozen corn along with the peas and carrots.

* Try grilling the pineapple (see page 105).

Skillet Corn Bread

There is something about cooking in cast iron that conjures images of our ancestors dining in their homestead under a starry sky. It might surprise you to learn that a campfire classic can be a health food! Corn is traditionally a revered crop by Native Americans, containing B vitamins, vitamins C and K, phytochemicals, and fiber. Serve topped with Roasted Squash Butter (page 264) or Chipotle Mayonnaise (page 273) alongside the Adzuki Bean Tempeh Chili (page 152).

TOTAL YIELD: 1 (10-INCH) CAST-IRON PAN OR 8 BY 8-INCH CASSEROLE DISH OF CORN BREAD

Serving Size: 1 slice
Number of Servings: 8
Prep Time: 10 minutes
Cook Time: 35 minutes
Total Time: 45 minutes

WET

3 tablespoons water
1 tablespoon chia seeds or ground flaxseeds
1½ cups soy milk
3 tablespoons coconut oil, vegan butter, or applesauce
1½ tablespoons freshly squeezed lime juice
1 cup fresh or frozen corn

DRY

1½ cups stone-ground cornmeal
¾ cup flour, such as a gluten-free flour blend (for homemade, see page 254), spelt, or whole wheat pastry
2 teaspoons baking powder
½ teaspoon sea salt

1. Preheat the oven to 325°F. Lightly oil a 10-inch cast-iron pan or 8 by 8-inch casserole dish and place in the oven while you prepare the rest of the recipe.
2. Begin to prepare the wet ingredients: Combine the water and chia seeds in a small bowl and stir well. Allow to sit for 10 minutes until a gel forms, stirring once or twice to make sure all the seeds are submerged in water.
3. Place the remaining wet ingredients in a bowl and mix well. Place the dry ingredients in a separate bowl and mix well. Add the wet ingredients and the chia seed mixture and mix well.
4. Carefully remove the cast-iron pan from the oven. Pour the batter (the entire mixture) into the pan and return it to the oven. Cook until a toothpick inserted into the center of the corn bread comes out dry, about 35 minutes. Enjoy warm or cold.

VARIATIONS

- Replace the chia and water with ¼ cup of aquafaba (see page 272).
- Replace the chia seeds and water with ½ cup of cooked and mashed sweet potato.
- Add ¼ cup of seeded and diced red bell pepper, 2 tablespoons of minced fresh cilantro, 1½ teaspoons of chili powder, and ⅛ teaspoon of chipotle powder to the dry ingredients.

Cheezy Artichoke Dip

Meet the secret weapon for convincing your guests they are eating a dairy-based spread. Spinach and artichokes make a perfect flavor as well as nutritional duo serving up plenty of iron, vitamin C, magnesium, and fiber, making this a nourishing dip rather than an overindulgent one. Serve at your next baby shower or cocktail party along with Cashew Cheese-Stuffed Sweet Peppers (page 179) and Curried Cauliflower Pakora (page 200).

TOTAL YIELD: 8 OUNCES
> Serving Size: 2 ounces
> Number of Servings: 4
> Prep Time: 15 minutes
> Cook Time: 30 minutes
> Total Time: 45 minutes

2 cups chopped spinach
½ cup vegan cream cheese or cashew cheese (for homemade, see page 179)
2 tablespoons nutritional yeast
2 teaspoons minced fresh dill
¾ teaspoon paprika (try smoked paprika)
½ teaspoon sea salt, or to taste
⅛ teaspoon ground black pepper
Pinch of crushed red pepper flakes (optional)
1 cup chopped artichoke hearts
Oil for ramekin (optional)
¼ cups bread crumbs (try gluten-free, optionally toasted in a small amount of olive oil) (optional)

1. Preheat the oven to 350°F. Place the spinach, vegan cream cheese, nutritional yeast, dill, paprika, salt, black pepper, and red pepper flakes, if using, in a food processor fitted with the S-blade and process until creamy. You can also mix these ingredients by hand in a large bowl.
2. Transfer to a bowl, add the artichoke hearts, and mix well.
3. Transfer to a lightly oiled or nonstick 8- or 10-ounce ramekin and top with the bread crumbs, if using. Place in the oven and bake for 30 minutes. Enjoy warm.

VARIATIONS

- Add ¼ cup of shredded vegan mozzarella or Cheddar cheese along with the vegan cream cheese.

- Replace the dill with 1 tablespoon of a Global Spice Blend, such as Italian, Cajun, or Moroccan (pages 249–252).

- Replace the spinach with arugula.

Loaded Nachos

Look no further for a party dish that always delivers, especially when your guests are famished. This loaded nacho plate is loaded with flavors and plant-based nutritional goodness! It's major comfort food satisfaction, without the heaviness or guilt. You can save time by using store-bought vegan cheese sauce and barbecued jackfruit (or make them in advance). Then, this dish can be ready in fifteen minutes or less . . . even prepared during a commercial break! Garnish with lime wedges and toasted pumpkin seeds and serve with Tart Cherry and Pomegranate Tonic (page 115).

TOTAL YIELD: 60 OUNCES

>   Serving Size: 10 ounces
>   Number of Servings: 6
>   Prep Time: 30 minutes
>   Cook Time: 45 minutes
>   Total Time: 60 minutes

1 recipe EZ Cheez Sauce (page 271)
   or 12 to 16 ounces store-bought vegan
   cheese sauce
1 recipe BBQ Jackfruit (page 217),
   Jackfruit Taco Filling (page 216),
   or 12 ounces store-bought
8 to 10 ounces vegan tortilla chips
1 (15-ounce) can black beans, drained well
   and rinsed, or 1½ cups cooked (see page
   102)
¾ cup salsa or chopped tomato
½ cup Vegan Sour Cream (page 274,
   or store-bought)
2 tablespoons roughly chopped fresh
   cilantro

1. After you make the recipes, keep the cheese sauce and jackfruit warm, set aside.
2. Build your plate: Place the tortilla chips on a large plate or platter. Top with the cheese sauce and jackfruit. Top with the black beans, salsa, vegan sour cream, cilantro, and any of the fixings listed in variations.

VARIATIONS

* Have a fiesta with your fixings: include ½ cup of diced tomato, ¼ cup diced red onion, 1 avocado cut into ½-inch cubes, or ½ cup of guacamole.

* Experiment with different tortilla chips. Out of chips? Serve with corn tortillas and have a soft taco night instead!

* Replace the black beans with pinto or refried beans.

Coconut Maple Glazed Sweet Potatoes with Toasted Walnuts

Creamy and decadent, this luscious dish is perfect to serve at your holiday feast. It's high in heart-healthy minerals, such as potassium, and immunity-boosting nutrients, such as vitamins A and C, and B vitamins. Try using garnet and purple sweet potatoes for the most vibrant colors and serve with Pecan Sage Holiday Loaf (page 244), Mushroom Leek Gravy (page 276), Lemony Herbed Cauliflower Roast (page 211), and Cranberry Apricot Sauce with Crystallized Ginger (page 268).

TOTAL YIELD: 2 POTATOES
>Serving Size: ½ potato
>Number of Servings: 4
>Prep Time: 5 minutes
>Cook Time: 55 minutes
>Total Time: 60 minutes

½ cup water

2 large sweet potatoes, sliced in half lengthwise

½ cup full-fat or light coconut milk

2 to 3 tablespoons pure maple syrup

½ teaspoon pure vanilla extract

½ teaspoon pumpkin pie spice

Pinch of sea salt

¼ cup chopped walnuts, optionally toasted in a 350°F oven for 10 minutes

1. Preheat the oven to 425°F. Place the water in a 9 by 13-inch casserole dish. Add the sweet potatoes, cut side up. Cover with aluminum foil, being sure not to have the foil in contact with the potatoes, and bake until just tender, about 45 minutes, depending on the size of the sweet potatoes. Remove from the oven.
2. Place the coconut milk, maple syrup, vanilla, pumpkin pie spice, and salt in a small bowl and whisk well.
3. Poke some holes in the sweet potatoes, using a fork. Pour the coconut milk mixture over the potatoes and return the casserole to the oven. Bake for an additional 10 minutes. Remove from the oven and place the potatoes on a serving dish.
4. Top with any of the coconut milk mixture left in the casserole, as well as the chopped walnuts, before serving.

VARIATIONS

- Add ¼ teaspoon of ground cardamom along with the pumpkin pie spice.

- Replace the walnuts with pecans or hazelnuts.

- Top with vegan butter if you feel like indulging.

- Replace the coconut milk with soy, rice, or almond milk.

- Experiment with different types of sweet potato, such as garnet, jewel, Japanese Hannah, or purple sweet potato.

Asian Couscous

Pearl couscous, popular in the Middle East, pairs wonderfully with wheat-free tamari, used extensively throughout Asia. While couscous is technically a pasta, it contains a substantial amount of protein. It blends well with heart-supportive shallots and peppers and nutrient powerhouses mushrooms and bok choy. Garnish with black and white sesame seeds and serve with Brazenly Braised Tempeh (page 219) or Black Gomasio Crusted Tofu (page 215), topped with Smoky Sweet Chili Garlic Sauce (page 263).

TOTAL YIELD: 36 OUNCES
> Serving Size: 8 to 10 ounces
> Number of Servings: 4
> Prep Time: 5 minutes
> Cook Time: 20 minutes
> Total Time: 25 minutes

1½ cups water or vegetable stock (for homemade, see page 248)

1 cup pearl couscous

¼ teaspoon sea salt (optional)

1 tablespoon sesame or coconut oil, or 3 tablespoons water

½ cup diced shallots

1 cup seeded and diced red bell pepper

1 cup quartered cremini or button mushrooms

2 cups chopped bok choy or baby bok choy (1-inch pieces)

2 teaspoons wheat-free tamari or other soy sauce, or to taste

3 tablespoons finely chopped fresh cilantro

1. Place the water, couscous, and salt, if using, in a 2-quart pot over high heat and bring to a boil. Lower the heat to low. Cover and cook until all the liquid is absorbed, about 15 minutes. Turn off the heat, keep covered, and allow to sit for 5 minutes. Fluff with a fork. Transfer to a large bowl.

2. Meanwhile, place a sauté pan over medium-high heat. Heat the oil. Add the shallots, bell pepper, and mushrooms and cook until the mushrooms are just tender, about 10 minutes, stirring frequently and adding small amounts of water or vegetable stock if necessary to prevent sticking. Add the bok choy and cook for 5 minutes, or until just tender, stirring frequently.

3. Add the tamari and cilantro and mix well. Transfer to the couscous and gently mix well before serving.

VARIATIONS

- Add 1 tablespoon of peeled and minced fresh ginger or minced garlic along with the shallots.

- Add ¼ teaspoon of crushed red pepper flakes and 1 teaspoon of Chinese five-spice powder along with the onion.

- Replace the bok choy with other greens, such as kale, chard, or collards.

- Go gluten-free and replace the couscous with millet, quinoa, rice, or rice pasta.

FIFTEEN

MARVELOUS MAIN DISHES

Congratulations on making it to the main event! For optimal digestion, it is generally recommended to enjoy your largest meal at lunch and have a lighter meal for dinner. Just something to keep in the back of your mind. For many people, their schedule doesn't allow them the luxury, so in the reputed last words of Buddha, "Do your best." (It's also a good idea to start with a salad, to balance out the potential for heaviness in the main course. See Chapter 13 for salad inspiration.)

With every meal, you have an opportunity to choose foods that will either increase your vitality and effectively lower your biological age, or lead you down the road of those common ailments that result in the inevitable decline seen too often with aging. With a balance of whole grains and legumes, an assortment of fresh organic veggies, and a little healthy fat, these main dishes use the power of the plate to bring us vitality. These are the meals that will sustain you, nourish your friends and family, and carry you together into a future of longevity.

First, here's the easiest way to create a powerful plant-based meal! The mantra for mains? "Monk Bowl." When you are in a pinch and are not sure what to prepare, the monk bowl can be your saving grace. Monk Bowls consist of a grain, a green, and a protein. You can create countless meals based on this simple formula.

- For the grain, rotate through different types of rice, millet, quinoa, brown rice pasta, and so on.
- The greens can consists of any vegetable or combination of vegetables that you love. They can be raw, steamed, roasted, grilled, sautéed, or a combination of different methods. Enjoy them perfectly as is, or have fun spiralizing or cutting them into fancy shapes.

- When it comes to veggies, think in terms of including as many colors as possible, with an emphasis on green.
- For plant proteins, rotate through different beans and legumes, tofu, tempeh, and seitan (for those who can tolerate gluten). Tofu or tempeh can be roasted, sautéed, or grilled and made with various marinades. Legumes can be boiled, refried, or made into patties.
- Global Spice Blends (see pages 249–252) can be added to your legumes to create even more variety.
- You may choose to boost your bowl by topping it with such extras as a few toasted seeds or nuts, sliced avocado, nutritional yeast, or sauerkraut.

TIMELESS TIPS: MAIN COURSE HACKS

- **Think leftovers.** Perhaps make a double batch of what you are preparing and come up with creative ways to enjoy it the following day with some simple tweaks.
- **Premade frozen meals** are a gift from heaven when you are totally pressed for time. Look for organic whenever possible. Vegan burritos, enchiladas, lasagne, curry bowls, pizza, and more are likely available in a store near you. Grab a handful of arugula or mixed salad greens and you are good to go.
- **Get saucy.** Make sauces from this book in advance, or stock up on some of your favorite store-bought sauces to have on hand in a pinch. You will be amazed at how simple it is to elevate your monk bowls, such as the Marvelous Macro Meal (page 226) with such sauces as BBQ, sweet-and-sour, or Thai peanut, to name a few.

Most Monk Bowls can be prepared from beginning to end within twenty to thirty minutes.

The main course is also where you can truly enjoy any world cuisine comfort food you desire. How about a Mushroom Risotto from Italy (page 233), or a Thai Red Coconut Curry (page 231) from . . . you guessed it, Thailand? The fun doesn't stop there: try Braised Mushroom Stroganoff (page 240) from Russia, Black Rice Sushi with Wasabi Mayo (page 222) from Japan, Spinach Chickpeas (page 213) from India, Garlicky Hummus (page 194) from the Middle East, Black-Eye Cabbage (page 212) from the southern United States, and even a vegan spin on a Philly cheese steak made with portobello mushrooms (page 232).

Finally, when holiday season hits, we have you covered. The Pecan Sage Holiday Loaf (page 244) topped with Mushroom Leek Gravy (page 276) will wow even the most omnivorous of your guests. Want to steal the show? Prepare the Lemony Herbed Cauliflower Roast (page 211), and top with Cranberry Apricot Sauce with Crystallized Ginger (page 268).

Lemony Herbed Cauliflower Roast

The ultimate in plant-based holiday roasts. Serve this as a decorative side dish or as the centerpiece. Gorgeous cauliflower certainly deserves center stage as one of the highest-nutrient and universally agreeable foods. The lemon and herb topping greatly helps increase absorption of all the nutrients it contains. Feel free to break out the electric carving knife for a dramatic effect when slicing. Top with Cranberry Apricot Sauce with Crystallized Ginger (page 268) or Chimichurri Topping (page 201).

TOTAL YIELD: 1 LARGE CAULIFLOWER
Serving Size: ¼ cauliflower
Number of Servings: 4
Prep Time: 5 minutes
Cook Time: 50 minutes
Total Time: 55 minutes

1 cup vegetable stock (for homemade, see page 248) or water

1 large cauliflower, leaves trimmed

3 to 4 tablespoons olive oil, divided (optional)

1½ teaspoons sea salt, divided

¼ teaspoon ground black pepper (try smoked)

2 tablespoons freshly squeezed lemon juice

2 tablespoons chiffonaded fresh basil

1 tablespoon finely chopped fresh flat-leaf parsley

1 tablespoon chiffonaded fresh sage

1 teaspoon garlic granules

½ teaspoon minced fresh rosemary

1. Preheat the oven to 425°F. Place the vegetable stock in an 8 by 8-inch casserole dish. Add the cauliflower. Drizzle with 1 to 2 tablespoons of the olive oil, if using, and top with ½ teaspoon of the salt and the black pepper. Use your (clean) hands to evenly coat the cauliflower.

2. Cover with aluminum foil, being sure not to let the foil contact the food, and bake until just tender all the way through, 45 to 50 minutes. Remove the foil.

3. Change the oven setting to HIGH broil. Broil for 5 minutes, or until the outside of the cauliflower turns a crispy brown. Remove from the oven.

4. Place the remaining ingredients in a small bowl. Baste the cauliflower well before showing off, slicing, and serving.

VARIATIONS

- Top with grated vegan cheese just before broiling.

- Drizzle with Zesty Lemon Sriracha Dressing (page 171) before serving.

- For a supreme **Tex-Mex Cauliflower Roast**, replace the lemon juice with lime juice; replace the basil, rosemary, parsley, and sage with 2 tablespoons minced fresh cilantro; and add 2 teaspoons of chili powder, 1 teaspoon of ground cumin, and ⅛ teaspoon of chipotle powder along with the salt and pepper before basting.

Black-Eye Cabbage

A family tradition in the Boudet household that goes back generations, this traditional New Year's dish features black-eyed peas for health and cabbage for wealth in the new year. They also make a hefty nutrient-dense combo with plenty of magnesium, potassium, copper, B vitamins, including B$_9$ (folate), and vitamins C and K to keep you clearheaded, strong, and balanced any day of the year. Top with a dollop of Vegan Sour Cream (page 274) and a sprinkle of Smoky Mushrooms (page 254), and serve along with Mushroom Risotto (page 233) or Quintessential Quinoa Pilaf (page 186), with Raw Choco-Cherry Bombs (page 281) for dessert.

TOTAL YIELD: 32 OUNCES
    Serving Size: 16 ounces
    Number of Servings: 2
    Prep Time: 10 minutes
    Cook Time: 15 minutes
    Total Time: 25 minutes

2 teaspoons olive or coconut oil, or 3 tablespoons water
½ cup diced yellow onion
½ cup diced carrot
½ teaspoon sea salt, or to taste
⅛ teaspoon ground black pepper
½ teaspoon Cajun Spice Mix (page 249, or store-bought)
1 (15-ounce) can black-eyed peas, or 1½ cups cooked (see page 102)
½ to ¾ teaspoon liquid smoke
6 cups chopped cabbage (½-inch pieces)
½ teaspoon wheat-free tamari or other soy sauce (optional)
2 tablespoons finely chopped fresh flat-leaf parsley

1. Place a medium-size pot over medium-high heat. Heat the oil. Add the onion, carrot, salt, pepper, and Cajun Spice Mix and cook for 5 minutes, stirring frequently and adding small amounts of water or vegetable stock if necessary to prevent sticking.
2. Add the black-eyed peas and liquid smoke and cook, stirring frequently, for 3 minutes. Add the cabbage and cook, stirring frequently, until just tender, about 5 minutes. Add the tamari, if using, and the parsley and mix well before serving.

VARIATIONS

- Add 1 tablespoon of freshly squeezed lemon juice along with the parsley.
- Add two pressed or minced garlic cloves along with the onion.
- Add ¼ cup of thinly sliced green onion along with the parsley.
- Top with crumbled store-bought tempeh bacon that has been baked or sautéed.

THE ULTIMATE AGE-DEFYING PLAN

Spinach Chickpeas

Spinach chickpeas, or *chana saag* for those in the know, is one of the easier traditional Indian dishes to veganize—simply substitute a plant-based milk, such as soy, almond, or coconut, for the dairy cream. These powerful peas in a bed of creamy garlic- and onion-infused spinach are a decadent way to absorb lots of iron, protein, calcium, magnesium, and of course, major antioxidant benefits! Serve along with Pilau Rice (page 198) and Curried Cauliflower Pakora (page 200).

TOTAL YIELD: 24 OUNCES
Serving Size: 8 ounces
Number of Servings: 3
Prep Time: 10 minutes
Cook Time: 20 minutes
Total Time: 30 minutes

1 cup unsweetened soy, coconut, or almond milk
½ cup diced white or yellow onion
3 to 4 cloves garlic, pressed or minced
1 tablespoon curry powder
1 (15-ounce) can chickpeas, or 1½ cups cooked (see page 102)
10 ounces frozen spinach (1 cup defrosted)
Pinch of cayenne pepper (optional)
½ teaspoon sea salt, or to taste
1 teaspoon wheat-free tamari or other soy sauce, or to taste (optional)
3 tablespoons freshly squeezed lemon juice
Minced fresh cilantro, for garnish

1. Place a medium-size pot over medium-high heat. Combine the soy milk, onion, garlic, and curry powder in the pot and cook for 5 minutes, stirring occasionally. Add the chickpeas and cook for 5 minutes, stirring occasionally.
2. Lower the heat to medium. Add the spinach and cayenne, if using, and cook for 10 minutes, stirring occasionally. Add the salt, tamari, if using, and lemon juice, and mix well. Garnish liberally with cilantro before serving.

VARIATIONS

- Add one 15-ounce can of diced fire-roasted tomatoes along with the spinach.
- Add 2 tablespoons of nutritional yeast along with the spinach.
- You can sauté the onion and garlic in sesame oil before adding other ingredients.
- Replace the chickpeas with cubed and roasted tofu or tempeh (see pages 104–105).
- Replace the frozen spinach with 4 cups fresh chopped spinach.

Himalayan Lentils and Greens

Red lentils are the pulse of choice for quick and easy chefs. High in protein, quick in preparation, and big on flavor, you might say it's the Everest of legumes. Lentils love your heart by providing lots of vitamin B$_9$ (folate) and magnesium, and soluble fiber. You can optionally top with a dollop of Vegan Sour Cream (page 274) or Coconut Yogurt (page 262) and serve with Coco Cauliflower (page 197) and Pilau Rice (page 198), or rice or quinoa (see page 101). If you are feeling adventurous, finish off with Mango Rice Pudding with Salted Caramel (page 293).

TOTAL YIELD: 48 OUNCES
 Serving Size: 12 ounces
 Number of Servings: 4
 Prep Time: 5 minutes
 Cook Time: 25 minutes
 Total Time: 30 minutes

4 cups water or vegetable stock (for homemade, see page 248)

¾ cup dried red lentils, rinsed and drained well

¾ cup diced yellow onion

1 tablespoon peeled and minced fresh ginger

¾ cup diced tomato or diced fire-roasted tomatoes

2 teaspoons curry powder

2 cups shredded greens, such as kale, chard, mustard or dandelion greens, or spinach

¾ to 1 teaspoon sea salt, or to taste

2 tablespoons finely chopped fresh cilantro

⅛ teaspoon cayenne pepper (optional)

1. Place the water, lentils, onion, ginger, tomato, and curry powder, in a medium-size pot over medium-high heat. Cook for 20 minutes, stirring occasionally.
2. Add the greens and cook for 5 minutes, stirring occasionally.
3. Add the salt, cilantro, and cayenne, if using, and stir well before serving.

VARIATIONS

- Add ½ teaspoon of ground cumin and/or ½ teaspoon of garam masala along with the curry powder.

- Add ½ teaspoon of wheat-free tamari or other soy sauce and/or 1 tablespoon of freshly squeezed lemon juice along with the cilantro.

- Replace the ginger with two to three pressed or minced garlic cloves and add ¾ cup of diced carrot or celery.

- Replace the red lentils with brown or black lentils or split peas and cook according to the instructions on pages 102–103.

Black Gomasio Crusted Tofu

Your koan of the day: *What's the sound of one tofu cutlet roasting?* Answer: *The sound of all of your body's protein needs being met on a plant-based diet!* Serve with Smoky Sweet Chili Garlic Sauce (page 263) over Quintessential Quinoa Pilaf (page 186) or Garlicky Whipped Parsnips (page 192) and Braised Kale with Shallots and Slivered Almonds (page 185) or Sunny Kale Salad (page 162).

TOTAL YIELD: 6 TOFU CUTLETS
    Serving Size: 2 cutlets
    Number of Servings: 3
    Prep Time: 20 minutes
    Marinate Time: 20 minutes
    Cook Time: 40 minutes
    Total Time: 60 minutes

14 ounces extra-firm tofu

2 tablespoons water

1 tablespoon wheat-free tamari or other soy sauce

2 teaspoons toasted sesame oil

¼ cup flour, such as a gluten-free flour blend (for homemade, see page 254), spelt, whole wheat pastry, or unbleached all-purpose

½ cup unsweetened soy, almond, or coconut milk

¼ cup plus 2 tablespoons Black Sesame Gomasio (page 253) or black sesame seeds

1 tablespoon white sesame seeds

⅛ teaspoon ground black pepper

1 teaspoon minced fresh cilantro

¼ teaspoon sea salt, only if using the black sesame seeds instead of the gomasio

1. Preheat the oven to 375°F. Slice the tofu widthwise into six cutlets. Place the water, tamari, and toasted sesame oil in a small baking sheet and mix well. Add the tofu cutlets. Allow to sit for 10 minutes. Flip and allow to sit 10 minutes.

2. Place in the oven and bake for 20 minutes. Remove from the oven and allow to cool until cool enough to handle.

3. Meanwhile, place the flour in a bowl. Place the soy milk in a separate bowl. Place the Black Sesame Gomasio, white sesame seeds, pepper, and cilantro (and salt, if using) in another bowl and mix well.

4. One at a time, dip the tofu cutlets in the flour mixture and coat well. Dip in the soy milk and coat well. Using your other hand, dip the cutlets in the gomasio mixture and coat well. Transfer to the baking sheet and bake for 10 minutes. Flip and cook for another 10 minutes. Serve warm.

VARIATIONS

- Replace the sesame seeds with finely ground nuts or seeds, such as cashews, pecans, macadamia nuts, or sunflower or pumpkin seeds.

- Add 1 tablespoon of a Global Spice Blend, such as Ethiopian, Cajun, Mexican, or Indian (pages 249–252) along with the sesame seeds.

- Replace the tofu with tempeh, Savory Baked Seitan (page 225), portobello mushrooms, cauliflower steaks, or thick slices of eggplant or zucchini.

- For an oil-free variation, replace the sesame oil with additional water.

Jackfruit Taco Filling

It behooves us to give a jack about how we can create healthy, plant-based alternatives to some of those foods that we know can send us to an early grave. Here it's jackfruit to the rescue, deliciously replacing the pork in your taquito. Walnuts also give a nice meatiness, as well as brain- and heart-boosting omega-3s, and important minerals, such as calcium, magnesium, potassium, and zinc. Serve as part of Loaded Nachos (page 206) or create the Jackfruit Tacos of your dreams by placing inside taco shells or soft tortillas, along with all of the fixings, such as shredded lettuce, minced red onion, avocado slices or guacamole, Vegan Sour Cream (page 274), and sprigs of cilantro.

TOTAL YIELD: 20 OUNCES
> Serving Size: 4 ounces
> Number of Servings: 5
> Prep Time: 10 minutes
> Cook Time: 20 minutes
> Total Time: 30 minutes

1 teaspoon olive oil, or 3 tablespoons water
¾ cup thinly sliced yellow onion
3 to 4 cloves garlic, pressed or minced
1 (14-ounce) can (1½ cups) young jackfruit, drained well (7.9 ounces dry weight)
½ teaspoon chipotle powder
½ cup chopped walnuts
1 cup diced fire-roasted tomatoes or small-chopped fresh tomato
2 teaspoons freshly squeezed lime juice
2 tablespoons finely chopped fresh cilantro
Sea salt and ground black pepper

1. Place a sauté pan over medium-high heat. Heat the oil. Add the onion and cook for 3 minutes, stirring frequently and adding small amounts of water if necessary to prevent sticking. Add the garlic and cook for 1 minute, stirring frequently.
2. Add the jackfruit and chipotle powder and cook for 5 minutes, stirring frequently and breaking up the larger pieces of jackfruit into smaller pieces as you stir. Lower the heat to medium. Add the walnuts and tomatoes and cook for 10 minutes, stirring frequently.
3. Add the lime juice and cilantro and stir well. Season with salt and pepper to taste before serving.

VARIATION
Replace the jackfruit with crumbled tempeh, tofu, or seitan.

BBQ Jackfruit

Smoky, tangy, and tender, this pig-free version of pulled pork will leave even confirmed porkavores extolling the virtues of jackfruit. It's a win-win to enjoy unmistakable barbecue while receiving heart-healthy nutrients minus the stress from an influx of fat and cholesterol. Serve as part of Loaded Nachos (page 206), or top with Sally's Super Simple Slaw (page 165) and Pickled Red Onion (page 261) and serve in a hoagie or along with Mac n Cheez (page 230).

TOTAL YIELD: 12 OUNCES
Serving Size: 4 ounces
Number of Servings: 3
Prep Time: 5 minutes
Cook Time: 45 minutes
Total Time: 50 minutes

1 (14-ounce) can (1½ cups) young jackfruit, drained well (7.9 ounces dry weight)
½ cup diced yellow onion
2 tablespoons olive oil, or ¼ cup water
2 teaspoons minced garlic
½ teaspoon liquid smoke
¼ teaspoon sea salt, or to taste
⅛ teaspoon chipotle powder
½ to ¾ cup store-bought barbecue sauce or Apricot BBQ Sauce (page 269)

1. Preheat the oven to 400°F. Place the jackfruit, onion, olive oil, garlic, liquid smoke, salt, and chipotle powder in a baking dish and mix well.
2. Cover, place in the oven, and bake for 30 minutes.
3. Add the barbecue sauce, mix well, and cook for 15 minutes. Stir well before serving.

VARIATIONS

- Add 1 tablespoon Cajun Spice Mix (page 249) along with the onion.

- If you have more time, you can lower the temperature to 350°F and double the cooking time.

- Replace the jackfruit with crumbled tempeh.

Classic Stir-fry

Need to whip together a meal in twenty-five minutes or less? Stir-fry is your secret weapon. With this dish, you will create a rainbow of veggies, ensuring you get a full balance of high-powered nutrients.

If you have a wok, break it out and we will wok you through the recipe. Use the firmest tofu you can find (see page 103). Enhance your stir-fry by adding sauces, such as Artful Almond Sauce (page 270), Smoky Sweet Chili Garlic Sauce (page 263), or Apricot BBQ Sauce (page 269). Top with nuts or seeds, and serve over quinoa or rice along with a large mixed green salad.

TOTAL YIELD: 32 OUNCES
> Serving Size: 16 ounces
> Number of Servings: 2
> Prep Time: 10 minutes
> Cook Time: 15 minutes
> Total Time: 25 minutes

1 tablespoon olive oil, or ½ cup water or vegetable stock (for homemade, see page 248)

¾ cup chopped red onion

½ cup chopped fennel bulb

14 ounces extra-firm or superfirm tofu, cut into ½-inch cubes

1 cup frozen peas and carrots

1½ cups shredded kale

1½ tablespoons wheat-free tamari or other soy sauce, or to taste

2 tablespoons finely chopped fresh cilantro

Hot sauce (optional)

1. Place a large sauté pan or wok over high heat. Heat the oil. Add the red onion and fennel and cook for 3 minutes, stirring frequently and adding small amounts of water or vegetable stock if necessary to prevent sticking.
2. Add the tofu and cook for 5 minutes, gently stirring frequently. Do your best not to break apart the tofu. Add the peas and carrots and cook for 5 minutes, gently stirring frequently. Add the kale and cook for 3 minutes, gently stirring frequently. (We think you got the "gently" part by now.)
3. Add the tamari, cilantro, and hot sauce to taste, if using, and gently stir well before serving.

VARIATIONS

- Replace the peas and carrots with chopped vegetables of your choosing, such as red cabbage, broccoli, cauliflower, or zucchini.
- Replace the kale with collards, chard, dandelion greens, or arugula.
- Add 1 tablespoon of a Global Spice Blend, such as Italian, Indian, or Cajun (pages 249–252), or adobe seasoning along with the onion.
- Replace the cilantro with fresh basil or parsley, or replace with 1 tablespoon of minced fresh dill, chervil, or summer savory.

Brazenly Braised Tempeh

With a nutty flavor and the ability to combine well with so many flavor profiles, tempeh is one of our go-to ingredients. Nutritionally, it contains all the amazing benefits of soy in an extra-gut-friendly form, with mood-boosting B vitamins as well. Top with your sauce du jour, such as Apricot BBQ Sauce (page 269), Chimichurri Topping (page 201), Artful Almond Sauce (page 270), or Smoky Sweet Chili Garlic Sauce (page 263).

TOTAL YIELD: 8 OUNCES
Serving Size: 4 ounces
Number of Servings: 2
Prep Time: 5 minutes
Cook Time: 20 minutes
Total Time: 25 minutes

1½ tablespoons olive oil, or 3 tablespoons water

8 ounces soy tempeh, sliced into 4 cutlets

¾ cup water or vegetable stock (for homemade, see page 248)

2 to 3 teaspoons wheat-free tamari or other soy sauce

2 teaspoons rice vinegar, or 1 tablespoon freshly squeezed lemon or lime juice

1 teaspoon Italian Spice Mix (page 251, or store-bought)

¼ teaspoon crushed red pepper flakes (optional)

Sea salt and ground black pepper

1. Place a medium-size sauté pan over medium-high heat. Heat the oil. Add the tempeh and cook for 3 minutes.
2. Flip and cook until golden brown, about 3 minutes, depending on the heat of the pan.
3. Add the remaining ingredients. Lower the heat to medium. Cook until all the liquid is absorbed, about 10 minutes. Flip the cutlets once or twice to ensure even cooking.

VARIATIONS

- Add 1 teaspoon of minced fresh dill, or 1 tablespoon of finely chopped fresh basil, parsley, or cilantro before serving.

- Add ½ teaspoon of liquid smoke along with the Italian Spice Mix.

- Replace the Italian Spice Mix with Cajun Spice Mix (page 249), Ethiopian Spice Mix (page 250), Indian Spice Mix (page 251), or Mexican Spice Mix (page 252).

- Replace the tempeh with extra-firm tofu, Savory Baked Seitan (page 225), or portobello mushrooms.

- For **Beer-Braised Tempeh**, replace the water with your favorite beer.

Herb-Roasted Tofu

Give people a block of tofu and you can feed them for a day. Show them how to make an herb-roasted tofu and you can feed them for a lifetime. Each bite can equip the immune, endocrine, metabolic, and cardiovascular cells with nutrients needed to thrive. So, give soy a chance. Top with toasted pine nuts and serve over cooked or raw greens, or as part of a Monk Bowl (see page 209), or along with Grilled Vegetables Extraordinaire (page 178) and Quintessential Quinoa Pilaf (page 186).

TOTAL YIELD: 12 OUNCES

Serving Size: 3 ounces
Number of Servings: 4
Prep Time: 10 minutes
Marinate Time: 10 minutes
Cook Time: 25 minutes
Total Time: 45 minutes

14 ounces extra-firm or superfirm tofu, cut into ½-inch cubes
2 teaspoons wheat-free tamari or other soy sauce
2 tablespoons water
2 teaspoons olive oil, or an extra tablespoon of water

HERB SAUCE

2 tablespoons chiffonaded basil
2 tablespoons finely chopped fresh flat-leaf parsley
2 tablespoons minced kalamata olives or your favorites
1 tablespoon nutritional yeast
2 teaspoons olive oil (optional)
1 teaspoon rice vinegar
Pinch of crushed red pepper flakes (optional)
Sea salt and ground black pepper

1. Preheat the oven to 375°F. Combine the tofu, tamari, water, and olive oil on a small baking sheet and mix well. Allow to sit for 10 minutes up to an hour, tossing once or twice to ensure even coating. Place in the oven and bake for 25 minutes, optionally stirring once after 10 minutes. Transfer to a bowl.

2. Meanwhile, place all the sauce ingredients in another bowl and mix well. Transfer to the bowl of tofu and mix well before serving.

VARIATIONS

- Replace the tofu with tempeh, cubed portobello mushroom, or cubed Savory Baked Seitan (page 225).

- Add one pressed or minced garlic clove to the Herb Sauce.

- Add ½ teaspoon of minced fresh rosemary and 1 teaspoon of dried oregano to the Herb Sauce.

- Add 2 teaspoons of Italian Spice Mix (page 251) to the Herb Sauce.

Roasted Tofu with Almond Sauce

Soy in its whole form, such as in tofu and tempeh, is great for meeting your daily protein needs. In fact, this dish gives you a double dose of protein, from the tofu and the almonds, which add even more healthy fats, fiber, magnesium, and vitamin E, all perfect for heart health and weight maintenance. Top with black and white sesame seeds and serve over rice noodles, or as part of a Marvelous Macro Meal (page 226) or on top of Garlicky Whipped Parsnips (page 192).

TOTAL YIELD: 12 OUNCES
  Serving Size: 4 ounces
  Number of Servings: 3
  Prep Time: 10 minutes
  Marinate Time: 10 minutes
  Cook Time: 30 minutes
  Total Time: 50 minutes

14 ounces extra-firm tofu, cut into 1-inch cubes

1 tablespoon water

2 teaspoons wheat-free tamari or other soy sauce

2 teaspoons olive oil, or additional water

2 teaspoons water

¾ cup Artful Almond Sauce (page 270) or peanut sauce (store-bought, or see variation on page 270)

¼ cup thinly sliced green onion

½ cup chopped almonds or peanuts

1. Preheat the oven to 375°F. Combine the tofu, water, tamari, and olive oil on a small baking sheet and mix well. Allow to sit for 10 minutes up to an hour, tossing once or twice to ensure even coating.
2. Place in the oven and bake for 15 minutes, optionally stirring once after 10 minutes.
3. Add the sauce and bake for 15 minutes. Top with the green onion and chopped almonds before serving.

VARIATIONS

⋙ Replace the tofu with tempeh, cubed portobello mushroom, or cubed Savory Baked Seitan (page 225).

⋙ Add 1 tablespoon of minced fresh cilantro along with the almond sauce.

⋙ For a pad thai–esque dish, transfer to a bowl, add 8 ounces of cooked rice noodles, and mix well. Top with mung bean sprouts and serve with a lime wedge.

Black Rice Sushi with Wasabi Mayo

Sushi night is on! This version is made with black "forbidden" rice. (Why is it called forbidden? We are forbidden to tell you. Okay . . . it was originally only served to the Chinese emperor and his inner circle. Now it is readily available at a natural food store near you.) Black rice has the highest antioxidant content of any rice. In fact, just the outside hull of the grain has one of the highest levels of anthocyanin antioxidants of any food! It is also low-glycemic, and a good source of fiber, iron, copper, and protein.

Use this recipe as a starting point and experiment with the variations. No time to make the wasabi mayo? No problem; simply serve with wheat-free tamari as a dipping sauce, with pickled ginger on the side. Serve with Domo Arigato Arame Salad (page 159) and Miso Roots Soup (page 142).

TOTAL YIELD: 4 ROLLS
  Serving Size: 1 roll
  Number of Servings: 4
  Prep Time: 15 minutes
  Cook Time: 40 minutes
  Total Time: 55 minutes

1 cup black forbidden rice
3 cups water or vegetable stock (for homemade, see page 248)
½ teaspoon sea salt, or to taste
2 teaspoons rice vinegar or mirin (optional)
4 nori sheets
1 avocado, peeled, pitted, and cut into thin slices
¾ cup seeded and julienned red bell pepper
1 carrot, cut into thin sticks, optionally steamed until just tender

WASABI MAYO
¼ cup vegan mayonnaise (for homemade, see page 273) or Vegan Sour Cream (page 274, or store-bought)
½ to 1 teaspoon wasabi powder
¼ teaspoon wheat-free tamari or other soy sauce (optional)
Sea salt and ground black pepper

1. Place the rice, water, salt, and rice vinegar, if using, in a 2-quart pot over high heat. Bring to a boil. Cover, lower the heat to low, and cook until all the liquid is absorbed, about 40 minutes. Stir well and allow to cool. Place in the refrigerator if you need to speed things up.
2. Meanwhile, prepare your fillings.
3. Prepare the Wasabi Mayo: Place all the ingredients in a small dish and mix well.
4. Have ready a small bowl of cold or room-temperature water. Place a bamboo rolling mat on a clean cutting board. (If not using a mat, simply place the nori on a clean, dry surface, such as a cutting board.) Place the nori sheet on the bamboo mat, shiny side down and with the long side parallel to the bottom edge of the cutting board.
5. Using a rice paddle or spatula and starting at the bottom edge of the sheet, spread about ¾ cup of the cooled rice on the nori sheet, leaving about 1½ inches at the top without any rice. Dip your hands in the water to prevent the rice from sticking to you. Spread half of the Wasabi Mayo over the rice.
6. Closely line up one-quarter each of the avocado, red pepper, and carrot on top of the rice, about 1½ inches from the bottom edge of the nori sheet. You can let some of the red pepper and carrot stick out the ends, for a creative presentation.
7. Grab the bottom edge and roll it up, applying pressure to keep the roll as tight as possible. Dip your fingers in the water, wet the exposed 1½-inch strip of bare nori, and keep rolling until that edge is on the bottom. Press firmly, and leave the roll seam side down while you move on to make the other three rolls.
8. When all four are rolled, start with the first roll and transfer to a cutting board.

Cut a diagonal line through the middle with a serrated knife, then cut straight lines halfway through each half. Give a hearty *domo arigato* and enjoy!

VARIATIONS

- Add a sprinkle of Black Sesame Gomasio (page 253) or hemp or sesame seeds, optionally toasted (see page 106), to your roll.

- Replace the black rice with sushi rice or brown rice (see page 101).

- Some ideas for fillings: raw or roasted asparagus spears; chopped Magical Mushroom Medley (page 184) or grilled and sliced portobello mushroom; mango slices; grilled pineapple slices; salad greens; chopped Braised Kale (page 185); sunflower sprouts; grated veggies, such as carrot, beet, daikon, or jicama.

- For a raw version, use untoasted nori sheets, Quick Cashew Cheese (page 179) instead of rice, and raw fresh veggies inside the wrap.

El Tortilla Pizza

A.k.a. the Busy Person's Pizza. The variations possible are as numerous as the tourists gazing upon the *Mona Lisa*. A fun way to pack in some phytonutrients, the tortilla creates a nice thin and crispy base to load up on all your favorite veggies. For a quick and easy feast, serve with a large organic mixed green salad, possibly topped with Rosemary Polenta Croutons (page 189), with your dressing of choice.

TOTAL YIELD: 2 (9-INCH) TORTILLA PIZZAS

> Serving Size: 1 pizza
> Number of Servings: 2
> Prep Time: 10 minutes
> Cook Time: 20 minutes
> Total Time: 30 minutes

2 (9-inch) tortillas

½ to ¾ cup tomato sauce (for homemade, see page 267)

½ cup arugula or chopped baby spinach

½ cup grated vegan cheese (for homemade, see page 179)

½ cup thinly sliced cremini or button mushrooms

¼ cup chopped artichoke hearts

2 tablespoons pitted and chopped olives

1. Preheat the oven to 350°F. Place the tortillas on a baking sheet. Spread the sauce on the tortillas.
2. Top with the arugula, cheese, mushrooms, artichoke hearts, and olives.
3. Transfer to the oven and bake for 20 minutes. Enjoy warm out of the oven!

VARIATIONS

- You can replace the tomato sauce with Pepita Pesto with Avocado (page 265) or a simple olive oil and minced garlic baste.

- Change up the green veggies to include kale, chard, collards, and whatever local greens are available.

- Change the veggies up to include chopped zucchini, asparagus, broccoli, or cauliflower.

- Replace the artichoke hearts with sustainably harvested hearts of palm.

- For a **Quesadilla Muy Simple**, sprinkle the tortilla with vegan cheese, add some veggies and shredded greens, and fold in half. Heat in a sauté pan on both sides until the cheese is melted.

- For a taste of India, replace the tomato sauce with Spinach Chickpeas (page 213). For a taste of the South, top with BBQ Jackfruit (page 217).

Savory Baked Seitan

Seitan, or "meat of wheat," consists almost entirely of gluten and is very high in protein. Those who can tolerate gluten on the occasion marvel at seitan's versatility. It is used to create a full spectrum of plant-based alternatives to meat. To get the full flavor of the dish, we recommend including the ingredients in the variations. Serve with Mushroom Leek Gravy (page 276) or Chunky Tomato Sauce (page 267), Garlicky Whipped Parsnips (page 192), and Sweet Chili Brussels Sprouts (page 190). Seitan . . . it's what's for dinner.

YIELD: 24 OUNCES
    Serving Size: 6 ounces
    Number of Servings: 4
    Prep Time: 15 minutes
    Cook Time: 1 hour 30 minutes
    Total Time: 1 hour 45 minutes

1¼ cups vital wheat gluten
½ cup nutritional yeast
½ cup garbanzo flour
1 cup water or vegetable stock (for homemade, see page 248)
2 tablespoons wheat-free tamari or other soy sauce
2 tablespoons olive oil (optional)
1 tablespoon onion flakes
1 tablespoon garlic flakes (optional)
1 teaspoon poultry seasoning
1½ teaspoons smoked paprika

1. Preheat the oven to 350°F. Place all the ingredients in a bowl and mix well. Knead with your hands for about 10 minutes; the mixture should be stretchable.
2. Form into an 8-inch log. Place in a loaf pan and cover with foil (make sure the foil does not contact the food). Bake for 45 minutes. Flip and bake, covered, for 45 minutes. Slice as needed and serve warm or cooled on its own, in sandwiches and wraps or in the serving suggestions listed above.

VARIATIONS

- Add a pinch of cayenne pepper along with the onion flakes.
- Add ¼ cup of ketchup and 1 teaspoon of vegan Worcestershire sauce along with the tamari.
- Add 1 tablespoon of a Global Spice Blend, such as Italian, Mexican, or Cajun (pages 249–252).

Marvelous Macro Meal

From the microcosm to the macrocosm, you can't but marvel at the elegant simplicity of this sustaining meal. The macrobiotic approach to eating looks at balancing the energetic qualities of food in a meal and emphasizes using local and seasonal ingredients whenever possible. This ensures the intake of necessary vitamins, minerals, and phytochemicals with optimal absorption, in line with nature's wisdom. Serve with Turmeric Tahini Dressing (page 172), Oil-Free Roasted Red Pepper Dressing (page 170), or Mushroom Leek Gravy (page 276) and a large mixed green salad.

TOTAL YIELD: 64 OUNCES

Serving Size: 32 ounces
Number of Servings: 2
Prep Time: 15 minutes
Cook Time: 45 minutes
Total Time: 60 minutes

2 cups water or vegetable stock (for homemade, see page 248)
1 cup uncooked short- or long-grain brown rice
½ teaspoon sea salt
½ cup dried arame or Domo Arigato Arame Salad (page 159)
2 teaspoons wheat-free tamari or other soy sauce, or to taste (optional if using arame salad)
2 teaspoons toasted sesame oil (optional if using arame salad)
4 cups assorted vegetables, chopped (try carrot, parsnip, broccoli, and/or cauliflower)
1 (15-ounce) can adzuki beans, or 1½ cups cooked (see page 102)
White and black sesame seeds

1. Place the water, rice, and salt in a 2-quart pot over high heat and bring to a boil. Cover, lower the heat to low, and cook until all the liquid is absorbed, about 45 minutes. Allow to sit for 5 minutes. Fluff with a fork.

2. Meanwhile, place the arame in a bowl with ample warm water to cover. Allow to sit until the arame is soft, about 20 minutes. Drain well. Add the tamari and toasted sesame oil and mix well. If using the arame salad, omit this step.

3. Meanwhile, place a steamer basket in a medium-size pot and fill with water until it reaches the bottom of the steamer basket. Cover, place over high heat, and bring to a boil.

4. Lower the heat to medium. Add the veggies and steam until the veggies are just tender, about 10 minutes, depending on the vegetables selected. Transfer to a bowl.

5. Place the adzuki beans in a small pot over medium-low heat. Cook until the beans are heated, about 5 minutes. Lower the heat to low.

6. Prepare your macro plate by arranging the rice, veggies, arame, and adzuki beans in a colorful palette. Garnish with sesame seeds before serving.

VARIATIONS

- Replace the brown rice with white basmati, or other grains, such as quinoa, millet, or buckwheat (see pages 100–101).

- Experiment with different veggies.

- Replace the adzuki beans with navy, black, or pinto beans or lentils.

- Add an extra cup of shredded greens, such as kale, collards, or chard, along with the veggies.

- Add roasted and sliced squash, such as kabocha, acorn, or buttercup (see page 105).

Sweet Potato Black Bean Sliders

Celebrate fall (and all the seasons, actually) with these Mexican-themed sweet potato sliders. The black bean and sweet potato combo is a perfect balance with herbs and spices to give an immediate boost to immunity and sustained energy. Not to mention, they make a lovely creative party dish. Add the ingredients listed in the variations for a spicy kick to your sliders. The optional garbanzo flour can give even more substance to your patties, and try gluten-free bread crumbs. Serve on vegan baguette slices, mushroom caps (see note), or vegan mini buns with Chipotle Mayonnaise (page 273) and all the fixings.

TOTAL YIELD: 20 OUNCES

Serving Size: 2 ounces
Number of Servings: 10
Prep Time: 15 minutes
Cook Time: 30 minutes
Total Time: 45 minutes

⅓ cup uncooked quinoa
⅔ cup water or vegetable stock (for homemade, see page 248)
1¼ teaspoons sea salt, or to taste, divided
1 large sweet potato, peeled and chopped
½ cup cooked black beans
¾ cup vegan bread crumbs
¼ cup thinly sliced green onion
2 tablespoons finely chopped fresh cilantro
2 teaspoons ground cumin
1 teaspoon wheat-free tamari or other soy sauce, or to taste (optional)
½ cup garbanzo flour (optional)
Olive or coconut oil for sautéing
Fixings: thinly sliced red onion, thinly sliced tomato, vegan cheese, sliced pickles, and your faves

1. Place the quinoa, water, and ½ teaspoon of the salt in a small pot over medium-high heat. Bring to a boil. Lower the heat to low, cover, and cook until all the liquid is dissolved, about 15 minutes. Remove from the heat and fluff with a fork. Keep covered until ready to use. This should yield about 1 cup of cooked quinoa.
2. Place the sweet potato in a separate pot, cover with water, and bring to a boil. Cook over high heat until the potato is just soft, about 20 minutes. Drain well, mash with a fork, and measure out 1½ cups for this recipe.
3. Combine the following in a large bowl and mix well: the cooked quinoa, cooked sweet potato, remaining ¾ teaspoon of sea salt, black beans, ¼ cup of the bread crumbs, green onion, cilantro, cumin, tamari, if using, and garbanzo flour, if using. If you wish, you can place this mixture in the refrigerator for 15 to 30 minutes.
4. Place the remaining ½ cup of bread crumbs in a small bowl. Form small patties of the sweet potato mixture (about ⅛ cup each) and coat with the bread crumbs.
5. Heat oil in a large sauté pan over medium-high heat. Place the patties in the pan and cook for 3 to 5 minutes on each side, until golden brown. Serve with the fixings and enjoy!

VARIATIONS

- Feel free to bake your sliders on a parchment paper–lined baking sheet in a 350°F oven for 20 minutes, flipping after 10 minutes.

- Add ¼ teaspoon of chipotle powder, ¼ teaspoon of crushed red pepper flakes, and ¼ teaspoon of ground black pepper along with the cumin.

- Replace the black beans with others, such as chickpeas or kidney or navy beans.

- For an Indian experience, add 1½ tablespoons of curry powder.

- Replace the quinoa with millet or rice (see page 101).

NOTE: FOR MUSHROOM CAPS

If serving with mushroom caps, select large cremini mushrooms and remove the stem. Be sure to form your sliders small enough that they can fit on top of the mushroom caps selected. Preheat the oven to 350°F. Place the empty mushroom caps on a baking sheet along with a small amount of water, drizzle with wheat-free tamari, and drizzle with lemon juice. Bake until just soft, 7 to 10 minutes, depending on the size of the mushrooms. Do not overcook. Remove the mushroom caps from the baking sheet and drain any liquid. To serve, place a cooked slider on top of a mushroom cap, then top with a dollop of Chipotle Mayonnaise (page 273) and a thin slice of your favorite vegan cheese. Layer on thinly sliced red onion, thinly sliced tomato, thinly sliced pickle, and a sprig of cilantro. Serve open faced, pierced with a toothpick. You can also optionally serve the sliders with a small piece of sautéed tempeh bacon as part of the fixings.

Mac n Cheez

Voted "Comfort Food of the Year" for five straight decades at the national comfort food convention, this vegan version of mac and cheese is for the child in all of us. Brazil nuts provide the right amount of selenium to support the thyroid in its hard work, while the cheez sauce ingredients have plenty of B vitamins and trace minerals to ensure a balanced mood at a cellular level. The addition of sweet green peas adds just the right touch of added protective phytosterols. For optimal creaminess, go with the coconut milk or soy milk option. Top with Smoky Mushrooms (page 254) and serve with BBQ Jackfruit (page 217), Sally's Super Simple Slaw (page 165), and a mixed green salad with dressing of choice.

TOTAL YIELD: 36 OUNCES
> Serving Size: 9 ounces
> Number of Servings: 4
> Prep Time: 10 minutes
> Cook Time: 15 minutes
> Total Time: 25 minutes

MAC CHEEZ SAUCE (MAKES 2 CUPS)
¾ cup chopped Brazil nuts or raw cashew pieces
1½ cups water, unsweetened soy milk, or coconut milk
3 tablespoons nutritional yeast
1½ teaspoons dehydrated onion
2 cloves garlic
3 tablespoons freshly squeezed lemon juice
¾ teaspoon salt, or to taste

PASTA
8 ounces uncooked elbow pasta
1 cup garden or sweet peas
¼ cup thinly sliced green onion (optional)
2 tablespoons finely chopped fresh flat-leaf parsley (optional)

1. Prepare the sauce: Place all the sauce ingredients in a blender and blend until creamy.
2. Cook the pasta according to the package instructions. Rinse and drain well.
3. Transfer to a bowl and add the sauce, peas, and green onion, if using. Mix well before serving and garnish with the parsley, if using.

VARIATIONS

- Go wild with different types of pasta, such as fusilli, penne, bowtie, and even alphabet.
- Add ¼ teaspoon of ground turmeric to the sauce for a golden color.
- Add 1 cup of shredded spinach, kale, or arugula along with the green onion.
- In a hurry? Substitute 2 cups of store-bought vegan cheese sauce for the Mac Cheez Sauce.

Thai Red Coconut Curry

Hold off on that fish sauce! This vegan version of the popular curry sauce is just as delicious (well, actually more delicious!) as the original. The red chiles in red curry paste keep your heart healthy and colds and flu away by their ability to really rev up circulation. Ginger, onion, red bell pepper, carrot, and cilantro all add further immunity-supporting and anti-inflammatory benefits. The coconut milk balances out the heat. Serve over jasmine rice or Pilau Rice (page 198) along with Miso Ginger Glazed Eggplant (page 202).

TOTAL YIELD: 16 OUNCES
  Serving Size: 8 ounces
  Number of Servings: 2
  Prep Time: 15 minutes
  Cook Time: 20 minutes
  Total Time: 35 minutes

1 tablespoon sesame oil, or 3 tablespoons water

1 cup thinly sliced yellow onion

1 tablespoon peeled and minced fresh ginger, and/or 1 tablespoon minced garlic

¾ cup thinly sliced carrot (⅛-inch slices)

¾ cup seeded and julienned red bell pepper

1 (13.5-ounce) can coconut milk

½ cup water

2 tablespoons vegan store-bought red curry paste

1½ tablespoons pure maple syrup or vegan granulated or brown sugar (optional)

1 teaspoon sea salt, or to taste

1½ tablespoons minced fresh cilantro

1. Place a large pot over medium-high heat. Heat the oil. Add the onion and cook for 2 minutes, stirring frequently. Add the ginger and carrot and cook for 3 minutes, stirring frequently. Add the bell pepper and stir well.
2. Lower the heat to medium, add the coconut milk, water, curry paste, maple syrup, if using, and salt, and cook for 15 minutes, stirring occasionally.
3. Garnish with cilantro before serving.

VARIATIONS

- Add 1 cup of cooked chickpeas along with the coconut milk.

- Be bold and add extra-firm or superfirm tofu, either roasted according to the instructions on pages 104–105 or sautéed. To sauté, place a sauté pan over medium-high heat. Add 1 tablespoon of coconut or sesame oil. Add the tofu and cook until it begins to crisp, about 7 minutes, gently stirring frequently. Add the tofu to the pot along with the veggies and gently stir well.

- Experiment with different veggies, such as snow peas, broccoli, eggplant, baby corn, asparagus, or your faves.

- Replace the coconut milk with unsweetened soy, rice, or almond milk.

- Replace the red curry paste with 1 tablespoon of curry powder or Indian Spice Mix (page 251).

Portobello Cheez Steak Stuffed Peppers

You would be hard pressed to find a street vendor near the Liberty Bell in Philly offering this plant-based version of the meat-based cheese steak . . . lovingly dubbed the "heart attack special" by many. Get your fix here with portobellos and all the veggie accompaniments—protecting your heart with plenty of potassium, magnesium, and B vitamins, including B_9 (folate), while still delivering that satisfying texture and delicious flavor you crave. Top with finely chopped flat-leaf parsley and serve with Mushroom Risotto (page 233) or Club Med Pasta Salad (page 168).

TOTAL YIELD: 4 BELL PEPPER HALVES, 8 OUNCES FILLING
  Serving Size: ½ bell pepper, 2 ounces filling
  Number of Servings: 4
  Prep Time: 10 minutes
  Cook Time: 30 minutes
  Total Time: 40 minutes

2 red, green, yellow, or orange bell peppers, or a combo

1 to 2 tablespoons olive oil, or ¼ cup water

1 cup thinly sliced yellow onion

3 to 4 cloves pressed or minced garlic

2 portobello mushrooms, gills removed and discarded, cut into ¼-inch slices (about 3 cups)

½ teaspoon sea salt, or to taste

¹⁄₁₆ teaspoon ground black pepper

¼ teaspoon smoked paprika or liquid smoke

1 tablespoon vegan steak sauce

¼ cup grated vegan cheese, or homemade (page 179)

1. Preheat the oven to 350°F. Slice the peppers in half lengthwise and remove the seeds. Lightly baste the peppers with oil and place on a baking sheet. You can omit the oil at this phase, if you wish. Roast for 20 minutes. Remove from the oven.

2. Meanwhile, place the remaining oil in a medium-size sauté pan over medium-high heat. Add the onion and cook for 3 minutes, stirring frequently and adding small amounts of water if necessary to prevent sticking. Add the garlic, portobello mushrooms, salt, and black pepper, and cook, stirring frequently, and chopping the portobello as you stir, until the portobellos are tender, about 5 minutes. Add the smoked paprika and steak sauce and mix well.

3. Transfer about ¼ cup of this mixture to each bell pepper half. Top with 1 tablespoon of vegan cheese per pepper and return the pan to the oven. Bake until the vegan cheese is melted, about 10 minutes.

VARIATIONS

- Replace the portobellos with chopped tempeh, tofu, or seitan.

- Go Mexican: Use poblano peppers instead of bell peppers. Add 1 tablespoon of Mexican Spice Mix (page 252) along with the salt, and add 1 tablespoon of minced fresh cilantro with the steak sauce. Top with vegan Jack cheese.

Mushroom Risotto

If you look closely at the ceiling of the Sistine Chapel, you may see an image of the cherubs dining on this creamy rice dish that is a staple in northern Italy. Typically made with arborio rice and continually stirred for optimum creaminess, it's the reason that Italian grandmothers have such strong flexor muscles. Savor the flavors and comfort, while enjoying the benefits of incredibly immunity-modulating beta-glucans, the healing compounds found in all edible mushrooms. Serve with Herb-Roasted Tofu (page 220) and Arugula Walnut Salad with Cashew Dill Dressing (page 161).

TOTAL YIELD: 24 OUNCES
   Serving Size: 8 ounces
   Number of Servings: 3
   Prep Time: 10 minutes
   Cook Time: 25 minutes
   Total Time: 35 minutes

3½ cups vegetable stock (for homemade, see page 248) or water

2 tablespoons olive oil, or ¼ cup water, divided

½ cup diced shallots

¾ teaspoon sea salt, or to taste, divided

½ teaspoon Italian Spice Mix (page 251, or store-bought)

⅛ teaspoon ground black pepper

¾ cup uncooked arborio rice

⅓ cup white wine (optional)

1½ cups thinly sliced mushrooms (try shiitake, cremini, and/or button)

Pinch of ground nutmeg (optional)

2½ tablespoons nutritional yeast

1½ tablespoons finely chopped fresh flat-leaf parsley

1. Place the vegetable stock in a medium-size pot over high heat. Bring to a boil. Lower the heat to low.

2. Place a large sauté pan over medium-high heat. Heat 1 tablespoon of the oil. Add the shallots, ½ teaspoon of the salt, and the Italian Spice Mix and pepper, and cook for 2 minutes, stirring constantly. Add the rice and the wine, if using, and cook for 2 minutes, stirring constantly. Lower the heat to medium.

3. Add ½ to ¾ cup of the warmed vegetable stock to the rice mixture and cook,

continues

stirring constantly, until the liquid is absorbed. Repeat until all the stock is used and the rice is just tender, about 20 minutes.

4. Meanwhile, place a small sauté pan over medium-high heat. Heat the remaining tablespoon of oil. Add the mushrooms, the nutmeg, if using, and the remaining ¼ teaspoon of salt and cook until the mushrooms are just tender, about 7 minutes, stirring frequently and adding small amounts of water if necessary to prevent sticking.

5. When the rice is done cooking, add the cooked mushrooms and the nutritional yeast and mix well. Garnish with the parsley before serving.

VARIATIONS

- Add ¼ teaspoon of crushed red pepper flakes along with the salt.

- Replace the mushrooms with spinach or other veggies, such as roasted squash or asparagus.

- You might get kicked out of the Vatican, but you can use a quick-cook method to cook the arborio rice. Place the following in a pot over high heat: the rice, 2½ cups of vegetable stock, and ½ teaspoon salt. Bring to a boil. Cover, lower the heat to low, and cook until all the liquid is absorbed, about 20 minutes. Remove from the heat and allow to sit for 10 minutes. Fluff with a fork. Add all the ingredients that are added to the rice in step 2 and mix well. Proceed to step 4.

- Indulge and add ½ cup of shredded vegan-style mozzarella or 2 tablespoons of vegan butter along with the parsley. Mix well before serving.

Quinoa Quiche

This quiche is actually a version of a Monk Bowl (see page 209), with quinoa as the grain, chickpeas as the protein, and spinach and tomato for the veggies. Huge on protein, iron, calcium, and all the important vitamins, this is certainly a vitality-building meal. Serve with a large salad and dressing of choice, or enjoy with a side of Sunny Kale Salad (page 162) and Baked Sesame Zucchini Fries (page 193).

TOTAL YIELD: 40 OUNCES FILLING,
1 (9½-INCH) PIE

> Serving Size: 1 slice
> Number of Servings: 8
> Prep Time: 15 minutes
> Cook Time: 60 minutes
> Total Time: 1 hour 15 minutes

1 vegan piecrust (page 236, or store-bought unsweetened crust)

1 cup water or vegetable stock (for homemade, see page 248)

½ cup uncooked quinoa

1½ teaspoons sea salt, divided

1 cup cooked chickpeas (see page 102)

1 cup finely chopped spinach or arugula

1 cup halved cherry tomatoes

1 cup chopped artichoke hearts

1 tablespoon Italian Spice Mix (page 251, or store-bought)

¼ teaspoon ground black pepper

Pinch of crushed red pepper flakes (optional)

1. Preheat the oven to 350°F. Poke a few holes in the bottom of the piecrust with a fork. Place the piecrust in the oven and bake for 5 minutes. Remove from the oven.

2. Meanwhile, place the water, quinoa, and ½ teaspoon of the salt in a small pot over high heat. Bring to a boil. Cover, lower the heat to low, and cook until all the liquid is absorbed, about 15 minutes. Allow to sit for 5 minutes.

3. Transfer to a bowl along with the remaining ingredients and mix well. Transfer to the piecrust, return the pie to the oven, and bake for 45 minutes.

VARIATIONS

> Add ½ cup of vegan cheese along with the artichoke hearts—highly recommended!

> Add ½ cup of cooked butternut squash along with the artichoke hearts.

> Replace the quinoa with millet or rice (see page 101).

Polenta Piecrust

A unique twist on the age-old piecrust, this version uses polenta to create an oil-free crust for your savory pie needs. If you don't have oat flour, don't worry! You can place rolled oats in a blender and blend until a flour is formed. High-fiber and mineral-boosting grains make this crust an energy-sustaining base for your favorite fillings. Use with Quinoa Quiche (page 235) and other savory pies. See the variations for a version you can use for The Great Pumpkin Cheez-cake (page 294).

TOTAL YIELD: 1 (9½-INCH) PIECRUST
  Serving Size: 1 slice
  Number of Servings: 8
  Prep Time: 10 minutes
  Cook Time: 55 minutes
  Cool Down Time: 10 minutes
  Total Time: 1 hour 15 minutes

3½ cups water

½ teaspoon sea salt, or to taste

1 cup polenta

¼ cup oat flour

1½ tablespoons Italian Spice Mix (page 251, or store-bought)

Oil for pie dish and basting crust (optional)

Melted vegan butter for basting crust (optional)

1. Preheat the oven to 375°F. Place the water and salt in a 2-quart pot and bring to a boil. Lower the heat to medium and carefully stir in the polenta. Cook for 10 minutes, stirring frequently and lowering the heat to low if necessary to prevent the polenta from bubbling up. (The worst burn Mark received in the kitchen was from polenta bubbling up . . . so be careful!) Add the oat flour and Italian Spice Mix, and mix well. Allow to cool until cool enough to handle.

2. Lightly oil a 9½-inch pie dish. (Or you can use a nonstick one, for an oil-free version.) Place the polenta mixture in the pie dish and using a spatula, or your hands if it's cool enough, press about the polenta to a ¼-inch depth along the bottom and sides of the dish. You can optionally baste the polenta at this point with olive oil or melted vegan butter.

3. Place in the oven and bake for 45 minutes. The crust will firm up the more it cools.

VARIATIONS

- Add ¼ cup of vegan butter or coconut oil along with polenta.

- For your sweet pies, add ¼ cup of vegan granulated sugar plus ½ teaspoon of ground cinnamon and ¼ teaspoon of ground nutmeg, or ¾ teaspoon of pumpkin pie spice.

Papas, Bean, and Greens Burritos

Papas means "potatoes," and in this case, papas refers to the potato tots (yes, tots!) that are included in this epic fiesta. This balanced meal of veggies, protein, and starch offers nutrition and satisfaction, perfected with an extra healthy boost from avocado. Add a dollop of Vegan Sour Cream (page 274) or Quick Cashew Cheese (page 179) and such fixings as diced red onion and cilantro sprigs to your burrito and serve with chips and Daikon with Avo Goddess Dressing (see page 160).

TOTAL YIELD: 4 BURRITOS
Serving Size: 1 burrito
Number of Servings: 4
Prep Time: 10 minutes
Cook Time: 20 minutes
Total Time: 30 minutes

20 ounces frozen potato tots or puffs (about 2 cups)
1 (15-ounce) can black beans, or 1½ cups cooked (see page 102)
1 teaspoon chili powder
Sea salt and ground black pepper
Wheat-free tamari or other soy sauce (optional)
2 cups chopped broccoli, zucchini, kale, cabbage, or green beans
4 large tortillas
½ cup salsa or chopped tomato
1 large avocado, peeled, pitted, and cut into thin slices

1. Cook the potato tots according to the package instructions. Set aside.
2. Meanwhile, place the beans and chili powder in a small pot over low heat. Add a pinch each of salt and pepper, and a splash of tamari, if using, and cook for 5 minutes, stirring frequently.
3. Place a steamer basket in a medium-size pot and fill with water until it reaches the bottom of the steamer basket. Cover, place over high heat, and bring to a boil.
4. Lower the heat to medium. Add the veggies and cook until just tender, about 5 minutes, depending on the vegetables selected. Transfer to a bowl. Be sure to drain off any excess water.
5. Lay out a tortilla. (Optionally, first warm the tortilla on a dry sauté pan over high heat until just warmed through.) Pretend there is an imaginary line going across

continues

continued

the center of the burrito. You are going to build the burrito, on and just under this line. Place about ½ cup of baked tots in the center of the tortilla. Smash down with a spoon or fork. Add one-quarter of the beans, veggies, salsa, and avocado.

6. Prepare to roll. First, pray to the burrito gods that your efforts will be successful. Once the burrito gods are appeased, proceed to the next step.

7. Fold the unfilled section beneath the line of filling to just cover the filling (not all the way across to the far edge). Then, one at a time, fold the sides of the tortilla toward the center. Once both sides are folded, proceed to tightly roll the burrito away from you. Voilà! Wasn't that easy! (Now you see why praying to the burrito gods was important.) Don't worry . . . it gets easier with practice!

8. Repeat rolling process for all four burritos.

VARIATIONS

- Add ½ teaspoon of ground cumin along with the chili powder.

- Add ¼ cup of shredded vegan cheese to the burrito before rolling.

- Replace the tots with cooked rice or quinoa (see page 101).

- Add ¼ cup of Jackfruit Taco Filling (page 216) to each burrito before rolling.

- For a **Breakfast Burrito**, add ½ cup of Tofu Rancheros (page 137) to each burrito and reduce the quantity or eliminate the black beans, depending on the size of the tortilla.

- Replace the black beans with pinto, navy, or kidney beans.

Hummus Panini with Balsamic Massaged Kale

Proteins, minerals, vitamins, and phytonutrients abound in this sandwich heaven. You can replace the hummus with Pepita Pesto with Avocado (page 265) or Cheezy Artichoke Dip (page 205) and serve with Smoky Truffled Baked Broccoli Fries (page 180), Baked Sesame Zucchini Fries (page 193), and a small side salad with dressing.

TOTAL YIELD: 2 PANINI
>   Serving Size: 1 panino
>   Number of Servings: 2
>   Prep Time: 15 minutes
>   Cook Time: 5 minutes
>   Total Time: 20 minutes

BALSAMIC MASSAGED KALE

1 cup shredded kale

2 teaspoons olive oil, or 1 tablespoon mashed avocado

1 teaspoon balsamic vinegar

1 teaspoon pure maple syrup (optional)

¼ teaspoon Dijon mustard (optional)

Pinch of sea salt

¼ cup vegan mayonnaise (for homemade, see page 273) or Sriracha Aioli (page 275) (optional)

2 ciabatta rolls or focaccia bread pieces, sliced in half horizontally

1 cup Garlicky Hummus (page 194, or store-bought)

4 thin slices red onion

2 thin slices tomato

½ avocado, peeled and cut into thin slices

Olive oil or melted vegan butter, for basting (optional)

1. Massage the kale: Place the kale in a bowl. Place the olive oil, balsamic vinegar, maple syrup, if using, Dijon mustard, if using, and salt in another small dish and whisk well.
2. Add to the kale and massage with clean hands until the kale softens and turns a dark green color. (Alternatively simply use shredded kale in the panini.)
3. Spread the vegan mayonnaise or aioli, if using, on the cut sides of each roll. Top the bottom of each roll with hummus, then onion, tomato, avocado, and kale. Top with the top piece of the roll.
4. Heat a panini press. You can optionally baste each assembled roll with olive oil or vegan butter on both sides before pressing. Place in the press and hold down with pressure on top of roll for 3 minutes, or until the roll is slightly toasted. Slice in half before enjoying.

VARIATIONS

- Experiment with different types of store-bought hummus and the variations listed in the Garlicky Hummus recipe (page 194).

- Replace the kale with mixed greens, spinach, chard, or arugula.

- Build out your panini by adding Smoky Mushrooms (page 254) and a slice of vegan cheese.

- If you do indulge in vegan lunch meats, we won't look if you add a few slices of that as well.

- Replace the rolls with tortillas or bread.

Braised Mushroom Stroganoff

When the desire for comfort food strikes, and the need for a health boost accompanies—mushrooms to the rescue! Even better with the added powers of onion, garlic, spices, and herbs to keep both immunity and mood balanced. Serve over rice, quinoa, or flat noodles (see variations). Top with Vegan Sour Cream (page 274) and serve with Braised Kale with Shallots and Slivered Almonds (page 185).

TOTAL YIELD: 40 OUNCES

    Serving Size: 8 ounces
    Number of Servings: 5
    Prep Time: 15 minutes
    Cook Time: 25 minutes
    Total Time: 40 minutes

3 tablespoons flour, such as a gluten-free flour blend (for homemade, see page 254), spelt, whole wheat pastry, or unbleached all-purpose

2½ tablespoons olive oil or water, divided

1 cup thinly sliced yellow onion

4 to 5 cloves garlic, pressed or minced

1½ teaspoons Herbes de Provence Spice Mix (page 250, or store-bought)

16 ounces cremini mushrooms, quartered (about 5 cups)

1½ teaspoons sea salt, or to taste

¼ teaspoon crushed red pepper flakes (optional)

⅛ teaspoon ground black pepper

½ cup red wine (optional)

2½ cups water or vegetable stock (for homemade, see page 248)

½ cup vegan mayonnaise (for homemade, see page 273) (optional)

3 tablespoons finely chopped flat-leaf parsley

1. Create a roux by combining the flour with 1½ tablespoons of olive oil in a small bowl and mix well, adding a small amount of water if necessary to remove any clumps of flour.

2. Place a medium-size pot or sauté pan over medium-high heat. Heat the remaining tablespoon of the olive oil. Add the onion, garlic, Herbes de Provence Spice Mix, mushrooms, salt, red pepper flakes, if using, and black pepper, and cook for 5 minutes, stirring frequently and adding small amounts of water or vegetable stock if necessary to prevent sticking. Add the red wine, if using, and cook for 2 minutes, stirring frequently.

3. Add the water, lower the heat to medium, and cook for 15 minutes, stirring occasionally. Add some of this cooking liquid to the roux and stir well. Add the roux as well as the vegan mayonnaise, if using, to the pot, and cook for 3 minutes, or until the liquid in the pot begins to thicken, stirring frequently. Add the parsley and stir well before serving.

VARIATIONS

- Add ⅛ teaspoon of ground nutmeg along with the mushrooms.

- Replace the mushrooms with 14 ounces of cubed extra-firm or superfirm tofu, or 8 ounces of cubed tempeh (optionally roasted; see pages 104–105).

- For the traditional flat noodles served with stroganoff, cook 12 ounces of dried pasta to yield 6 cups of cooked pasta.

- Add 2 tablespoons of vegan butter along with the parsley, if you feel like indulging.

Roasted Butternut Squash Penne with Sage

A favorite of pastaterians everywhere, the butternut squash adds a creamy and buttery flavor while the earthiness of the sage brings it all home. In addition to flavor bliss, butternut plus plenty of herbs is always an immunity-happy combo. For a gluten-free dish, use a rice pasta. Serve with Arugula Walnut Salad with Cashew Dill Dressing (page 161) and Cashew Cheese–Stuffed Sweet Peppers (page 179).

TOTAL YIELD: 48 OUNCES
> Serving Size: 12 ounces
> Number of Servings: 4
> Prep Time: 10 minutes
> Cook Time: 30 minutes
> Total Time: 40 minutes

10 ounces frozen butternut squash

3½ tablespoons olive oil, or ¼ cup water, divided

1 teaspoon sea salt, divided

¼ teaspoon ground black pepper, divided

8 ounces penne rigate (try rice pasta)

1½ tablespoons minced garlic

½ teaspoon Italian Spice Mix (page 251, or store-bought)

⅛ teaspoon crushed red pepper flakes (optional)

2 tablespoons chiffonaded fresh sage or basil

2 tablespoons nutritional yeast

1½ tablespoons finely chopped fresh flat-leaf parsley

1. Preheat the oven to 400°F. Place the butternut squash, 1½ tablespoons olive oil, ¼ teaspoon of the salt, and ⅛ teaspoon of the black pepper on a baking sheet and mix well. Place in the oven and roast for 30 minutes or until squash is browned.

2. Meanwhile, bring a pot of water, optionally salted with 1 teaspoon of salt, to a boil. Add the penne and cook until just tender, 6 to 8 minutes, or according to the package instructions. Rinse and drain well.

3. Meanwhile, combine the remaining olive oil, garlic, Italian Spice Mix, remaining ¾ teaspoon of salt, remaining ⅛ teaspoon of black pepper, crushed red pepper flakes, if using, in a small pot over low heat and cook for 10 minutes, stirring occasionally. Add the sage and nutritional yeast and cook for 5 minutes, stirring occasionally.

4. Place all the ingredients in a large bowl and gently toss well. Garnish with the parsley before serving.

VARIATIONS

- Replace the penne with your favorite pasta, such as angel hair, rotini, or fettuccine.

- Replace the butternut squash with other squash, such as acorn, kabocha, or buttercup.

- Replace the butternut squash with roasted sweet potatoes or Rainbow Roasted Roots (page 196).

- Replace the olive oil with vegan butter.

- Add ½ teaspoon of minced fresh rosemary and 2 teaspoons of minced fresh oregano or marjoram along with the sage.

Brats and Kraut

A plant-based version of what is aptly called *Wurst* (worst for your health that is!), vegan sausages actually are a thing. Add some good-for-your-gut sauerkraut and fresh arugula, with mood-balancing olives and lighter rice noodles, and we say, "Why not?!" Serve on its own or drizzle with Oil-Free Roasted Red Pepper Dressing (page 170) or Zesty Lemon Sriracha Dressing (page 171), alongside a glass of Tart Cherry and Pomegranate Tonic (page 115).

TOTAL YIELD: 40 OUNCES
   Serving Size: 10 ounces
   Number of Servings: 4
   Prep Time: 10 minutes
   Cook Time: 20 minutes
   Total Time: 30 minutes

6 ounces thin rice noodles (2 cups cooked)

1 tablespoon olive oil, or ¼ cup water

14 ounces vegan sausage (try Field Roast, Tofurky, or Beyond Sausage brand), cut into ½-inch slices

2 cups baby arugula

¼ cup chopped kalamata olives or your favorites

¼ cup sauerkraut or Ruby Kraut (page 259)

2 tablespoons hemp or flaxseed oil (optional)

1½ tablespoons stone-ground, Dijon, or yellow mustard

2 tablespoons nutritional yeast

1. Cook the noodles according to the package instructions. Rinse and drain well. Set aside.
2. Meanwhile, place a small sauté pan over medium-high heat. Heat the oil. Add the vegan sausage and cook for 5 minutes, stirring frequently and adding small amounts of water or vegetable stock if necessary to avoid sticking. Set aside.
3. Place the arugula in a large bowl. Add the noodles, vegan sausage, olives, sauerkraut, hemp oil, if using, and mustard, and mix well. Top with the nutritional yeast before serving.

VARIATIONS

- Add 2 tablespoons of finely chopped fresh flat-leaf parsley or cilantro along with the arugula.

- Replace the arugula with spinach or mixed organic greens.

- For a gluten-free version, replace the vegan sausage with 14 ounces of extra-firm tofu or 8 ounces of cubed tempeh.

- Replace the rice noodles with another form of pasta, or rice, quinoa, or millet (see page 101).

Pecan Sage Holiday Loaf

What better way to express our gratitude for the bounty of nature than by creating a plant-based centerpiece for our holiday feasts? You, too, can pardon a turkey and serve this satisfying, savory and nutty loaf instead. The sage adds a savory aromatic flavor, helpful with digestion of proteins. The pecan is a perfect warming and sweet choice for maintaining immunity and mood-boosting, with essential fats and B vitamins as well as antioxidant beta-carotene. We recommend using all the optional ingredients for the ultimate loaf experience! Serve with Mushroom Leek Gravy (page 276), Braised Kale with Shallots and Slivered Almonds (page 185), and Lemony Herbed Cauliflower Roast (page 211) with Cranberry Apricot Sauce with Crystallized Ginger (page 268). Save room for The Great Pumpkin Cheezcake (page 294).

TOTAL YIELD: 60 OUNCES
Serving Size: 10 ounces
Number of Servings: 6
Prep Time: 10 minutes
Cook Time: 1 hour 30 minutes
Total Time: 1 hour 40 minutes

1 cup uncooked brown rice

2¾ cups vegetable stock (for homemade, see page 248) or water

2 teaspoons sea salt, or to taste

1 tablespoon olive oil, plus more for casserole dish, or 3 tablespoons water

1 cup diced yellow onion

¾ cup thinly sliced celery

5 cloves garlic, pressed or minced (optional)

1 cup finely chopped pecans, optionally toasted in a 350°F oven for 10 minutes

1 (15-ounce) can chickpeas, liquid reserved, or 1½ cups cooked (see page 102)

2 tablespoons minced fresh sage

2 tablespoons finely chopped fresh flat-leaf parsley (optional)

1 tablespoon Italian Spice Mix (page 251, or store-bought)

¼ teaspoon ground black pepper

1½ tablespoons wheat-free tamari or other soy sauce (optional)

1 teaspoon smoked paprika, or ¼ teaspoon crushed red pepper flakes (optional)

½ cup vegan gluten-free bread crumbs (optional)

1. Preheat the oven to 350°F. Place the rice, vegetable stock, and ½ teaspoon of sea salt in a 2-quart pot over medium-high heat. Bring to a boil. Lower the heat to a simmer, cover, and cook until all the liquid is absorbed, about 45 minutes.

2. Meanwhile, heat a small sauté pan over medium-high heat. Heat the oil. Add the onion, celery, and ½ teaspoon salt and cook for 3 minutes, stirring frequently and adding small amounts of water if necessary to prevent sticking. Add the garlic, if using, and cook for 3 minutes, stirring frequently.

3. Transfer to a bowl along with remaining ingredients, except the oil, and including the remaining 1 teaspoon of salt, and mix well. Add the cooked rice and stir well.

4. Transfer to a well-oiled or nonstick 8 by 8-inch casserole dish and press down firmly. Top with the bread crumbs, if using, and bake for 40 minutes.

5. Remove from the oven and allow to cool slightly before slicing and serving.

VARIATIONS

- For an oil-free version, omit the oil and use ¼ water or vegetable stock (for homemade, see page 248) to sauté the onion, celery, and garlic.

- Add 1 cup of diced mushrooms along with the onion and celery.

- Add ½ teaspoon of minced fresh rosemary and 2 tablespoons of nutritional yeast with the sage.

- Add one 15-ounce can of pure pumpkin puree and/or cooked lentils along with the pecans.

SIXTEEN

CUTTING-EDGE CONDIMENTS AND SAUCES

So often, the flavor of a memorable dish all comes down to the accoutrements. In this chapter, we reveal the delicious secret—it's all about the sauce. Such sauces as Smoky Sweet Chili Garlic Sauce (page 263), EZ Cheez Sauce (page 271), Apricot BBQ Sauce (page 269), and Artful Almond Sauce (page 270) are versatile tools in your vegan arsenal. Pour them over steamed veggies (see page 106), roasted or grilled veggies, Savory Baked Seitan (page 225), or roasted tofu and tempeh (see pages 104–105).

When it comes to condiments, black is the new green. Your guests will be thoroughly impressed when you break out the Black Sesame Gomasio (pages 104–105).

We are also including some core condiment recipes from our companion book, *Healing the Vegan Way*. Be sure to create your own Salt-Free Seasoning (page 253), Global Spice Blends (pages 249–252), and Vegan Sour Cream (page 274), both a cooked and raw version.

And did you ever imagine you could be making your own jam (Chia Peach Pepper Jam, page 258), or yogurt (Coconut Yogurt, page 262)? How

> ## TIMELESS TIPS: CONDIMENT AND SAUCÉ HACKS
>
> One of the biggest quick and easy kitchen hacks is to create your own Global Spice Blends. This is crucial for the seven-ingredient kitchen, as one blend can deliver on several flavors at once. Make your own, or stock up on store-bought varieties.
>
> Keep a stock of your favorite condiments and sauces on hand. Nutritional yeast, which lends a cheeselike flavor to foods and is a good source of vitamin B_{12} and protein, is a top condiment we always travel with.

about homemade pickled vegetables (Pickled Red Onion, page 261) or sauerkraut (Ruby Kraut, page 259). Welcome to the new you!

Soup Stock

Bring depth to your soups and stews, and even your grain dishes. You can use your stock in any savory recipe that calls for water, including the water sauté method discussed on page 106.

Avoid the packaging and potential for lots of sodium in store-bought versions by creating your own.

For a simple soup stock, save the clippings and scraps of vegetables used in preparing other recipes. Place them in a large, heavy-bottomed stockpot over low heat with water to cover and simmer until all the veggies are completely cooked. Cook until the liquid is reduced to 75 to 50 percent of the original volume. The vegetables' flavor will be imparted to the broth. Experiment with different vegetables and herbs until you discover your favorite combinations. In general, you are looking to create a relatively neutral stock that can be used for all of your soup needs. Strain well, and add salt and freshly ground pepper to taste to the liquid.

Try using trimmings from potatoes, celery, carrots, tomatoes, onions, parsley, mushrooms, parsnips, zucchini, leeks, corn cobs, and garlic. Many avoid using vegetables that become bitter, such as bell peppers, radishes, turnips, broccoli, cauliflower, and Brussels sprouts.

Small amounts of herbs, such as parsley, are okay. You can use a few sprigs of other herbs, such as thyme, fennel, oregano, dill, basil, or marjoram. Keep in mind that too much of these herbs can overpower the stock. Also, be sure to add them toward the end of the cooking process, to avoid bitterness. The stock may be frozen and defrosted for future use. You can even pour it into ice cube trays, freeze, and use as needed.

If you find that you do not have so many trimmings to use, you can keep a bag or small bucket in the freezer to save the trimmings. Once you have enough accumulated to fill a stockpot, get your soup stock going.

Global Spice Blends

Spice blends allow you to create global variations to your dishes. Start by adding a small amount of the blend and increase the quantity to taste. Remember that it will take some time for the flavors to absorb, so use sparingly at first.

Cajun Spice Mix

TOTAL YIELD: 4 OUNCES
  Serving Size: 1½ teaspoons
  Number of Servings: 16
  Prep Time: 5 minutes
  Total Time: 5 minutes

1½ tablespoons paprika
1½ tablespoons chili powder
1½ teaspoons ground black pepper
1½ teaspoons onion powder
1½ teaspoons garlic powder
1½ teaspoons dried thyme leaves
1½ teaspoons ground coriander
1½ teaspoons dried basil (optional)
1½ teaspoons dried oregano
½ teaspoon cayenne pepper (optional)

Place all the ingredients in a medium-size bowl and mix well. Store in a glass jar and use within 1 month.

Ethiopian Spice Mix, a.k.a. Berbere

TOTAL YIELD: 4 OUNCES
　Serving Size: 1½ teaspoons
　Number of Servings: 16
　Prep Time: 5 minutes
　Total Time: 5 minutes

2 tablespoons paprika
2 tablespoons ground ginger
1 tablespoon ground coriander (optional)
1½ teaspoons ground allspice
1½ teaspoons ground cinnamon
1½ teaspoons ground fenugreek (optional)
¾ teaspoon ground nutmeg
¾ teaspoon ground cloves
¾ teaspoon cayenne pepper

Place all the ingredients in a medium-size bowl and mix well. Store in a glass jar and use within 1 month.

Herbes de Provence Spice Mix

Create your own blend of this classic French herb combination. Feel free to leave out an ingredient or two (or three), if necessary. You can even experiment with different quantities of the same ingredients, based upon your personal preference.

TOTAL YIELD: 6 OUNCES
　Serving Size: 1½ teaspoons
　Number of Servings: 24
　Prep Time: 5 minutes
　Total Time: 5 minutes

2 tablespoons dried thyme
2 tablespoons dried summer savory (optional)
2 tablespoons dried marjoram
1 tablespoon dried rosemary
1 tablespoon dried tarragon
1 tablespoon dried oregano
1 tablespoon dried basil
1 tablespoon dried sage
2 teaspoons crushed culinary-grade lavender flowers (optional)
2 teaspoons fennel seeds (optional)

Place all the ingredients in a medium-size bowl and mix well. Store in a glass jar and use within 1 month.

Indian Spice Mix

TOTAL YIELD: 4 OUNCES
    Serving Size: 1½ teaspoons
    Number of Servings: 16
    Prep Time: 5 minutes
    Total Time: 5 minutes

3 tablespoons curry powder

2 tablespoons ground cumin (optionally toasted; see page 106)

1 tablespoon ground coriander

1 tablespoon brown mustard or fennel seeds

1 teaspoon ground ginger

½ teaspoon ground cardamom

¼ teaspoon ground cloves

Place all the ingredients in a medium-size bowl and mix well. Store in a glass jar and use within 1 month.

Italian Spice Mix

TOTAL YIELD: 4 OUNCES
    Serving Size: 1½ teaspoons
    Number of Servings: 16
    Prep Time: 5 minutes
    Total Time: 5 minutes

3 tablespoons dried basil

2 tablespoons dried marjoram

1 tablespoon dried oregano

1 tablespoon dried sage

2 teaspoons dried thyme

1 teaspoon garlic powder

Place all the ingredients in a medium-size bowl and mix well. Store in a glass jar and use within 1 month.

Mexican Spice Mix

TOTAL YIELD: 4 OUNCES
    Serving Size: 1½ teaspoons
    Number of Servings: 16
    Prep Time: 5 minutes
    Total Time: 5 minutes

¼ cup chili powder
2 tablespoons ground cumin (optionally toasted; see page 106)
1 tablespoon dried oregano
½ teaspoon ground cinnamon
½ teaspoon chipotle powder

Place all the ingredients in a medium-size bowl and mix well. Store in a glass jar and use within 1 month.

Moroccan Spice Mix

TOTAL YIELD: 4 OUNCES
    Serving Size: 1½ teaspoons
    Number of Servings: 16
    Prep Time: 5 minutes
    Total Time: 5 minutes

2 tablespoons ground cumin
2 tablespoons ground coriander
1½ tablespoons paprika
1 tablespoon ground turmeric
1 teaspoon ground ginger
1 teaspoon ground cinnamon
1 teaspoon ground allspice
½ teaspoon cayenne pepper (optional)

Place all the ingredients in a medium-size bowl and mix well. Store in a glass jar and use within 1 month.

Salt-Free Seasoning

From *Healing the Vegan Way*

Are you on a sodium-restricted diet? This salt-free seasoning includes naturally salty celery and sea vegetables. Use whenever salt is called for in a recipe.

TOTAL YIELD: 2 OUNCES
Serving Size: ½ teaspoon
Number of Servings: 24
Prep Time: 5 minutes
Total Time: 5 minutes

¼ cup kelp granules
1 teaspoon celery seeds
1 teaspoon onion powder
1 teaspoon garlic powder
½ teaspoon freshly ground black pepper

Place all the ingredients in a medium-size bowl and mix well. Store in a glass jar and use within 1 month.

Black Sesame Gomasio

This is not proven scientifically, but a friend swears that his hair is regaining its color after eating 1 tablespoon of black sesame seeds a day. This may be because the black ones have a significant amount of the trace mineral copper, which has a role in the continued production of melanin in the body. Black sesame seeds are also a great way to get a little boost of bone-protective calcium and magnesium, and healthy fiber. Sprinkle on dishes whenever salt is called for, to give an extra mineral boost. We love it on toast and on salads.

TOTAL YIELD: 4 OUNCES
Serving Size: 1 teaspoon
Number of Servings: 24
Prep Time: 5 minutes
Total Time: 5 minutes

½ cup black sesame seeds
½ teaspoon sea salt

Combine the sesame seeds and salt in a blender or coffee grinder and pulse a few times so some of the seeds are pulverized and most remain whole. Store in a glass jar at room temperature and use within 1 month.

VARIATIONS
- Change the black sesame seeds to brown or white or a combination.
- Experiment with different types of salt, such as smoked salt.

Gluten-Free Flour Mix

Use this blend to replace wheat flour in the recipes. Combine these gluten-free flours and starches in the following ratio: 1 part sorghum flour; 1 part fine brown rice flour; 1 part tapioca flour (the same as tapioca starch) or ½ part potato starch (not potato flour), and ½ part tapioca flour or arrowroot powder.

Total Time: 5 minutes

1. Combine these gluten-free flours and starches in the above ratio, to obtain the necessary quantity of flour substitute.
2. When using this mix to replace wheat flour, add ¼ teaspoon of xanthan or guar gum for each cup of flour for cookies, and ½ teaspoon per cup of flour for cakes and brownies.

Smoky Mushrooms

We would like to introduce you to the bacon of the fungi kingdom, the virtues of which are extolled by Babe, Wilbur, and Porky Pig, among many others. Enjoy the earthy goodness of this amazing food in a tasty, fun, and versatile condiment. Warning: These are highly addictive and since the mushrooms cook down, you may want to double or triple the batch! If you have the time, and want some seriously addictive crispy mushrooms, keep them in the oven (on the middle rack) for 2 to 2½ hours instead of the 60 minutes called for in the recipe. Serve over Black-Eye Cabbage (page 212), Smashed Avocado Toast Supreme (page 127), Braised Kale with Shallots and Slivered Almonds (page 185), and as part of a MLT that includes lettuce, tomato, and Sriracha Aioli (page 275).

TOTAL YIELD: 8 OUNCES
Serving Size: 1 ounce
Number of Servings: 8
Prep Time: 10 minutes
Marinate Time: 10 minutes
Cook Time: 60 minutes
Total Time: 1 hour 20 minutes

8 ounces cremini mushrooms, cleaned well with stem on, thinly sliced into about 1/16-inch slices (about 3 cups)

2 tablespoons warm water

2 teaspoons wheat-free tamari or other soy sauce

1 tablespoon olive or coconut oil, or an extra tablespoon of water

1½ teaspoons liquid smoke

2 teaspoons pure maple syrup

1 teaspoon raw apple cider vinegar

1 teaspoon garlic powder

1 teaspoon onion granules

⅛ teaspoon sea salt, or to taste

⅛ teaspoon cayenne pepper (optional)

⅛ teaspoon ground black pepper

1. Preheat the oven to 250°F. Remove the very bottom portion of the stem of the mushrooms if dirty. Place in a shallow bowl.
2. Place all the remaining ingredients in a small bowl and whisk well. Add to the mushrooms and coat well. Marinate for 10 minutes.
3. Transfer to the oven and bake for 60 minutes, stirring occasionally.

VARIATIONS

- For a lower-sodium version, use a low-sodium tamari or other soy sauce.
- Replace the mushrooms with an equivalent amount of medium-soft coconut meat.
- Replace the mushrooms with large dried coconut flakes and cook until crispy, about 10 minutes.

Marinades

Creating marinades is a key technique in vegan food preparation, especially when working with tofu, which will take on the flavor of the marinade. Place vegetables and tofu in the marinade for a minimum of ten minutes. The longer they sit in the marinade, the more of its flavors they will acquire. These are simple marinades that make enough for 14 ounces of tofu or tempeh or two servings of vegetables.

Use the following recipes as a starting point to create a vast array of flavorful marinades. Some of our go-to marinade ingredients include toasted sesame oil, mirin, stone-ground or Dijon mustard, brown rice vinegar, horseradish, minced garlic or ginger, pure maple syrup, balsamic vinegar, red or white wine, sherry, liquid smoke, truffle oil, hot sauce, sriracha, and a variety of spices and herbs.

Smoky Maple Marinade

TOTAL YIELD: 4 OUNCES
    Serving Size: 4 ounces
    Number of Servings: 1
    Prep Time: 5 minutes
    Total Time: 5 minutes

¼ cup filtered water

3 tablespoons wheat-free tamari or other soy sauce

2 tablespoons olive oil (optional)

1 tablespoon pure maple syrup, coconut nectar, or date syrup (for homemade, see page 109)

2 teaspoons balsamic vinegar (optional)

½ teaspoon liquid smoke, or 1 teaspoon smoked paprika

1 teaspoon minced garlic or peeled and minced fresh ginger

Pinch of chipotle powder

Place all the ingredients in a medium-size bowl and whisk well.

Cilantro Lime Marinade

TOTAL YIELD: 4 OUNCES
    Serving Size: 4 ounces
    Number of Servings: 1
    Prep Time: 5 minutes
    Total Time: 5 minutes

¼ cup freshly squeezed lime juice

¼ cup filtered water

2 tablespoons minced fresh cilantro

1½ teaspoons Dijon or stone-ground mustard

½ teaspoon sea salt

¼ teaspoon ground black pepper

1 tablespoon olive oil (optional)

½ teaspoon chili powder

⅛ teaspoon cayenne pepper or crushed red pepper flakes

Place all the ingredients in a medium-size bowl and whisk well.

VARIATIONS

🥄 Replace the lime juice with lemon juice.

🥄 Replace the cilantro with mixed fresh herbs, such as parsley, basil, rosemary, thyme, oregano, and/or dill.

🥄 Add 2 teaspoons of a Global Spice Blend, such as Italian, Indian, Mexican, or Cajun (pages 249–252).

Sweet and Spicy Pumpkin Seeds

Add a sweet, spicy, and salty crunch to your salads, stir-fries, and vegan soufflés.

Pumpkin seeds can be a man's best friend, known for their benefit to prostate health by providing a strong source of zinc, vitamin E, and a hormone-balancing healthy fat profile—great for women, too.

TOTAL YIELD: 8 OUNCES
Serving Size: 1 ounce
Number of Servings: 8
Prep Time: 5 minutes
Cook Time: 20 minutes
Total Time: 25 minutes

1 cup pumpkin seeds
1 tablespoon coconut or olive oil (optional)
2 teaspoons pure maple syrup
¾ teaspoon garam masala
¼ teaspoon chipotle powder
1 teaspoon wheat-free tamari or other soy sauce
Pinch of sea salt

1. Preheat the oven to 300°F. Combine all the ingredients in a medium-size bowl and mix well.
2. Transfer to a lightly oiled or parchment paper–lined baking sheet and bake for 20 minutes, stirring once or twice to ensure even cooking.
3. Remove from the oven and allow to cool, stirring occasionally to prevent sticking.

VARIATIONS

- Replace the pumpkin seeds with seeds and nuts of your choosing. Try sunflower seeds, hazelnuts, slivered almonds, or walnuts.

- Add 1 teaspoon of a Global Spice Blend, such as Moroccan, Cajun, Indian, or Ethiopian (pages 249–252).

Balsamic Reduction

From *Healing the Vegan Way*

Balsamic vinegar is a reduction itself—white sweet grapes boiled down to a syrup. Balsamic hails from Italy, where it is produced in the regions of Modena and Reggio. It has a rich, complex flavor with a hint of sweetness from the grapes. Reduce it even further via the addition of another grape product—heart-healthy red wine. Drizzle this over salads and for garnishing your culinary creations!

YIELD: 4 OUNCES
Serving Size: 2 teaspoons
Number of Servings: 12
Prep Time: 5 minutes
Cook Time: 30 minutes
Total Time: 35 minutes

1 cup balsamic vinegar
¼ cup red wine (try Chianti) (optional)
2 tablespoons white balsamic vinegar (optional)
1 tablespoon coconut sugar, Sucanat, or vegan granulated sugar (optional)

1. Place all the ingredients in a small saucepan over medium heat.
2. Cook for 30 minutes, or until the liquid is reduced in half, stirring occasionally and being careful not to boil.
3. Allow the mixture to cool before transferring to a squeeze bottle. Store in the fridge for up to 2 weeks.

Chia Peach Pepper Jam

Spice it up! We be jammin' with jalapeño and chia seeds in this simple spread that will elevate your breakfast or snacking experience. Plenty of vitamin C-rich ingredients, plus all the extra nutrient power of chia make this a brain-, heart-, and immune system-friendly jam. Serve over Superseed Baked French Toast (page 136), toast or bagel of choice, and on your vegan cheese board along with crackers.

TOTAL YIELD: 14 OUNCES
Serving Size: 1 ounce
Number of Servings: 14
Prep Time: 5 minutes
Chill Time: 60 minutes
Total Time: 1 hour 5 minutes

½ cup chopped fresh peaches
1 cup water or fruit juice
3 tablespoons chia seeds
1 tablespoon seeded and diced jalapeño pepper
½ teaspoon garam masala
¼ teaspoon ground cinnamon
Pinch of cayenne pepper
3 to 4 tablespoons pure maple syrup or other sweetener to taste, depending on sweetness of the peaches

Place all the ingredients in a blender or small food processor and blend until smooth. Taste and add more sweetener, if necessary, to reach desired level of sweetness. Allow to chill in the refrigerator for 60 minutes up to overnight to solidify.

VARIATIONS

- Replace the peaches with other fresh or frozen fruit, such as strawberries, cherries, blueberries, apricots, or mangoes.
- Try different fruit juices, such as orange, peach, or dark cherry.
- Replace the garam masala with ¼ teaspoon of ground cardamom or nutmeg.
- Feel free to leave out the jalapeño.

Ruby Kraut

Long live purple cabbage! And long live those who consume it! Including cultured foods, like kraut, in your diet is one of the best ways to strengthen your microbiome and ensure a long and healthy life. The ruby red kraut gets its color from this superstar cruciferous veggie and the extra-superpowerful red beet. Be sure to save some of the outer cabbage leaves when you prepare the recipe, as they will be used in our fermenting method to create a seal over the kraut. Get your kraut on and serve with your salads and as a condiment for as many meals as you can, including Sweet Potato Black Bean Sliders (page 228), BBQ Jackfruit (page 217) on top of Brazenly Braised Tempeh (page 219), and in your Black Rice Sushi with Wasabi Mayo (page 222).

TOTAL YIELD: 28 OUNCES
Serving Size: 2 ounces
Number of Servings: 14
Prep Time: 15 minutes
Culture Time: 3 to 4 days
Total Time: 3 to 4 days

continues

continued

4½ cups shredded red cabbage, divided, 1 or 2 outer leaves reserved

½ cup water

¾ teaspoon sea salt, or to taste

2 cups peeled and shredded beet

2 tablespoons peeled and minced fresh ginger

2 teaspoons peeled and minced fresh turmeric (optional)

1 teaspoon seeded and diced hot chile pepper, or ¼ teaspoon crushed red pepper flakes (optional)

1½ teaspoons caraway or coriander seeds

1. Place 1 cup of the red cabbage, the water, and the salt in a blender and blend until slightly liquefied. Transfer to a bowl along with the rest of the cabbage (except the reserved leaves), beet, ginger, turmeric, if using, and hot chile pepper, if using, and caraway seeds, and mix well.
2. Transfer to a very clean 1-quart mason jar and press down firmly. Top with the reserved outer leaves of the cabbage and press down firmly. Add more water if necessary to have the leaves completely submerged. Cover with a lid and leave in a warm, dark place.
3. Remove the lid once or twice a day to "burp" the kraut and allow the naturally forming gasses to release.
4. Ferment until tangy, 2 to 4 days, depending on the temperature. Remove and discard the outer leaves, and place the jar in the refrigerator. Enjoy within a couple of weeks.

VARIATION

🍃 Replace the red cabbage with green cabbage or napa cabbage. Add other veggies, such as fresh ginger, shredded carrot, thinly sliced daikon radish, hot chile pepper, or garlic.

Pickled Red Onion

Want to be pickled pink? Look no further than the Bermuda, or red, onion, which will take on a pinkish hue. Pickling is an ancient way of preserving the bounty of harvest season. It also increases digestion and nutritional absorption by stimulating digestive enzymes when we eat it as a snack or alongside a meal. Serve on salads, such as Sunny Kale Salad (page 162), or on your Sweet Potato Black Bean Sliders (page 228).

TOTAL YIELD: 32 OUNCES
Serving Size: 2 ounces
Number of Servings: 16
Prep Time: 5 minutes
Cook Time: 5 minutes
Pickling Time: 12 hours
Total Time: 12 hours 10 minutes

2 teaspoons coriander seeds

2 teaspoons fennel seeds

2 teaspoons brown mustard seeds

1 teaspoon allspice berries

1 star anise, or 2 bay leaves

1 cup apple cider vinegar

1 teaspoon sea salt, or to taste

4 cups loosely packed thinly sliced red onion

1. Place a dry small sauté pan or pot over medium-high heat. Place the coriander, fennel, and mustard seeds in the pan and cook for 3 minutes, or until the seeds begin to pop, stirring constantly.
2. Lower the heat to low. Add the allspice berries, star anise, vinegar, and salt and stir well. Simmer for 5 minutes. Transfer to a clean 1-quart mason jar.
3. Add the onion and seal tightly with a lid. Allow to sit at room temperature for 12 hours. Place in the refrigerator. Enjoy the following day. Keeps for up to 3 weeks.

VARIATIONS

- You can vary the ingredients you use in the pickling spice mixture, such as by including 1 teaspoon of juniper berries, a sprig of rosemary, two bay leaves or kaffir lime leaves, and/or 1 teaspoon of cardamom pods.

- Replace the onion with other veggies, such as carrot, cauliflower, cabbage, daikon, bell pepper, cucumber, and/or okra.

Coconut Yogurt

You won't believe how easy it is to create your own yogurt. Use any vegan acidophilus capsule to start the magic. You can get a daily dose of positive probiotic friends while enjoying a subtly sweet coconut flavor, not to mention the immunity-supportive lauric acid compounds specific to coconut. Serve as part of your breakfast bowls, on top of granola or fresh fruit, or in any recipe that calls for yogurt.

TOTAL YIELD: 14 OUNCES
Serving Size: 2 ounces
Number of Servings: 7
Prep Time: 5 minutes
Culturing Time: 3 days
Total Time: 3 days

1 (13.5-ounce) can full-fat coconut milk
½ teaspoon vegan acidophilus culture (1 or 2 capsules)

1. Combine the coconut milk and acidophilus in a small bowl and whisk well.
2. Transfer to a clean mason jar. Cover with cheesecloth or a mesh bag. Place in a warm, dark place and allow to sit for 2 to 3 days, tasting daily for tanginess. You want there to be some tang, but not so much that it becomes overwhelming.
3. After 3 days, place a lid on the jar and keep in the refrigerator for up to 5 days.

VARIATION

- Blend with your favorite fruit after culturing. Try with blueberries, mangoes, peaches, or strawberries.

Smoky Sweet Chili Garlic Sauce

Many commercial brands of Asian sauces contain fish. Here is a certified fish sauce-free way to take the flavors of your dishes to the next level. Now you can enjoy all the sweet, spicy, pungent flavors without any mystery ingredients. Serve as part of Sweet Chili Brussels Sprouts (page 190), or over roasted or grilled tofu (see pages 104–105), or Black Gomasio Crusted Tofu (page 215), or as a dipping sauce for Curried Cauliflower Pakora (page 200). You can store leftovers, if there are any, in a jar in the fridge and reheat for serving.

TOTAL YIELD: 8 OUNCES
 Serving Size: 2 ounces
 Number of Servings: 4
 Prep Time: 10 minutes
 Cook Time: 20 minutes
 Total Time: 30 minutes

½ cup plus 2 tablespoons water, divided
½ cup rice vinegar
4 to 5 garlic cloves, pressed or minced
1 tablespoon wheat-free tamari or other soy sauce
3 tablespoons pure maple syrup, coconut nectar, vegan granulated or brown sugar, or date syrup (for homemade, see page 109)
½ teaspoon chipotle powder
1 tablespoon arrowroot powder

1. Place a small pot over medium-low heat. Add ½ cup of the water and the rice vinegar, garlic, tamari, maple syrup, and chipotle powder and stir well. Cook for 15 minutes, stirring frequently.
2. Place the arrowroot powder and remaining 2 tablespoons of water in a small bowl and stir well.
3. Add to the pot and stir well. Cook until the sauce thickens, about 3 minutes, stirring constantly. Serve warm or cooled.

VARIATIONS

- Replace the garlic with fresh ginger.
- Up the heat by adding 1 teaspoon of seeded and diced hot chile pepper.
- Add ¼ cup of apricot preserves.

Roasted Squash Butter

Did you know you can create a creamy, buttery spread using a roasted squash? Which is fantastic, because any way you get more immunity-boosting, high-antioxidant squash, you are doing yourself a favor. Serve as a spread on crusty bread, mix with roasted tofu or tempeh (see pages 104–105), or add to your Papas, Bean, and Greens Burritos (page 237). You can also use this as a substitute for the cheese in Mac n Cheez (page 230).

TOTAL YIELD: 8 OUNCES
Serving Size: 2 ounces
Number of Servings: 4
Prep Time: 10 minutes
Cook Time: 30 minutes
Total Time: 40 minutes

1 medium-size butternut or buttercup squash
¼ cup tahini
½ teaspoon smoked paprika
¼ teaspoon sea salt, or to taste
⅛ teaspoon ground black pepper

1. Preheat the oven to 400°F. Carefully slice the squash in half and remove the seeds. Place about ½ inch of water in a small, rimmed baking sheet. Add the squash, cut side down, and cook until a knife can pass easily through the thickest portion, about 30 minutes, depending on the size of the squash. Allow to cool. Scoop out 1 cup, tightly packed, of the squash for use in this recipe.

2. Transfer the cooked squash to a food processor with the remaining ingredients and process until smooth. Store in a glass container in the fridge and use within 1 week.

VARIATIONS

- Experiment with different varieties of squash and even sweet potatoes.

- Add 2 tablespoons of hemp, flax, or olive oil.

- Add 2 teaspoons of a Global Spice Blend, such as Italian, Moroccan, Mexican, or Cajun (pages 249–252).

Pepita Pesto with Avocado

This vegan pesto will get the seal of approval from even the most ardent pesto fans. The secret ingredient? Nutritional yeast to create the cheesy flavor traditionally provided by Parmesan cheese. The gorgeous color produced by this pesto is a reminder of the gifts of nature from these health-sustaining seeds, herbs, spices, and amazing avocado as well! Enjoy with pasta, as a topping for Cashew Cheese–Stuffed Sweet Peppers (page 179), mixed with Roasted Cauliflower and Broccoli (page 181), or Grilled Vegetables Extraordinaire (page 178), and as a dipping sauce for Baked Cajun Veggie Fritters (page 187).

TOTAL YIELD: 4 OUNCES
> Serving Size: 1 ounce
> Number of Servings: 4
> Prep Time: 15 minutes
> Total Time: 15 minutes

½ cup tightly packed fresh basil
¼ heaping cup raw or toasted pepitas
¼ heaping cup mashed avocado
1 tablespoon nutritional yeast
1 clove garlic, pressed or minced
2 tablespoons freshly squeezed lemon juice
2 tablespoons minced red or green onion
¼ teaspoon sea salt, or to taste
⅛ teaspoon ground black pepper
Pinch of crushed red pepper flakes
   (optional)

Place all the ingredients in a small food processor and process until creamy. You can also process in a blender, though you may need to double the recipe, or add water (or olive oil), for it to blend well.

VARIATIONS

- Replace the avocado with olive oil.

- Replace the basil with fresh cilantro or flat-leaf parsley.

- Replace the pumpkin seeds with pine nuts, pecans, pistachios, macadamia nuts, or cashews.

Smoky Cashew Cream

Further proof that vegans can enjoy all the flavors of dairy-based products without all the detrimental health effects! This dairy-free, oil-free cream delivers on cashews' promise of mood-enhancing B vitamins as well as enough concentration of essential minerals to prevent deficiency diseases with regular consumption. Depending on the size of your blender, you may want to double this recipe so there are enough ingredients to completely cover the blender blade, allowing for a creamy texture. Serve whenever sour cream is called for. Add to Braised Mushroom Stroganoff (page 240) or Loaded Nachos (page 206), or use on top of Jackfruit Tacos (see page 216) or baked potatoes.

TOTAL YIELD: 6 OUNCES
  Serving Size: 1 ounce
  Number of Servings: 6
  Prep Time: 5 minutes
  Soak Time: 20 minutes
  Total Time: 25 minutes

½ cup raw cashew pieces
½ cup water
2 teaspoons freshly squeezed lemon juice
¼ teaspoon smoked paprika
Pinch of cayenne pepper or crushed red pepper flakes

1. Place the cashews in a bowl with ample water to cover. Allow to sit for 20 minutes up to a few hours. Drain and rinse well.
2. Transfer to a blender along with the remaining ingredients, including the ½ cup of water, and blend until creamy.

VARIATIONS

- Replace the cashews with Brazil or macadamia nuts.
- For a taste of Oaxaca, replace the lemon juice with lime juice and add 1 teaspoon of chile powder and 2 teaspoons of minced fresh cilantro.

Chunky Tomato Sauce

Sicily is for lovers . . . specifically, pasta sauce lovers. Maybe it's the heart-healthy antioxidant lycopene, which give the tomatoes their red hue, that will have you singing "That's *amore*" before your second helping. Serve over pasta, roasted or grilled tofu and tempeh, Savory Baked Seitan (page 225), or Cauliflower Steaks (page 201).

TOTAL YIELD: 24 OUNCES

   Serving Size: 4 ounces
   Number of Servings: 6
   Prep Time: 10 minutes
   Cook Time: 25 minutes
   Total Time: 35 minutes

1 tablespoon olive oil, or 3 tablespoons water
¾ cup diced yellow onion
¼ teaspoon sea salt, plus to taste
1 tablespoon Italian Spice Mix (page 251, or store-bought)
1½ cups chopped cremini or button mushrooms
3 to 4 garlic cloves, pressed or minced
¼ cup red wine (optional)
1 (15-ounce) can diced fire-roasted tomatoes, or 1½ cups diced tomato
½ cup water
2 teaspoons balsamic vinegar
2 tablespoons finely chopped basil and/or flat-leaf parsley
Ground black pepper
Pinch of crushed red pepper flakes (optional)

1. Place a 2-quart pot over medium-high heat. Heat the oil. Add the onion, sea salt, and Italian Spice Mix, and cook for 3 minutes, stirring frequently and adding small amounts of water or vegetable stock if necessary to prevent sticking. Add the mushrooms and cook for 3 minutes, stirring frequently. Add the garlic, and cook for 2 minutes, stirring frequently. Add the red wine, if using.

2. Lower the heat to medium. Add the tomatoes and water and cook for 15 minutes, stirring occasionally.

3. Add the balsamic vinegar and basil and mix well. Season to taste with additional salt, black pepper, and red pepper flakes, if using, before serving.

VARIATIONS

- Add 1 tablespoon of nutritional yeast along with the basil.

- Add 8 ounces of crumbled tempeh or 14 ounces of crumbled tofu for a Bolognese sauce.

- Add ¼ cup of chopped olives along with the basil.

- For a smoother sauce, transfer to a blender or blend with an immersion blender until your desired consistency is attained.

Cranberry Apricot Sauce with Crystallized Ginger

One of the dishes that will make you go "Ho Ho Ho," serve this sweet and tart sauce to your sweetheart and other loved ones at your holiday meal. The digestive benefits from all three main ingredients of this twist on traditional cranberry sauce make it a perfect starter or addition to a special meal. Serve as a spread on baguette slices or over Lemony Herbed Cauliflower Roast (page 211) and Pecan Sage Holiday Loaf (page 244).

TOTAL YIELD: 14 OUNCES
 Serving size: 2 ounces
 Number of Servings: 7
 Prep Time: 5 minutes
 Cook Time: 20 minutes
 Total Time: 25 minutes

10 ounces frozen cranberries, or 3 cups fresh

½ cup chopped dried apricots

½ teaspoon orange zest

½ cup freshly squeezed orange juice

½ cup water

¼ cup diced crystallized ginger

½ teaspoon ground cinnamon

¼ teaspoon ground cardamom

1 tablespoon pure maple syrup, coconut nectar, or date syrup (for homemade, see page 109) (optional)

¼ teaspoon crushed red pepper flakes (optional)

¼ to ½ cup water (optional)

1. Place the cranberries in a small pot over medium-high heat. Cook for 5 minutes, stirring frequently.
2. Add the remaining ingredients and cook for an additional 15 minutes, stirring frequently. All the cranberries should be broken apart. Add small amounts of additional water to create your desired consistency. Serve warm or at room temperature.

VARIATIONS

- Add ⅛ teaspoon of ground nutmeg along with cinnamon.
- Replace the apricots with figs, dates, or cherries.

Apricot BBQ Sauce

Down-home tangy goodness awaits with this exceptionally exquisite entourage of flavors. Apricots are not only a fun choice to add a little sweetness, they also bring in lots of beta-carotene, healthy fiber, and vitamin C, and are known to release powerful antioxidants for maintaining optimal vision, healthy skin, and protection against lung and other cancers. Serve as part of BBQ Jackfruit (page 217), over Skillet Corn Bread (page 204), Brazenly Braised Tempeh (page 219), or roasted tofu (see pages 104–105).

TOTAL YIELD: 14 OUNCES
 Serving Size: 2 ounces
 Number of Servings: 7
 Prep Time: 5 minutes
 Soak Time: 20 minutes
 Cook Time: 5 minutes
 Total Time: 30 minutes

1½ cups water
¼ cup chopped dried apricots
6 ounces tomato paste
2 tablespoons molasses
1 tablespoon apple cider vinegar
1 teaspoon chili powder
¾ teaspoon liquid smoke
½ teaspoon chipotle powder
2 teaspoons wheat-free tamari or
 other soy sauce (optional)
Sea salt and ground black pepper

1. Place the water and apricots in a bowl and allow to soak for 20 minutes.
2. Transfer the apricots and their soak water to a blender with the remaining ingredients and blend until smooth.
3. Transfer to a pot over low heat and cook until warm, stirring occasionally, about 5 minutes.

VARIATIONS

- Omit the apricots and add pure maple syrup to taste.

- Replace the tomato paste with ketchup.

- Vinegar lovers can increase the vinegar to 2 tablespoons.

Artful Almond Sauce

When the peanut sauce craving hits—and believe us, it will—you can turn to this more healthful nut to deliver on the creamy and delectable flavors you are looking for. Almonds provide plenty of calcium as well as healthy fats, fiber, protein, magnesium, and vitamin E. They help lower blood sugar and cholesterol levels and reduce blood pressure. And they are just good, especially when ground into a creamy butter. Serve as part of Roasted Tofu with Almond Sauce (page 221), or as a dipping sauce for Curried Cauliflower Pakora (page 200).

TOTAL YIELD: 14 OUNCES

Serving Size: 2 ounces
Number of Servings: 7
Prep Time: 10 minutes
Total Time: 10 minutes

½ cup almond butter

½ cup coconut, soy, or almond milk

½ cup water

1 tablespoon freshly squeezed lime juice

2 teaspoons wheat-free tamari or other soy sauce, or to taste

2 teaspoons pure maple syrup, or to taste

¼ teaspoon crushed red pepper flakes (optional)

1 teaspoon minced fresh cilantro

¼ teaspoon sea salt, or to taste

1. Place all the ingredients in a bowl and whisk well. Depending on the consistency of the almond butter and coconut milk, you may wish to add small amounts of water if necessary to reach your desired consistency.
2. Transfer to a small pot over low heat and cook until just warm, about 5 minutes, stirring frequently.

VARIATIONS

- Add ½ teaspoon of tamarind paste.
- Every now and then, we love to replace the almond butter with peanut butter.

EZ Cheez Sauce

Cheese—the last frontier for many in making the switch to a fully plant-based lifestyle. The good news is that it has never been easier to create the satisfying, creamy, and, well . . . cheesy flavors with plants. Easy on digestion, and loaded with flavor and nutrition while lower in calories, this cheez may change your life! Serve with Loaded Nachos (page 206), over tofu or tempeh cutlets (see page 104), Steamed Supreme (page 176), or any recipe where a creamy cheese is called for.

TOTAL YIELD: 16 OUNCES
>   Serving Size: 4 ounces
>   Number of Servings: 4
>   Prep Time: 10 minutes
>   Cook Time: 15 minutes
>   Total Time: 25 minutes

1¼ cups peeled and chopped white potato (½-inch pieces)

½ cup peeled and chopped carrot (½-inch pieces)

½ cup diced yellow onion

4 to 5 cloves garlic

1 cup water or vegetable stock (for homemade, see page 248)

3 tablespoons nutritional yeast

2 tablespoons olive oil (optional)

1 tablespoon freshly squeezed lemon juice

½ teaspoon sea salt, or to taste

¼ teaspoon chipotle powder

⅛ teaspoon ground black pepper, or to taste

1. Place the potato, carrot, onion, and garlic in a medium-size pot and add ample water to cover. Place over medium-high heat and cook until tender, about 15 minutes, stirring occasionally. Drain well and reserve 1 cup of the cooking liquid.

2. Place the cooked vegetables in blender along with the remaining ingredients, including the reserved 1 cup of water, and blend until creamy. Add more water if necessary to reach desired consistency. Proceed to indulge!

VARIATIONS

- Add ¼ cups of soaked and drained raw cashews to the blender.

- Add ¼ to ½ teaspoon of truffle oil.

- Add 2 teaspoons of a Global Spice Blend, such as Cajun, Mexican, Italian, or Indian (pages 249–252).

Aqua Mayo

The liquid from cooked chickpeas, affectionately known as aquafaba, is rocking the foundation of the vegan culinary world. It's used in both sweet dishes—see Vegan Fluff (page 283)—and in savory dishes as an egg-white replacer. Use wherever mayo is called for, as an alternative to the cholesterol-laden mayonnaise made from eggs.

TOTAL YIELD: 12 OUNCES
  Serving Size: 1 ounce
  Number of Servings: 12
  Prep Time: 15 minutes
  Total Time: 15 minutes

¼ cup aquafaba (see headnote)
¼ teaspoon cream of tartar
¾ cup safflower or grapeseed oil
1 teaspoon freshly squeezed lemon juice
1 teaspoon apple cider vinegar
¼ teaspoon Dijon mustard
¼ teaspoon sea salt, or to taste

1. Place the aquafaba in a medium-size mixing bowl or stand mixer fitted with the whisk attachment. If using the mixing bowl, get your hand mixer ready to rock.
2. Add the cream of tartar and mix on high speed until medium peaks begin to form, about 10 minutes.
3. Slowly add the remaining ingredients and mix for an additional 5 minutes. Transfer to a glass jar in the refrigerator and use within a week or so.

VARIATION

🌿 Add 1 teaspoon of vegan granulated sugar along with the vinegar.

Vegan Mayonnaise

From *Healing the Vegan Way*

While debate rages over whether it's legal to refer to anything as mayonnaise without eggs, we are going to go out on a limb and sing the praises of this vegan version. It is made with safflower seeds, similar to sunflower seeds, which contain an abundance of vitamin E and monounsaturated fat. Use wherever vegan mayonnaise is called for.

TOTAL YIELD: 18 OUNCES
    Serving Size: 1 ounce
    Number of Servings: 18
    Prep Time: 15 minutes
    Total Time: 15 minutes

1½ cups safflower oil
¾ cup soy milk (see note)
2 teaspoons raw coconut nectar or agave nectar (optional)
¾ teaspoon Dijon mustard
¾ teaspoon sea salt, or to taste
2 teaspoons freshly squeezed lemon juice

1. Combine all the ingredients, except the lemon juice, in a blender and blend until smooth.
2. Slowly add the lemon juice through the top while blending, until the mixture thickens.

Note: Some brands of soy milk will emulsify better than others. For best results, shake the soy milk well and use at room temperature.

VARIATION

⚶ For an oil-free version, replace the oil with soaked and drained raw cashew pieces or macadamia nuts.

Chipotle Mayonnaise

Insider secret: Mark travels internationally with his chipotle powder. Always delivering on a smoky flavor and just the right amount of heat, chipotle is made from smoked red jalapeño peppers. Hot peppers also have a natural pain-reducing property and help maintain healthy circulation in all blood vessels. Serve as a spread on wraps, sandwiches, Hummus Panini with Balsamic Massaged Kale (page 239) or Sweet Potato Black Bean Sliders (page 228), schmeared on your Skillet Corn Bread (page 204), or a dollop on Adzuki Bean Tempeh Chili (page 152).

TOTAL YIELD: 6 OUNCES
    Serving Size: 0.5 ounce
    Number of Servings: 12
    Prep Time: 5 minutes
    Total Time: 5 minutes.

¾ cup vegan mayonnaise (for homemade, see page 273)
2 teaspoons freshly squeezed lime juice
½ teaspoon chipotle powder, or 1 fresh chipotle pepper (see variation)
¼ teaspoon chili powder

Place all the ingredients in a small bowl and whisk well.

VARIATION

⚶ Turn up the heat by adding one dried chipotle chile, soaked in warm water until soft, then seeded. Place in a food processor with the other ingredients and puree until smooth.

Vegan Sour Cream

From *Healing the Vegan Way*

Pssst. Vegans like sour cream, too! Serve a dollop to add creamy magic to your Black-Eye Cabbage (page 212), Loaded Nachos (page 206), Papas, Bean, and Greens Burrito (page 237), Jackfruit Tacos (see page 216), and Braised Mushroom Stroganoff (page 240).

YIELD: 12 OUNCES
  Serving Size: 1 ounce
  Number of Servings: 12
  Prep Time: 5 minutes
  Total Time: 5 minutes

¾ cup vegan mayonnaise (for homemade, see page 273)
1 tablespoon freshly squeezed lemon juice
½ teaspoon fresh dill (optional)
Pinch of sea salt

Place all the ingredients in a medium-size bowl and whisk well.

Raw Cashew Sour Cream

From *Healing the Vegan Way*

Keep your sour cream raw by using cashews as a base instead of vegan mayo. This version delivers on essential minerals and vitamin C. Enjoy on the same dishes as the cooked version, and add a dollop to your raw dishes, such as Raw Chilled Strawberry Soup (page 141).

TOTAL YIELD: 14 OUNCES
  Serving Size: 1 ounce
  Number of Servings: 14
  Prep Time: 35 minutes
  Total Time: 35 minutes

1 cup raw cashew pieces
2 tablespoons plus 2 teaspoons freshly squeezed lemon juice
½ to ¾ cup water
2 teaspoons olive oil (optional)
1 teaspoon minced fresh dill (optional)
¼ teaspoon sea salt, or to taste

1. Place the cashews in a bowl with ample water to cover. Allow to sit for 25 minutes, or up to 3 hours.
2. Rinse and drain well.
3. Place in a blender with all the remaining ingredients, including ½ cup of the water, and blend until creamy. Add additional water, if necessary, to reach your desired consistency. This will be determined by the strength of your blender.

Sriracha Aioli

Spicy garlicky goodness awaits with this easy way to take your vegan mayo experience to the next level. Garlic and lemon produce a detoxifying and balancing effect, while sriracha's chili pepper has a blood-moving benefit. Let your imagination run wild with creative ways that you can incorporate this burst of flavors into your culinary creations. Serve as a dipping sauce for Curried Cauliflower Pakora (page 200), Coco Jackfruit Nuggets (page 183), or as a spread on your Hummus Panini with Balsamic Massaged Kale (page 239) and even Black Rice Sushi with Wasabi Mayo (page 222).

TOTAL YIELD: 4 OUNCES
 Serving Size: 0.5 ounce
 Number of Servings: 8
 Prep Time: 5 minutes
 Cook Time: 30 minutes
 Total Time: 35 minutes

1 head garlic

½ teaspoon olive oil (optional)

¼ teaspoon sea salt, or to taste

Pinch of ground black pepper

½ cup vegan mayonnaise (for homemade, see page 273)

1 to 2 tablespoons sriracha, or to taste

1 teaspoon freshly squeezed lemon juice

½ teaspoon Italian Spice Mix (page 251, or store-bought)

1. Preheat the oven to 400°F. Slice off the very top of the garlic head. Brush with olive oil, if using, and sprinkle with a pinch of salt and pepper. Place in a ramekin or small baking dish, optionally covering with foil.
2. Roast until the garlic is just soft, about 30 minutes. Squeeze the cloves out of the skin and chop well.
3. Transfer to a bowl along with the remaining ingredients and mash well.

VARIATIONS

- For an oil-free version, replace the mayonnaise with ½ cup of soaked and drained raw cashews (soak for 15 minutes up to a few hours) and ½ cup of water. Adjust the seasonings to taste.

- Replace the Italian Spice Mix with Cajun Spice Mix (page 249), Indian Spice Mix (page 251), or Moroccan Spice Mix (page 252).

- Add ¼ cup of roasted red bell pepper and puree in food processor.

Mushroom Leek Gravy

A long-held conspiracy theory is that vegans serve a vegan gravy at holiday feasts, and never tell their guests it's vegan. Join the resistance and give this one a try. You can't go wrong with immunity-boosting shiitakes bathed in pure whole food flavor. Sweeter than onion, leeks add the benefits of allium plus extra vitamin K. Serve over Pecan Sage Holiday Loaf (page 244), Rainbow Roasted Roots (page 196), tofu or tempeh cutlets (see page 104), Garlicky Parsnips (page 192) . . . actually, pretty much everything!

TOTAL YIELD: 32 OUNCES

> Serving Size: 4 ounces
> Number of Servings: 8
> Prep Time: 5 minutes
> Cook Time: 20 minutes
> Total Time: 25 minutes

1 tablespoon olive oil, or 3 tablespoons water

¾ cup thinly sliced leek, rinsed and drained well

4 to 5 garlic cloves, pressed or minced

¾ cup thinly sliced shiitake mushrooms

4 cups water or vegetable stock (for homemade, see page 248), divided

2 tablespoons wheat-free tamari or other soy sauce, or to taste

¼ cup nutritional yeast

3 tablespoons arrowroot powder

2 tablespoons finely chopped fresh flat-leaf parsley

Sea salt and ground black pepper

Pinch of cayenne pepper (optional)

1. Place a medium-size pot or sauté pan over medium-high heat. Heat the oil. Add the leek and cook for 3 minutes, stirring frequently and adding small amounts of water or vegetable stock if necessary to prevent sticking.
2. Add the garlic and mushrooms and cook for 5 minutes, stirring frequently. Add 3½ cups of the water and the tamari and nutritional yeast and cook for 5 minutes, stirring occasionally.
3. Combine the arrowroot powder and ½ cup of cold water in a small bowl and stir well. Add to the pot. Cook until the gravy thickens, about 5 minutes, stirring constantly.
4. Add the parsley and mix well. Season with salt and black pepper to taste and the cayenne, if using, before serving.

VARIATIONS

🌿 Replace the leeks with yellow onion.

🌿 Replace the shiitakes with mushrooms of your choosing, such as oyster, button, or cremini.

🌿 Instead of using the arrowroot mixture, you can replace it with a roux made with ¼ cup of flour and 3 tablespoons of oil. Place the flour and oil in a small bowl and mix well. Add in step 3.

SEVENTEEN

DEATH-DEFYING DESSERTS AND SNACKS

How sweet it is to indulge without guilt! Although refined sugar deservedly gets a bad rap, we are wired to gravitate toward the sweet. Tasting sweetness has an effect on pleasure hormones dopamine and serotonin, and glucose can provide that quick needed energy boost, especially during high-endurance sports or when your brain is working overtime.

We like to view the world of sweeteners on a spectrum. On one side, there's the evil empire, consisting of refined white sugar and high-fructose corn syrup. They are the addictive culprits in causing inflammatory damage to your joints, gut, and brain as well as challenging heart health by increasing triglycerides and slowing insulin responsiveness over time. Please minimize your consumption of these sweeteners. On the other end of the spectrum, we have apples and other whole fresh fruit—full of life-giving antioxidants, vitamins, and minerals as well as heart-healthy fiber!

When you do indulge, it is best to gravitate toward fruit to satisfy your sweet craving, and use "healthier" concentrated sweeteners in moderation. Please see the sweetener chart on page 107 for a list of some of the more healthful sweeteners; also see our recipe for a fruit-sweetened date syrup (page 109) that can replace concentrated sweeteners, such as agave or coconut nectar or maple syrup. (For those on a sugar-restricted diet, remember sugar is sugar, regardless of the source.)

We adhere to a theory of relativity when it comes to dessert. Is a vegan gluten-free chocolate brownie, sweetened with coconut nectar or maple syrup, healthy? Relative to a shot of wheatgrass, probably not. Relative to a brownie that is made with eggs, butter, and refined white sugar? You betcha!

Don't leave home without your vegan survival kit. This can include a superfood trail mix, such as Brain Health Trail Mix (page 280), vegan energy bars, seed or nut butter with apple slices or celery sticks, chia seeds (simply add a plant-based milk and your trail mix, and you have a high energy meal on the run), rice crackers, and other staples to take the edge off if you find yourself far from a vegan haven in your travels.

Stock up on some of the healthier store-bought items for when the sweet craving hits: vegan dark chocolate, granola bars, and other healthy treats will be there for you when you need them most.

You'll find lots here to satisfy your cravings. Save room for Raw Peppermint Patty Fudge Brownies (page 291), Superfood Chocolate Bark (page 284), Walnut Flapjacks (page 286), and The Great Pumpkin Cheezcake (page 294).

By the way, making Vegan Fluff with Aquafaba (page 283) may very well be the coolest thing you have ever seen in a kitchen.

Gourmet Popcorn

How about upping your movie night game? The mere mention of truffle oil and popcorn in the same sentence will do the trick. Organic popcorn is a great choice for a high-fiber snack that can be a perfect medium for tasty superfood additions. Cozy up and include this simple, yet oh-so-elegant and addictive snack along with your favorite flick. Sprinkle with Black Sesame Gomasio (page 253) and serve with a tall glass of Tart Cherry and Pomegranate Tonic (page 115).

TOTAL YIELD: 80 OUNCES
Serving Size: 10 ounces
Number of Servings: 8
Prep Time: 5 minutes
Cook Time: 10 minutes
Total Time: 15 minutes

1 to 2 tablespoons olive or coconut oil
½ cup unpopped popcorn kernels
Drizzle of truffle oil
3 tablespoons nutritional yeast
½ to 1 teaspoon maca powder (optional)
1 teaspoon garlic flakes
1 teaspoon onion flakes
¼ to ½ teaspoon sea salt

1. Place a large pot over high heat. Add olive oil. Add three kernels of popcorn to the pot and cover with a lid.
2. As soon as the popcorn pops, add the remaining kernels, cover with the lid, and shake vigorously over (not on) the burner until all the corn is popped, about 3 minutes.
3. Transfer to a clean paper bag, add the truffle oil, and shake well. Add the remaining ingredients and shake, transfer to a bowl, and enjoy immediately.

VARIATIONS

- Add ⅛ teaspoon of chipotle powder along with the nutritional yeast.

- You can omit the maca, garlic, and onion and add 2 teaspoons of chlorella along with the nutritional yeast.

- Add 1 tablespoon of a Global Spice Blend, such as Cajun, Italian, Mexican, or Indian (pages 249–252).

- Of course, you can air-pop the popcorn and proceed to step 3.

Brain Health Trail Mix

Feel your body creating new brain cells with every bite of this high-energy snack. So many nutrients for cognitive function are covered here—healthy omega-3 fats, minerals, antioxidants, and a nice little buzz of pure vitamin power. Include in your snack arsenal to fight off hunger in between meals or on long travel days.

TOTAL YIELD: 24 OUNCES

Serving Size: 2 ounces
Number of Servings: 12
Prep Time: 10 minutes
Total Time: 10 minutes

½ cup walnuts
½ cup pumpkin seeds
½ cup chopped Brazil nuts (½-inch pieces)
¼ cup goji berries
½ cup dried currants
¼ cup large coconut flakes
¼ cup cacao nibs

Combine all the ingredients in a medium-size bowl and mix well.

VARIATIONS

- There's no end to the superfood mixes you can create. Replace the walnuts with other nuts, such as hazelnuts, pecans, almonds, or cashews. Replace the pumpkin seeds with sunflower seeds.

- Replace the goji berries and currants with raisins and other chopped dried fruit, such as figs, apricots, mango, or papaya.

- Add other dried superfood fruits, such as mulberries or golden berries.

- You can optionally toast the nuts and seeds until just golden brown and aromatic (see page 106).

Raw Choco-Cherry Bombs

Peace bombs, of course! Ready for a glimpse of fruit-sweetened nirvana? Surrounding the glorious cherry with the goodness of cacao, dates, pecans, coconut, and more, makes this an immunity-boosting, brain-healthy, anti-inflammatory, body-balancing supertreat! Pack up a few in a glass container for an energy burst when on the road.

TOTAL YIELD: 10 BALLS
> Serving Size: 1 ball
> Number of Servings: 10
> Prep Time: 20 minutes
> Total Time: 20 minutes

¾ cup chopped raw pecans

½ cup pitted and chopped Medjool dates

3 tablespoons cacao nibs, or 2 tablespoons unsweetened cacao powder

¼ teaspoon ground cinnamon

⅛ teaspoon ground cardamom

10 pitted fresh or frozen cherries (if frozen, thawed and drained)

10 drops cherry extract (optional)

3 tablespoons shredded unsweetened coconut

1. Place the pecans in a food processor and process until smooth, like a nut butter consistency. Add the dates, cacao nibs, cinnamon, and cardamom and process until smooth. Some pieces of cacao nibs are okay.
2. Form ten small balls. Make an indentation with a finger or teaspoon in the center of a ball. Add the cherry and a drop of the cherry extract, if using, and reform the ball so that the cherry is in the center. Repeat to complete the other nine bombs.
3. Roll in the coconut before serving.

VARIATIONS

- Replace the pecans with walnuts or sunflower or pumpkin seeds. Or any nut or seed, for that matter.

- Replace the Medjool dates with another variety of date. You may need to soak the dates to soften before using in the recipe if they are very dry. Replace the dates with dried figs, apricots, raisins, or prunes.

- Add 2 tablespoons of raw coconut nectar, pure maple syrup, or date syrup (for homemade, see page 109) for an extra-sweet sensation.

- Replace the cherry with blueberries, raspberries, or blackberries.

- Add 1 teaspoon of pure vanilla extract.

- Replace the coconut with hemp or sesame seeds, or raw cacao powder.

Raw Fig Thumbprint Cookies

If you have a Sicilian family, you know about fig cookies! But no need for nostalgia for those dense butter- and flour-filled morsels—our raw vegan version is bursting with vitality. These truly honor the flavor and goodness of figs, delivering a brain- and heart-healthy delightful treat that even Sicilian grandmas would enjoy! This recipe actually makes enough filling for two batches, since a single batch would be too small for most food processors to effectively process. Top with shredded coconut, and serve as part of a raw food snack pack along with Raw Choco-Cherry Bombs (page 281) and a luxurious glass of Pumpkin Seed Milk (page 116) or Oat Milk (see page 116).

TOTAL YIELD: 10 COOKIES
    Serving Size: 1 cookie
    Number of Servings: 10
    Prep Time: 5 minutes
    Soak Time: 15 minutes
    Chill Time: 20 minutes
    Total Time: 40 minutes

FILLING
½ cup chopped Turkish or Calimyrna figs
½ cup water or fruit juice
¼ teaspoon ground cinnamon

BASE
¾ cup chopped walnuts
¼ cup rolled oats
⅓ cup finely chopped dates
⅛ teaspoon ground cardamom

1. Place the filling ingredients in a bowl and allow to sit for 15 to 30 minutes. Transfer to a blender or small food processor and blend until smooth.
2. Meanwhile, place the base ingredients in a food processor fitted with the S-blade and process until uniform. Form ten cookies, using a tablespoon or small scoop, and make an indentation in the center of each cookie, using the bottom of a teaspoon.
3. Fill each indentation with the blended filling ingredients. Refrigerate for 20 minutes or longer before serving.

VARIATIONS
- Replace the figs with apricots, prunes, raisins, or dried cherries.
- Replace the walnuts with pecans, pistachio nuts, or almonds.
- Add 1 teaspoon of orange zest along with the figs.
- Experiment with different fruit juices instead of water. Try with orange, apple, pineapple, or mango.
- Replace the filling with an equivalent amount of Berry Mousse (page 290).

Vegan Fluff with Aquafaba

They say that all great culinary discoveries are made on the shoulders of those who came before us. Not so with aquafaba, the liquid from cooked beans, in this case chickpeas. Who knew that we have been throwing away the wrong part of the can for all of these years (just kidding . . . chickpeas are awesome!). We guarantee that it will be one of the most amazing things you witness in the kitchen, when the chickpea liquid transforms itself into white fluffy meringue before your very eyes. Go with unsalted or low-sodium chickpeas if you can find them. Adding the optional guar gum allows the fluff to stay stable for longer in the fridge, up to a week or longer. Serve on top of The Great Pumpkin Cheezcake (see page 294), Fruit Compote (page 287), Berry Mousse (page 290), and any other dessert you can think of. You won't be disappointed!

TOTAL YIELD: 48 OUNCES
    Serving Size: 4 ounces
    Number of Servings: 12
    Prep Time: 15 minutes
    Total Time: 15 minutes

¾ cup unsalted or low-salt chickpea brine (from one 15-ounce can of unsalted or low-sodium chickpeas)
¼ teaspoon cream of tartar
½ teaspoon pure vanilla extract
¼ to ½ cup vegan granulated sugar
½ teaspoon guar gum (optional)

1. Place the chickpea brine and cream of tartar in a stand mixer. Beat on high speed until medium-soft peaks form, about 10 minutes. Alternatively, you can also use a large bowl and an old-fashioned eggbeater.
2. Add the vanilla and sugar and beat on high speed until firm peaks form, about 5 minutes. For a sweeter fluff, feel free to add more sugar to taste.
3. Add the guar gum, if using, and beat on high speed for 5 minutes.

VARIATION

For vegan macaroons, please see our instructional video at www.doctorchefresources.com.

Superfood Chocolate Bark

Who knew that something so simple can taste so good? Considered a basic food group by vegans, dark chocolate has many surprising benefits, including being one of the highest antioxidant foods as well as an excellent source of highly important magnesium. Also makes a lovely bed for superfood seeds, berries, ginger, and coconut, to up the nutrition, or used in whatever other way you like. You can speed up the chill time by allowing the bark to chill in the freezer instead of the refrigerator. Store in a refrigerator for up to 2 weeks if you can restrain yourself. (PS: The candy cane version will make you very popular during holiday party season.)

TOTAL YIELD: 12 OUNCES
>   Serving Size: 2 ounces
>   Number of Servings: 6
>   Prep Time: 20 minutes
>   Cook Time: 15 minutes
>   Chill Time: 30 minutes
>   Total Time: 50 to 65 minutes, including chill time

1 cup vegan dark chocolate chips
⅓ cup chopped crystallized ginger (¼-inch pieces)
¼ cup goji berries or dried currants, divided
¼ cup pumpkin seeds, divided
½ teaspoon peppermint extract
1 tablespoon coconut flakes
1 tablespoon hemp seeds

1. Place a small pot of water over medium heat. Place a medium-size metal or glass bowl over the pot (it should not touch the water). Add the chocolate chips to the bowl. Heat until melted, about 10 minutes.
2. Add the crystallized ginger, 2 tablespoons each of the goji berries and pumpkin seeds, and the peppermint extract, and stir well.
3. Transfer to a parchment paper–lined baking sheet and spread into a ¼-inch-thick layer. Top with the remaining 2 tablespoons each of goji berries and pumpkin seeds, the coconut flakes, and the hemp seeds. Use another sheet of parchment paper to press down to create a uniform thickness.
4. Place in the refrigerator and chill until the chocolate is firm enough to cut, about 20 minutes. Cut into your desired shapes with a knife or pizza cutter. Return the pan to the refrigerator for an additional 10 minutes to harden. Store in a glass jar in the fridge for up to 2 weeks.

VARIATIONS

- Holiday season? Try crushing up a couple of candy canes and add along with the pumpkin seeds.

- Replace the currants with dried cranberries or mulberries.

- Replace the pumpkin seeds with sunflower seeds or chopped pecans, walnuts, cashews, or macadamia nuts.

- Add 1 teaspoon of pure vanilla extract or another flavor of extract, such as hazelnut, orange, or coffee. Alternatively, replace it with a teaspoon of rum or liqueur, such as Kahlúa or Cointreau, which are both vegan.

Plantain Cranberry Chocolate Chip Cookies

One of the superheroes of the tropics, plantains can be featured in both savory and sweet dishes.

Plantains' high fiber and mineral content add a balancing touch to this superfood delicacy.

Feel free to substitute ripe bananas for the plantains. Enjoy with a glass of Brazil nut milk (see page 116 in the variations) or Choco-Cherry Berry Smoothie (page 121).

TOTAL YIELD: 12 OUNCES
Serving Size: 1 ounce
Number of Servings: 12
Prep Time: 15 minutes
Cook Time: 15 minutes
Total Time: 30 minutes

2 black-ripe plantains, mashed (1 cup)
⅔ cup flour, such as a gluten-free flour blend (for homemade, see page 254), spelt, whole wheat pastry, or unbleached all-purpose
2 to 3 tablespoons pure maple syrup or coconut nectar (optional, depending on sweetness of plantains)
¼ teaspoon ground cinnamon
⅛ teaspoon ground allspice
¼ cup dried cranberries
¼ cup vegan dark chocolate chips

1. Preheat the oven to 350°F. Place all the ingredients in a bowl and mix well to create the dough. Place in the refrigerator for 15 minutes.
2. Form twelve cookies (1 heaping tablespoon of the dough each) and press down slightly.
3. Bake for 15 minutes. Allow to cool slightly before enjoying.

VARIATIONS

- Replace the chocolate chips with chopped crystallized ginger, walnuts, pecans, or macadamia nuts.

- Replace the cranberries with raisins, dried currants, or chopped dates.

- Add 2 tablespoons of coconut flakes along with the chocolate chips.

Walnut Flapjacks

According to Arthurian legend, flapjacks were the secret to the endurance of the Knights of the Round Table on their search for the holy grail. Not to be confused with American flapjacks, a.k.a. pancakes, these rolled oat-based desserts are popular throughout the United Kingdom. Prunes add chewiness and moisture, along with healthy doses of vitamin K, potassium, and beta-carotene. If you feel like indulging, you can schmear a bit of vegan butter on the flapjack while still warm. Serve with a cuppa Rosemary Star Anise Tea (page 113) or warmed Cacao Turmeric Elixir (page 120).

TOTAL YIELD: 1 (8-INCH) SQUARE CASSE-ROLE DISH, 24 OUNCES BATTER
>   Serving Size: 1 (2-inch) square piece
>   Number of Servings: 16
>   Prep Time: 10 minutes
>   Soak Time: 15 minutes
>   Cook Time: 40 minutes
>   Total Time: 1 hour 5 minutes

2 tablespoons ground flaxseeds or chia seeds

1 cup pitted and chopped prunes, divided

1¼ cups plus 2 tablespoons water

½ cup pure maple syrup (optional)

¾ cup rolled oats

¾ cup oat flour

½ cup chopped walnuts

½ teaspoon ground cinnamon

1 teaspoon baking powder

Oil for casserole dish (optional)

1. Preheat the oven to 350°F. Place the flax-seeds, ½ cup of the prunes, and water in a bowl. Allow to sit for 15 minutes, stirring occasionally. Transfer to a blender along with the maple syrup, if using, and blend until smooth.
2. Meanwhile, place the remaining ½ cup of prunes and remaining ingredients, except the oil, in a large bowl and mix well. Add the blended prune mixture and mix well.
3. Transfer to a well-oiled, nonstick, or parchment paper–lined 8 by 8-inch casserole dish. Bake for 40 minutes. Serve warm or at room temperature.

VARIATIONS

- Replace ½ cup of the prunes and the cup of water with ½ cup of oil, such as safflower.
- Replace ½ cup of the chopped prunes with other dried fruit, such as raisins or chopped dates or figs.
- Add ¼ cup of vegan dark chocolate chips.
- Replace 1 cup of the water with freshly squeezed orange juice. Add ½ teaspoon of orange zest along with the walnuts.
- Replace the oat flour with flour of your choosing, such as a gluten-free flour blend (for homemade, see page 254), spelt, whole wheat pastry, or unbleached all-purpose.

Fruit Compote

Warming, spiced fruits make a wonderfully nourishing fall or winter treat, and a perfect way to continue enjoying highly beneficial fruit throughout the year. Enjoy warm or cold on its own or topped with Vegan Coco Whip (page 289) or Coconut Yogurt (page 262). You didn't hear it here, but you can also top it with your favorite vegan ice cream. The adventurous can take the next step and use the compote as the fruit filling in a Fruit Cobbler (page 288).

TOTAL YIELD: 24 OUNCES
Serving Size: 6 ounces
Number of Servings: 4
Prep Time: 10 minutes
Cook Time: 15 minutes
Total Time: 25 minutes

1½ cups diced pineapple
1 cup diced pear
1 cup diced peach
½ cup blackberries
½ cup freshly squeezed orange juice
½ cup finely chopped dates
½ teaspoon ground cinnamon

Place all the ingredients in a medium-size pot over medium heat. Cook until the fruit breaks down and begins to thicken, about 15 minutes, stirring frequently.

VARIATIONS

- Add 1 teaspoon of orange zest and 2 tablespoons of pure maple syrup, or desired sweetener to taste.
- Add ½ teaspoon pumpkin pie spice and ¼ teaspoon of ground cardamom.
- Add ½ cup of chopped crystallized ginger.
- Replace the fruit with your favorite fresh or frozen fruits, such as mango, nectarine, strawberries, blueberries, mixed berries, plum, and yes, even banana.
- Replace the dates with prunes or dried apricots or figs.
- Replace the orange juice with another fruit juice, such as apple or pineapple.

Fruit Cobbler

Take your fruit compote to the next level by including it in this simple cobbler. The humble oat, surprisingly nutrient dense, blends with dried coconut for a tasty topping to our antioxidant-rich treat—enjoy as a dessert or as part of a special breakfast along with a glass of Pumpkin Seed Milk (page 116).

TOTAL YIELD: 1 (8-INCH) SQUARE CASSEROLE DISH

> Serving Size: 1 (2-inch) square piece
> Number of Servings: 16
> Prep Time: 10 minutes
> Cook Time: 45 minutes
> Total Time: 55 minutes

1 recipe Fruit Compote (page 287), cooked and left in its pot, or 24 ounces fresh or frozen fruit, cooked in a pot over low heat until just soft

1 tablespoon arrowroot powder

¼ cup water

½ cup coconut nectar or pure maple syrup (optional)

Oil for casserole

TOPPING: DRY

¾ cup rolled oats

½ cup flour, such as a gluten-free flour blend (for homemade, see page 254), spelt, or whole wheat pastry

¼ cup dried coconut

TOPPING: WET

¼ cup vegan granulated sugar (optional)

Pinch of sea salt

¼ teaspoon cinnamon or pumpkin pie spice

¼ cup almond milk (for homemade, see variation on page 116)

2 tablespoons melted coconut oil or vegan butter (optional)

1. Dissolve the arrowroot powder in the water and add to the pot of cooked compote. Cook for 5 minutes, stirring frequently. For added sweetness, add the coconut nectar, if desired. Transfer to a lightly oiled or nonstick 8 by 8-inch casserole dish.

2. Combine the dry ingredients in a bowl and mix well. Combine the wet ingredients in a separate bowl and mix well. Add the wet to the dry and mix well. Crumble on top of the fruit compote. Bake for 45 minutes in a 350°F oven.

Coco Berry Delight

Further proof that you don't need to sacrifice flavor when indulging in a dairy-free whipped cream. Here's a healthy and luscious way to enhance all the benefits of one of the top protective foods—berries! Plan ahead so you can place your coconut milk in the fridge for at least 12 hours for this recipe. Granulated sugar works best, though the sugar is actually optional. You might love it with just the natural sweetness of the coconut milk. You can serve the Vegan Coco Whip on top of your favorite vegan ice cream or on top of The Great Pumpkin Cheezcake (page 294), Berry Mousse (page 290), or Fruit Compote (page 287).

TOTAL YIELD: 16 OUNCES FRUIT, 8 OUNCES WHIP

   Serving Size: 4 ounces fruit, 2 ounces whip
   Number of Servings: 4
   Prep Time: 15 minutes
   Total Time: 15 minutes

VEGAN COCO WHIP

1 (14-ounce) can coconut milk

½ teaspoon pure vanilla extract

2 tablespoons vegan granulated sugar, or to taste (optional)

Pinch of ground cardamom

Pinch of ground cinnamon

2 cups assorted berries

¼ cup cacao nibs

1. Place the can of coconut milk in the refrigerator for at least 12 hours. Open the can and scoop out just the solid cream and place in a mixing bowl or stand mixer fitted with the whisk attachment, discarding the liquid portion or saving for use in soups or in rice dishes.

2. Add the vanilla, sugar, if using, cardamom, and cinnamon and whip (use an eggbeater if whisking manually) until a whipped cream consistency is attained, about 10 minutes.

3. Place the berries in bowls and top with the whip and cacao nibs before serving. Get ready to indulge!

4. Serve immediately. If necessary, you can refrigerate. Rewhip before serving.

VARIATIONS

- Replace the berries with fresh fruit of your choosing.

- Top with additional superfoods, such as chia seeds, goji berries, or hemp seeds.

Berry Mousse

We sincerely hope that you will enjoy this berry good recipe. As we may have mentioned, the more berries you eat, the better off your heart, brain, skin, and digestion will be! The cashew base adds even more heart, brain, mood, and skin benefits with its B vitamins, vitamin E, protein, and mineral content. Top with Vegan Coco Whip (page 289) or Vegan Fluff with Aquafaba (page 283) and fresh berries.

TOTAL YIELD: 16 OUNCES
  Serving Size: 4 ounces
  Number of Servings: 4
  Soak Time: 20 minutes
  Prep Time: 5 minutes
  Total Time: 25 minutes

¾ cup raw cashew pieces

1 cup blueberries

¾ cup vanilla almond or soy milk

1 teaspoon pure vanilla extract

¼ teaspoon ground cardamom

2 tablespoons pure maple syrup (optional)

1. Place the cashews in a bowl with ample water to cover. Allow to sit for 20 minutes up to a few hours. Drain and rinse well.
2. Transfer to a strong blender or food processor along with the remaining ingredients and blend until creamy.

VARIATIONS

- To keep this recipe raw, use homemade almond milk (see variation, page 116).
- Replace the blueberries with strawberries, mango, or peach.
- Replace the cashews with macadamia or Brazil nuts.
- Add ½ cup of just-ripe avocado (if it's too ripe, it will impart an avocado flavor).

Raw Peppermint Patty Fudge Brownies

What more can we say? Sometimes the name alone is sufficient to instantly activate cravings. This brownie has all the elements: fudgy, chocolaty, nutty, and a creamy mint filling, made with a base of all whole food ingredients to keep your energy sustained without a sugar crash. Get a double dose of brain-boosting magnesium with the cacao and the dates. If you want this to be 100 percent fruit sweetened, use date syrup (for homemade, see page 109) as the sweetener. You can also omit the peppermint filling for a straight-on raw fudge brownie. Enjoy with a glass of Pumpkin Seed Milk (page 116) or Creamy Tropical Bliss (page 118).

TOTAL YIELD: 24 OUNCES
> Serving Size: 2 ounces
> Number of Servings: 12
> Soak Time: 20 minutes
> Prep Time: 20 minutes
> Freeze Time: 3 hours
> Total Time: 3 hours 40 minutes—shorter if you omit the Creme Filling.

CREME FILLING
1 cup raw cashew pieces
½ cup water
¼ cup coconut nectar, pure maple syrup, date syrup (for homemade, see page 109), or agave nectar. (Note that clear agave nectar will yield the whitest cream.)
½ teaspoon peppermint extract

BROWNIES
1 cup hazelnuts
¾ cup tightly packed pitted Medjool dates
¼ cup water or fruit juice
½ cup unsweetened cacao powder
¼ cup almond butter
2 tablespoons raw coconut nectar, pure maple syrup, or date syrup (for homemade, see page 109) (optional)
½ teaspoon ground cinnamon (optional but recommended)
Pinch of sea salt
Oil for casserole dish (optional)

1. Prepare the filling: Place the cashews in a bowl with ample water to cover. Allow to sit for 20 minutes, up to a few hours. Rinse and drain well. Transfer to a blender along with the remaining filling

continues

continued

ingredients and blend until creamy. Set aside.

2. Prepare the brownies: Place the hazelnuts in a food processor and process until smooth. Add the remaining brownie ingredients, except the oil, and process until smooth.

3. Lightly oil an 8 by 8-inch casserole dish, or use a nonstick pan. Spread the brownie mixture in the pan. Top with the Creme Filling. Place in the freezer until solid enough to cut, about 3 hours.

4. To serve, slice into small squares. Enjoy! Keep any leftovers refrigerated and eat within a week.

VARIATIONS

- Replace the hazelnuts with almonds, pecans, cashews, or sunflower seeds.

- Replace the cashews with macadamia nuts.

- Add ½ teaspoon of pure vanilla extract and ¼ teaspoon of ground cardamom along with the dates.

- Want to create a double layer brownie, with the cream layer in the center? Then, reduce the water in the cream layer to ¼ cup and use a small loaf pan instead of an 8 by 8-inch pan. Place half of the brownie mixture in the bottom of the pan. Top with the cream layer. Freeze for 2 hours. Place the remaining half of the brownie mixture on top of the cream layer and freeze for 1 hour.

Mango Rice Pudding with Salted Caramel

This recipe was passed down by Krishna himself as a gift for those of us who like to enjoy a sweet dessert every now and then. Vitamin C–packed mango is like a kiss from the sun, not to mention it helps with hydration and building collagen in tissues. A known aura cleanser, the salted caramel puts this over the top. Top with toasted coconut and serve with Digestive Support Tea (page 122).

TOTAL YIELD: 32 OUNCES
  Serving Size: 8 ounces
  Number of Servings: 4
  Prep Time: 5 minutes
  Cook Time: 25 minutes
  Total Time: 30 minutes

1¾ cups water

1¼ cups uncooked white basmati rice

1 (13-ounce) can coconut milk, divided

1 teaspoon plus ⅛ teaspoon sea salt, divided

1 cup chopped fresh or frozen and defrosted mango (small chop)

¼ cup vegan granulated or brown sugar or desired sweetener to taste

¼ teaspoon ground cinnamon

¼ teaspoon ground cardamom

⅓ cup chopped macadamia or pistachio nuts, optionally toasted (see page 106), for garnish

1. Place the water, rice, 1 cup of the coconut milk, and ⅛ teaspoon of the sea salt in a medium-size pot over high heat. Bring to a boil. Stir well, cover, lower the heat to low, and cook until all the liquid is absorbed, about 20 minutes. Remove from the heat, leave the cover on, and allow to sit for 5 minutes. Fluff with a fork. Add the mango and stir well.

2. Meanwhile, create the salted caramel sauce. Place the remaining ¾ cup of coconut milk, remaining 1 teaspoon of sea salt, and the sugar, cinnamon, and cardamom in a small pot over low heat. Cook for 10 minutes, stirring frequently. Keep warm until ready to serve.

3. To serve, portion out the rice into individual bowls or use one large serving bowl. Drizzle with the caramel sauce and top with the chopped macadamia nuts before serving.

VARIATIONS

- Add ½ cup of raisins along with the rice.

- Replace the coconut milk with soy, almond, rice, or pumpkin seed milk (for homemade, see page 116).

- Replace the basmati rice with black "forbidden" rice and add an extra cup of water. Cook until all the liquid is absorbed.

The Great Pumpkin Cheezcake

Even Charlie Brown would rave about this vegan, cashew-based cheesecake. Versatile, beta-carotene-rich golden pumpkin keeps the skin and immune system superhealthy, and has far-reaching nutritional benefits to keep you healthy both inside and out. Nutritional yeast gives the cheesy flavor and a boost of nutrients, including vitamin B_{12}. Top with Vegan Coco Whip (page 289) or Vegan Fluff with Aquafaba (page 283) and serve after your holiday feast if you have any room!

TOTAL YIELD: 24 OUNCES FILLING,
1 (9-INCH) PIECRUST

Serving Size: 1 (3-ounce) slice
Number of Servings: 8
Prep Time: 5 minutes
Soak Time: 20 minutes
Cook Time: 60 minutes
Total Time: 1 hour 25 minutes

1 piecrust (store-bought or homemade [see variation of Polenta Piecrust, page 236])

¾ cup raw cashew pieces

½ cup vanilla soy or almond milk

½ to ¾ cup pure maple syrup, coconut nectar, date syrup (for homemade, see page 109), or desired sweetener to taste

1 (15-ounce) can pure pumpkin puree, or freshly roasted (see page 153)

3 tablespoons nutritional yeast

¼ cup freshly squeezed lemon juice

2 teaspoons pumpkin pie spice

¼ teaspoon sea salt

1. Preheat the oven to 350°F. Poke a few holes in the bottom of the piecrust with a fork. Place the piecrust in the oven and bake for 5 minutes. Remove.
2. Place the cashew pieces in a bowl with ample water to cover. Allow to sit for 20 minutes to up to a few hours. Rinse and drain well. Transfer to a blender along with the soy milk and maple syrup and blend well. Add the remaining ingredients to the blender and blend until creamy.
3. Transfer to the piecrust. Place in the oven and bake for 50 minutes or until the top is golden brown with cracks appearing on the surface.

VARIATIONS

🔸 Add 2 teaspoons of pure vanilla extract along with the lemon juice.

🔸 For a **Pumpkin Meringue Cheezcake**, top with one recipe Vegan Fluff with Aquafaba (page 283). Set the oven to HIGH broil. Broil for 5 minutes, or until the top begins to brown. If you are feeling a bit more pyromaniacal, you can break out the crème brûlée torch and go to town.

ACKNOWLEDGMENTS

This book would not be possible without the loving support of our families. Without the babysitting help of grandparents Bill and Cathy Boudet, and Roberta Reinfeld, you may not be holding this book in your hands now. We are grateful for all of you.

We also give thanks to the countless individuals who have pioneered the research regarding the benefits of a plant-based diet for our health and for creating a sustainable future for humanity. They have cleared the way for the cultural shift of the main-streaming of veganism that we are now experiencing. *Viva la révolution!*

Many thanks, props, and respect always to our teachers and mentors. Special thanks go to our rock star literary agent, Marilyn Allen, and for our dear friend Daniel Rhoda. We count our lucky stars that we are able to publish another book with Da Capo and our editors Katie McHugh Malm, Iris Bass, Claire Schulz, and Renée Sedliar. Thank you once again for believing in us.

Thanks to the stellar team of recipe testers and food photographers, including Elizabeth Arraj, Suzanne Prendergast, Lisa Portnoff, Lisa Parker, Roland Barker, and Olivia Wallace. Thanks to Helena Long and Hailey Haddox for your help with editing. Special thanks also to the Fountain of Youther contributors. You are inspiring the next generation!

NOTES

Chapter One: Live Longer, Live Better

3   **A recent study reported that the average life expectancy:** CDC current life expectancy: https://www.cnn.com/2017/12/21/health/us-life-expectancy-study/index.html.

3   **A six-year study by the Centers for Disease Control:** E. S. Ford et al., "Healthy Lifestyle Behaviors and All-Cause Mortality Among Adults in the United States," *Preventive Medicine* 55, no. 1 (July 2012): 23–27.

3   **a large ten-year observational study:** Rosalind Chia-Yu Chen et al., "Cooking Frequency May Enhance Survival in Taiwanese Elderly," *Public Health Nutrition* 15, no. 7 (July 2012): 1142–1149, published online May 11, 2011.

4   **The National Council on Aging recently outlined:** https://www.ncoa.org/blog/10-common-chronic-diseases-prevention-tips/.

5   **vegetarians live on average almost eight years longer:** https://www.huffingtonpost.com/kathy-freston/plant-based-diet_b_1981838.html.

6   **A 2012 paper found that the amino acid leucine:** B. C. Melnik, "Leucine Signaling in the Pathogenesis of Type 2 Diabetes and Obesity," *World Journal of Diabetes* 3, no. 3 (March 15, 2012): 38–53.

7   **In 2008, Dr. Dean Ornish teamed up:** D. Ornish et al., "Increased Telomerase Activity and Comprehensive Lifestyle Changes: A Pilot Study," *Lancet Oncology* 9, no. 11 (November 2008): 1048–1057.

7   **In a 2013 follow-up study:** Dean Ornish et al., "Effect of Comprehensive Lifestyle Changes on Telomerase Activity and Telomere Length in Men with Biopsy-Proven Low-Risk Prostate Cancer: 5-Year Follow-up of a Descriptive Pilot Study," *Lancet Oncology* 14 (September 17, 2013): 1112–1120.

8   **In a 2003 eight-week dietary intervention study:** S. K. Bøhn et al., "Blood Cell Gene Expression Associated with Cellular Stress Defense Is Modulated by Antioxidant-Rich Food (Kiwi) in a Randomised Controlled Clinical Trial of Male Smokers," *BMC Medicine* 8 (September 16, 2010): 54.

9   **Measuring the effects of a plant-based diet:** Monica H. Carlsen et al., "The Total Antioxidant Content of More Than 3100 Foods, Beverages, Spices, Herbs and Supplements Used Worldwide," *Nutrition Journal* 9 (2010): 3, published online January 22, 2010.

9   **Studies have shown that pterostilbene:** Resveratrol and pterostilbene: https://www.nutraingredients-usa.com/Article/2011/11/21/Resveratrol-may-boost-mental-functions-but-pterostilbene-may-be-even-better-Animal-studies#.

10   **whether omega-3 polyunsaturated fatty acid:** J. K. Kiecolt-Glaser et al., "Omega-3 Fatty Acids, Oxidative Stress, and Leukocyte Telomere Length: A Randomized Controlled Trial," *Brain Behavior and Immunity* 28 (February 2013): 16–24, published online September 23, 2012.

10   **In a Harvard study published in *JAMA*:** Mingyang Song et al., "Association of Animal and Plant Protein Intake with All-Cause and Cause-Specific Mortality," *JAMA Internal Medicine* 176, no. 10 (October 2016): 1453–1463, doi: 10.1001/jamainternmed.2016.4182.

10   **people who ate the most whole grains:** Geng Zong et al., "Whole Grain Intake and Mortality from All Causes, Cardiovascular Disease, and Cancer: A Meta-analysis of Prospective Cohort Studies," *Circulation* 133 (2016): 2370–2380.

10   **overall cognition in seniors:** M. C. Morris et al., "Nutrients and Bioactives in Green Leafy Vegetables and Cognitive Decline: Prospective Study," *Neurology* 90, no. 3 (January 16, 2018): e214–e222, published online December 20, 2017.

Chapter Two: Brain Health—Stay Mentally Sharp: Combat Cognitive Decline

12   **But a National Institutes of Health (NIH) study:** Dale E. Bredesen, "Reversal of Cognitive Decline: A Novel Therapeutic Program (MEND Study)," *Aging* (Albany, NY) 6, no. 9 (September 2014): 707–717, published online September 27, 2014, doi: 10.18632/aging.100690.

14   **Globally, the lowest validated rates of Alzheimer's:** J. E. Galvin, "Pass the Grain; Spare the Brain," *Neurology* 69, no. 11 (September 11, 2007): 1072–1073.

14   **And, in a new book on brain health:** Dean and Ayesha Sherzai, *The Alzheimer's Solution: A Breakthrough Program to Prevent and Reverse the Symptoms of Cognitive Decline at Every Age* (New York: HarperOne, 2017).

16   **supplementing with DHA and EPA omega-3s:** Joel Fuhrman, "Omega-3 Fatty Acids, DHA and EPA, Are Crucial for Brain Health Through All Stages of Life," *Eat to Live* (blog), September 18, 2017, https://www.drfuhrman.com/library/eat-to-live-blog/149/omega -3-fatty-acids-dha-and-epa-are-crucial-for-brain-health-through-all-stages-of-life.

17   **Deficiency in any one B vitamin:** David O. Kennedy, "B Vitamins and the Brain: Mechanisms, Dose and Efficacy—A Review," *Nutrients* 8, no. 2 (February 2016): 68, published online January 28, 2016, doi: 10.3390/nu8020068.

17   **More than a third of psychiatric admissions:** E. Reynolds, "Vitamin B12, Folic Acid, and the Nervous System," *Lancet Neurology* 5 (2006): 949–960, doi: 10.1016/S1474-4422(06) 70598-1.

19   **twelve weeks of supplementation:** Robert Krikorian et al., "Blueberry Supplementation Improves Memory in Older Adults," *Journal of Agricultural and Food Chemistry* 58, no. 7 (April 14, 2010): 3996–4000.

21   **Wendy Suzuki describes:** Wendy Suzuki with Billie Fitzpatrick, *Healthy Brain, Happy Life: A Personal Program to Activate Your Brain & Do Everything Better* (New York: Dey Street Books, 2015).

21   **dancing has the most profound effect:** Kathrin Rehfeld et al., "Dancing or Fitness Sport? The Effects of Two Training Programs on Hippocampal Plasticity and Balance Abilities in Healthy Seniors," *Frontiers in Human Neuroscience* (June, 15 2017), https://doi.org/10.3389 /fnhum.2017.00305.

21   **A 1992 Japanese study:** Masashichi M. Kawano, Koichi Mimura, and Mitsuo Kaneko, "The Effect of Table Tennis Practice on Mental Ability Evaluated by Kana-Pick-Out Test," *International Journal of Table Tennis Sciences* (1992), 1: 57–62.

22   **Reading a novel:** Gregory S. Berns et al., "Short- and Long-Term Effects of a Novel on Connectivity in the Brain," *Brain Connectivity* 3, no. 6, published online December 9, 2013, https://doi.org/10.1089/brain.2013.0166.

22   **brain cells shrink while you sleep?:** Lulu Xie et al., "Sleep Drives Metabolite Clearance from the Adult Brain," *Science* 342, no. 6156 (October 18, 2013): 373–377, doi: 10.1126/science.1241224.

23   **A 2006 study:** P. D. Larsen and D. C. Galletly, "The Sound of Silence Is Music to the Heart," *Heart* 92, no. 4 (April 2006): 433–434, published online December 9, 2005, doi: 10.1136/hrt.2005.071902.

24   **can directly prevent age-related macular degeneration:** Francis E. Cangemi, "TOZAL Study: An Open Case Control Study of an Oral Antioxidant and Omega-3 Supplement for Dry AMD," *BMC Ophthalmology* 2007: 3.

24   **daily dietary supplementation with the berries:** Peter Bucheli et al., "Goji Berry Effects on Macular Characteristics and Plasma Antioxidant Levels," *Optometry and Vision Science* 88, no. 2 (2011): 257–262.

24   **ginkgolides—antioxidants that help protect:** Konstantin Tziridis et al., "Protective Effects of *Ginkgo biloba* Extract EGb 761 Against Noise Trauma-Induced Hearing Loss and Tinnitus Development," *Neural Plasticity* (2014).

24   **exercising provides the best protection:** Chul Han et al., "Effects of Long-Term Exercise on Age-Related Hearing Loss in Mice," *Journal of Neuroscience* 36, no. 44 (November 2, 2016): 11308–11319, doi: https://doi.org/10.1523/JNEUROSCI.2493-16.2016.

Chapter Three: Aging Takes Guts!: Optimize Your Digestion

29   **small intestines to absorb what you eat:** E. Britton and J. T. McLaughlin, "Aging and the Gut," *Proceedings of the Nutrition Society* (UK) (November 2012): 1–5.

31   **the top three risk factors:** Martha L. Slattery et al., "Eating Patterns and Risk of Colon Cancer," *American Journal of Epidemiology* 148, no. 1 (1998).

33   **in the 2011 *New England Journal of Medicine*:** Dariush Mozaffarian et al., "Changes in Diet and Lifestyle and Long-Term Weight Gain in Women and Men," *New England Journal of Medicine* (June 23, 2011), https://www.nejm.org/doi/full/10.1056/Nejmoa1014296.

34   **People who ate just ¾ cup of beans:** Russell de Souza, "Eating Beans, Peas, Chickpeas or Lentils May Help Lose Weight and Keep It Off," *American Journal of Clinical Nutrition* (March 30, 2016).

35   **Getting fewer than seven hours of sleep:** Andrew D. Calvin et al., "Effects of Experimental Sleep Restriction on Caloric Intake and Activity Energy Expenditure," *Chest* 144, no. 1 (July 2013): 79–86, published online February 7, 2013, doi: 10.1378/chest.12-2829.

36   **Discontinue using antibacterial soaps:** J. V. Ribaldo et al., "Household Triclosan and Triclocarban Effects on the Infant and Maternal Microbiome," *EMBO Molecular Medicine* 9, no. 12 (December 2017): 1732–1741, doi: 10.15252/emmm.201707882.

43   **Having healthy muscle mass essentially protects:** Byunghun So et al., "Exercise-Induced Myokines in Health and Metabolic Diseases," *Integrative Medicine Research* 3, no. 4 (December 2014): 172–179.

44   **Other hormones secreted by muscle:** Myokines are cytokines produced within skeletal muscle cells and released into the circulation can induce downstream cytokine-mediated events and possibly influence further the cytokine and immune system. It has been suggested that cytokines and other muscle-derived peptides that are expressed, produced, and released by muscle fibers and exert paracrine or endocrine effects should be classified as "myokines." It appears that skeletal muscle has the capacity to express several myokines, such as IL-6, IL-8, IL-15, and leukemia inhibitory factor, while these muscle contraction–induced myokines can mediate direct endocrine anti-inflammatory effects. https://www.sciencedirect.com/topics/neuroscience/myokine, https://www.sciencedirect.com/science/article/pii/S2213422014000705.

44   **building lean muscle mass:** Tyna Moore, "Muscle As Medicine: A Most Naturopathic Anti-Aging Medicine," *Naturopathic Doctor News & Review*, posted May 1, 2017, https://ndnr.com/anti-aging/muscle-as-medicine-a-most-naturopathic-anti-aging-medicine/.

44   **One small study looked at ten female:** N. F. Taylor et al., "Progressive Resistance Exercise for People with Multiple Sclerosis," *Disability Rehabilitation* 38, no. 18 (September 30, 2006): 1119–1126.

Chapter Five: Protect Your Heart for the Long Run

52   **can melt away atherosclerotic plaques:** H. S. Dod et al., "Effect of Intensive Lifestyle Changes on Endothelial Function and on Inflammatory Markers of Atherosclerosis," *American Journal of Cardiology* 105, no. 3 (February 1, 2010): 362–367.

52   **This has been shown in many studies since the 1970s:** F. R. Ellis and T. A. Sanders, "Angina and Vegan Diet," *American Heart Journal* 93, no. 6 (June 1977): 803–805.

52   **a plant-based diet can reduce angina attacks:** R. A. Vogel, M. C. Coretti, and G. D. Plotnick, "Changes in Flow-Mediated Brachial Artery Vasoactivity with Lowering of Desirable Cholesterol Levels in Healthy Middle-Aged Men," *American Journal of Cardiology* 77, no. 1 (January 1996): 37–40; M. F. McCarty, "A Shift in Myocardial Substrate, Improved Endothelial Function, and Diminished Sympathetic Activity May Contribute to the Anti-anginal Impact of Very-Low-Fat Diets," *Medical Hypotheses* 62, no. 1 (2004): 62–71; J. A. Frattaroli et al., "Angina Pectoris and Atherosclerotic Risk Factors in the Multisite Cardiac Lifestyle Intervention Program," *American Journal of Cardiology* 101, no. 7 (April 1, 2008): 911–918.

54   **over 32 million Americans:** Qiuping Gu et al., "Prescription Cholesterol-Lowering Medication Use in Adults Aged 40 and Over: United States, 2003–2012," NCHS Data Brief No. 177, December 2014.

55   **plant-based diet may decrease your cholesterol levels:** Philip J. Tuso et al., "Nutritional 54 for Physicians: Plant-Based Diets," *Permanente Journal* 17, no. 2 (Spring 2013): 61–66.

55   **Dr. Esselstyn's arrest and reversal study:** C. B. Esselstyn Jr., "Updating a 12-Year Experience with Arrest and Reversal Therapy for Coronary Heart Disease," *American Journal of Cardiology*

84, no. 3 (August 1999): 339–341, A8; Caldwell B. Esselstyn Jr., "We Can Prevent and Even Reverse Coronary Artery Heart Disease," *Medscape General Medicine* 9, no. 3 (2007): 46, published online August 31, 2007; C. Esseltyn et al., "A Way to Reverse CAD," *Journal of Family Practice* 63, no. 7 (July 2014): 356–364.

55   **his strict whole food, plant-based protocol:** Caldwell B. Esselstyn Jr., *Prevent and Reverse Heart Disease: The Revolutionary, Scientifically Proven, Nutrition-Based Cure* (New York: Avery Books: 2018).

55   **Framingham Heart Study:** Syed S. Mahmood et al., "The Framingham Heart Study and the Epidemiology of Cardiovascular Diseases: A Historical Perspective," *Lancet* 383, no. 9921 (March 15, 2014): 999–1008, published online September 29, 2013, doi: 10.1016/S0140-6736(13)61752-3, http://www.framinghamheartstudy.org/.

56   **Nitric oxide is critical to healthy arterial function:** https://nutritiongenome.com/nitric-oxide-a-key-understanding-of-inflammation/.

56   **top way to increase nitric oxide:** T. Otsuki, K. Shimizu, and S. Maeda, "Changes in Arterial Stiffness and Nitric Oxide Production with Chlorella-Derived Multicomponent Supplementation in Middle-Aged and Older Individuals," *Journal of Clinical Biochemistry and Nutrition* 57, no. 3 (November 2015): 228–232, doi: 10.3164/jcbn.15-86, published online October 17, 2015.

56   **your blood flow is sixteen times as great!:** Poiseuille's law: The quantity of a liquid flowing through a tube increases by the fourth power of the increase of the radius of the tube. Increase the radius by a factor of 2, the flow increases by the fourth power of the radius, that is, by a factor of 2 * 2 * 2 * 2—by a factor of 16 times!

56   **choline from plant-based sources:** M. R. Olthof and P. Verhoef, "Effects of Betaine Intake on Plasma Homocysteine Concentrations and Consequences for Health," *Current Drug Metabolism* 6, no. 1 (February 2005): 15–22.

56   **can also be metabolized into trimethylamine oxide:** "Choline, TMAO and Heart Health," Cleveland HeartLab (blog), May 8, 2017, http://www.clevelandheartlab.com/blog/choline-tmao-heart-health/.

57   **What they found is that those with low levels:** Shoaib Afzal and Børge G. Nordestgaard, "Vitamin D and Risk of Cardiovascular Disease," *Arteriosclerosis, Thrombosis, and Vascular Biology* 37 (2017): 1981–1982.

57   **Hawthorn berry is now being studied:** Jie Wang, Xingjiang Xiong, and Bo Feng, "Effect of *Crataegus* Usage in Cardiovascular Disease Prevention: An Evidence-Based Approach," *Evidence Based Complementary Alternative Medicine* 2013 (2013): 149363, published online December 29, 2013.

58   **Green tea contains a powerful antioxidant:** Pon Velayutham, Anandh Babu, and Dongmin Liu, "Green Tea Catechins and Cardiovascular Health: An Update," *Current Medicinal Chemistry* 15, no. 18 (2008): 1840–1850.

58   **In a Tufts University study:** Diane L. McKay et al., "Hibiscus Sabdariffa L. Tea (Tisane) Lowers Blood Pressure in Prehypertensive and Mildly Hypertensive Adults," *Journal of Nutrition* 140, no. 2 (February 1, 2010): 298–303.

59   **electron deficiency from lack of connection:** Gaétan Chevalier et al., "Earthing: Health Implications of Reconnecting the Human Body to the Earth's Surface Electrons," *Journal of Environmental and Public Health* 2012 (2012): 291541, published online January 12, 2012.

59 **At least a dozen studies have shown:** James L. Oschman, Gaétan Chevalier, and Richard Brown, "The Effects of Grounding (Earthing) on Inflammation, the Immune Response, Wound Healing, and Prevention and Treatment of Chronic Inflammatory and Autoimmune Diseases," *Journal of Inflammation Research* 8 (2015): 83–96, published online March 24, 2015, doi: 10.2147/JIR.S69656.

59 **book *HeartMath Solution*:** Doc Childre and Howard Martin, *The HeartMath Solution: The Institute of HeartMath's Revolutionary Program for Engaging the Power of the Heart's Intelligence* (New York: HarperOne, 1999).

59 **people who practice meditation:** Robert Schneider et al., "Effects of Stress Reduction on Clinical Events in African Americans with Coronary Heart Disease: A Randomized Controlled Trial," *Circulation* 120 (2009): S461.

59 **Dr. Dean Ornish's work:** Dean Ornish, *Dr. Dean Ornish's Program for Reversing Heart Disease* (New York: Random House, 1990), https://www.ornish.com/undo-it/.

Chapter Six: Kidney Health Is Key

65 **Research shows promise in the use:** Oscar H. Franco et al., "Use of Plant-Based Therapies and Menopausal Symptoms, A Systematic Review and Meta-analysis," *JAMA* 315, no. 23 (2016): 2554–2563, published online June 21, 2016, doi: 10.1001/jama.2016.8012; P. Sunita and S. P. Pattanayak, "Phytoestrogens in Postmenopausal Indications: A Theoretical Perspective," *Pharmacognosy Review* 5, no. 9 (January–June 2011): 41–47; Sukanya Jaroenporn et al., "Improvements of Vaginal Atrophy Without Systemic Side Effects After Topical Application of *Pueraria mirifica*, a Phytoestrogen-Rich Herb, in Postmenopausal Cynomolgus Macaques," *Journal of Reproduction and Development* 60, no. 3 (2014): 238–245, published online April 21, 2014, doi: 10.1262/jrd.2013-144; M.-N. Chen, C.-C. Lin, and C.-F. Liu, "Efficacy of Phytoestrogens for Menopausal Symptoms: A Meta-analysis and Systematic Review," *Climacteric* 18, no. 2 (March 2015): 260–269, published online December 1, 2014.

66 **Nettle leaf . . . enlarged prostate:** M. R. Safarinejad, "Urtica dioica for Treatment of Benign Prostatic Hyperplasia: A Prospective, Randomized, Double-Blind, Placebo-Controlled, Crossover Study," *Journal of Herbal Pharmacotherapy* 5, no. 4 (2005): 1–11; T. Schneider and H. Rübben, "Stinging Nettle Root Extract (Bazoton-uno) in Long Term Treatment of Benign Prostatic Syndrome (BPS): Results of a randomized, Double-Blind, Placebo Controlled Multicenter Study After 12 Months," *Urologe A* 43, no. 3 (March 2004): 302–306.

66 **saw palmetto . . . inflamed or enlarged prostate:** S. A. Kaplan, "Serenoa repens for Lower Urinary Tract Symptoms/Benign Prostatic Hyperplasia: Current Evidence and Its Clinical Implications in Naturopathic Medicine," *Journal of Urology* 199, no. 6 (June 2018): 1372–1373, published online March 20, 2018.

67 **Phytoestrogenic foods . . . kidney function:** T. Ranich, S. J. Bhathena, and M. T. Velasquez, "Protective Effects of Dietary Phytoestrogens in Chronic Renal Disease," *Journal of Renal Nutrition* 11, no. 4 (October 2001): 183–193.

67 **soy specifically . . . protective effect:** Esther Walser-Domjan et al., "Association of Urinary Phytoestrogen Concentrations with Serum Concentrations of Prostate-Specific Antigen in the

National Health and Nutrition Examination Survey," *Nutrition and Cancer* 65, no. 6 (2013): 813–819, doi: 10.1080/01635581.2013.801999.

Chapter Seven: Look Younger: Secrets of Skin Health

73   **safer sunscreen brands:** https://www.ewg.org/sunscreen/report/executive-summary/#.WzLgZxIzrOQ.

75   **Eating silica- and other mineral-rich foods:** Silke K. Schagen et al., "Discovering the Link Between Nutrition and Skin Aging," *Dermatoendocrinology* 4, no. 3 (July 1, 2012): 298–307.

75   **Coconut oil contains lauric acid:** T. Nakatsuji et al., "Antimicrobial Property of Lauric Acid Against Propionibacterium Acnes: Its Therapeutic Potential for Inflammatory Acne Vulgaris," *Journal of Investigative Dermatology* 129, no. 10 (October 2009): 2480–2408, doi: 10.1038/jid.2009.93, published electronically April 23, 2009.

75   **Eating food sources of beta-carotene:** M. L. Slattery et al., "Carotenoids and Colon Cancer," *American Journal of Clinical Nutrition* 71, no. 2 (February 2000): 575–582.

76   **Vitamin C also helps with skin cell repair:** Juliet M. Pullar, Anitra C. Carr, and Margreet C. M. Vissers, "The Roles of Vitamin C in Skin Health," *Nutrients* 9, no. 8 (August 2017): 866.

76   **Dark-colored fruits . . . anthocyanidins:** Ruža Pandel et al., "Skin Photoaging and the Role of Antioxidants in Its Prevention," *ISRN Dermatology* (2013): 930164.

76   **Berries . . . ellagic acid:** Beomyeol Baek et al., "Ellagic Acid Plays a Protective Role Against UV-B-Induced Oxidative Stress by Up-Regulating Antioxidant Components in Human Dermal Fibroblasts," *Korean Journal of Physiology Pharmacology* 20, no. 3 (May 2016): 269–277.

76   **One study adding avocado oil to your diet:** M. J. Werman, "The Effect of Various Avocado Oils on Skin Collagen Metabolism," *Connective Tissue Research* 26, no. 1–2 (1991): 1–10.

76   **Green tea . . . epigallocatechin gallate:** Lesley E. Rhodes et al., "Oral Green Tea Catechin Metabolites Are Incorporated into Human Skin and Protect Against UV Radiation-Induced Cutaneous Inflammation in Association with Reduced Production of Pro-inflammatory Eicosanoid 12-hydroxyeicosatetraenoic Acid," *British Journal of Nutrition* (September 14, 2013): 891–900.

77   **According to a 2010 study:** G. G. Hillebrand et al., "New Wrinkles on Wrinkling: An 8-Year Longitudinal Study on the Progression of Expression Lines into Persistent Wrinkles," *British Journal of Dermatology* (May 20, 2010).

78   **Castor oil packs:** W. A. McGarey, *The Oil That Heals* (Virginia Beach, VA: A.R.E. Press, 1993); Grady Harvey, "Immunomodulation Through Castor Oil Packs," *Journal of Naturopathic Medicine* 7, no. 1:84–89 (n.d.), https://drprincetta.com/wp-content/uploads/2016/01/Castor-Oil-Packs-Immunomodulation.pdf; Todd A. Born, "Topical Use of Castor Oil, What Does the Science Say?" *Dermatology, Naturopathic Doctor News and Review* (May 5, 2015).

79   **2012 study in the *Biological Trace Research Journal*:** Zuzanna Sabina Goluch-Koniuszy, "Nutrition of Women with Hair Loss Problem During the Period of Menopause," *Prz Menopauzalny* 15, no. 1 (March 2016): 56–61, published online March 29, 2016, doi: 10.5114/pm.2016.58776.

84 **intracellular lipid inhibits:** M. Roden et al., "Mechanism of Free Fatty Acid–Induced Insulin Resistance in Humans," *Journal of Clinical Investigation* 97, no. 12 (June 15, 1996): 2859–2865; Neal Barnard, Susan Levin, and Caroline Trapp, "Meat Consumption as a Risk Factor for Type 2 Diabetes," *Nutrients* 6, no. 2 (February 2014): 897–910.

86 **Men can eat a bunch of red grapes:** M. Emília Juan et al., "Trans-resveratrol, a Natural Anti-oxidant from Grapes, Increases Sperm Output in Healthy Rats," *Journal of Nutrition* 135, no. 4 (April 1, 2005): 757–760.

86 **resveratrol, which makes for hardier sperm:** S. Shin et al., "Trans-resveratrol Relaxes the Corpus Cavernosum ex Vivo and Enhances Testosterone Levels and Sperm Quality in Vivo," *Archives of Pharmacal Research* 31, no. 1 (January 2008): 83–87.

88 **Such herbs as licorice root:** S. Azmathulla, A. Hule, and S. R. Naik, "Evaluation of Adaptogenic Activity Profile of Herbal Preparation," *Indian Journal of Experimental Biology* 44, no. 7 (July 2006): 574–579.

90 **Many industrial chemicals:** Evanthia Diamanti-Kandarakis et al., "Endocrine-Disrupting Chemicals: An Endocrine Society Scientific Statement," *Endocrine Reviews* 30, no. 4 (June 2009): 293–342.

93 **Check the Environmental Working Group:** https://www.ewg.org/consumer-guides# .WzMKdhIzrOQ.

RESOURCES

Want to Know More?

Consider checking out the Doctor and the Chef Wellness Programs (www.doctorandchef.com) offered by Ashley Boudet, ND, and Chef Mark Reinfeld. We offer seasonal wellness weekends, free online events, a Facebook community, and a membership program where you have ongoing access to Ashley and Mark to receive all of the support you need to succeed on a plant-based lifestyle. The Doctor and Chef help make healthy living easy.

Mark's company, Vegan Fusion, promotes the benefits of plant-based cuisine for our health, the preservation of our planet, and to create a more peaceful world. In addition to award-winning cookbooks, we offer workshops, chef trainings and immersions, a plant-based chef certification program, and vegan culinary retreats around the world. We also offer consulting services, and can assist in menu and recipe development with this innovative global cuisine. For inspiration surrounding the vegan lifestyle, to check out our online culinary course, and to sign up for our free online newsletter, please visit www.veganfusion.com.

Further Reading

Explore this section to deepen your knowledge of the information illuminated in *The Ultimate Age-Defying Plan.*

Health and Wellness

Barnard, Neal D., MD. *Dr. Neal Barnard's Program for Reversing Diabetes: The Scientifically Proven System for Reversing Diabetes without Drugs.*

———. *Power Foods for the Brain: An Effective 3-Step Plan to Protect Your Mind and Strengthen Your Memory.*

———. *The Cheese Trap: How Breaking a Surprising Addiction Will Help You Lose Weight, Gain Energy, and Get Healthy.*

Brazier, Brendan. *Thrive: The Plant-Based Whole Foods Way to Staying Healthy for Life.*

Campbell, T. Colin, and Howard Jacobson. *Whole: Rethinking the Science of Nutrition.*

Campbell, T. Colin, and Thomas M. Campbell II. *The China Study: The Most Comprehensive Study of Nutrition Ever Conducted and the Startling Implications for Diet, Weight Loss, and Long-Term Health.*

Esselstyn, Caldwell B. Jr., MD. *Prevent and Reverse Heart Disease: The Revolutionary, Scientifically Proven, Nutrition-Based Cure.*

Fuhrman, Joel, MD. *Eat to Live: The Revolutionary Formula for Fast and Sustained Weight Loss.*

———. *The End of Diabetes: The Eat to Live Plan to Prevent and Reverse Diabetes.*

Greger, Michael, and Gene Stone. *How Not to Die: Discover the Foods Scientifically Proven to Prevent and Reverse Disease.*

Hever, Julieanna. *The Complete Idiot's Guide to Plant-Based Nutrition.*

———. *The Vegiterranean Diet.*

Kahn, Joel K., MD. *The Whole Heart Solution: Halt Heart Disease Now with the Best Alternative and Traditional Medicine.*

Klaper, Michael, MD. *Vegan Nutrition: Pure and Simple.*

Ornish, Dean. *Dr. Dean Ornish's Program for Reversing Heart Disease: The Only System Scientifically Proven to Reverse Heart Disease Without Drugs or Surgery.*

Pierre, John. *The Pillars of Health.*

Pitchford, Paul. *Healing with Whole Foods.*

Fitness

Brazier, Brendan. *Thrive Fitness: The Vegan-Based Training Program for Maximum Strength, Health & Fitness.*

Cheeke, Robert. *Vegan Bodybuilding & Fitness.*

Frasier, Matt, and Matthew Ruscigno. *No Meat Athlete: Run on Plants and Discover Your Fittest, Fastest, Happiest Self.*

Frey, Rea. *Power Vegan: Plant-Fueled Nutrition for Maximum Health and Fitness.*

Greene, Ben, and Brett Stewart. *The Vegan Athlete: Maximizing Your Health and Fitness While Maintaining a Compassionate Lifestyle.*

Jones, Ellen Jaffe. *Vegan Fitness for Mortals: Eat Your Veggies, Be Active, Avoid Injury, and Get Healthy for Life.*

Lifestyle

Adams, Carol J., Patti Breitman, and Virginia Messina. *Never Too Late to Go Vegan: The Over-50 Guide to Adopting and Thriving on a Plant-Based Diet.*

Barnard, Neal, MD. *Breaking the Food Seduction: The Hidden Reasons Behind Food Cravings—and 7 Steps to End Them Naturally.*

Davis, Brenda, RD, and Vesanto Melina, MS, RD. *The Complete Guide to Adopting a Healthy Plant-Based Diet.*

Day, Jackie. *The Vegan Way: 21 Days to a Happier, Healthier Plant-Based Lifestyle That Will Transform Your Home, Your Diet, and You.*

Foer, Jonathan Safran. *Eating Animals.*

Hicks, J. Morris. *Healthy Eating, Healthy World.*

Jacobson, Michael F., PhD. *Six Arguments for a Greener Diet: How a Plant-Based Diet Could Save Your Health and the Environment.*

Joy, Melanie. *Why We Love Dogs, Eat Pigs, and Wear Cows: An Introduction to Carnism.*

Jurek, Scott. *Eat & Run: My Unlikely Journey to Marathon Greatness.*

Lyman, Howard F., with Glen Merzer. *Mad Cowboy: Plain Truth from the Cattle Rancher Who Won't Eat Meat.*

Marcus, Erik. *Vegan: The New Ethics of Eating.*

Messina, Virginia, and J. L. Fields. *Vegan for Her: The Woman's Guide to Being Healthy and Fit on a Plant-Based Diet.*

Moran, Victoria. *The Good Karma Diet: Eat Gently, Feel Amazing, Age in Slow Motion.*

Moran, Victoria, with Adair Moran. *Main Street Vegan: Everything You Need to Know to Eat Healthfully and Live Compassionately in the Real World.*

Muelrath, Lani. *Mindful Vegan: A 30-Day Plan for Finding Health, Balance, Peace, and Happiness.*

Norris, Jack, and Virginia Messina. *Vegan For Life: Everything You Need to Know to Be Healthy and Fit on a Plant-Based Diet.*

Robbins, John. *Diet for a New America.*

———. *Healthy at 100.*

———. *No Happy Cows: Dispatches from the Frontlines of the Food Revolution.*

———. *The New Good Life: Living Better Than Ever in an Age of Less.*

Roll, Rich. *Finding Ultra: Rejecting Middle Age, Becoming One of the World's Fittest Men, and Discovering Myself.*

Stone, Gene. *Forks Over Knives: The Plant-Based Way to Health.*

Stuart, Tristram. *The Bloodless Revolution: A Cultural History of Vegetarianism from 1600 to Modern Times.*

Tuttle, Will, PhD. *World Peace Diet: Eating for Spiritual Health and Social Harmony.*

Cookbooks

Challis, Tess, *Food Love: Nourishing Yourself, Your Family, and the Planet.*

Prussack, Steven. *Juice Guru: Transform Your Life by Adding One Juice a Day.*

Prussack, Steven, and Bo Rinaldi. *The Complete Idiot's Guide to Juice Fasting.*

Reinfeld, Mark. *Healing the Vegan Way.*

———. *The 30-Minute Vegan: Soup's On!*

———. *The 30-Minute Vegan's Taste of Europe.*

Reinfeld, Mark, and Bo Rinaldi. *Vegan Fusion World Cuisine.*

Reinfeld, Mark, Bo Rinaldi, and Jennifer Murray. *The Complete Idiot's Guide to Eating Raw.*

Reinfeld, Mark, and Jennifer Murray. *The 30-Minute Vegan*.

Reinfeld, Mark, and Jennifer Murray. *The 30-Minute Vegan's Taste of the East*.

Rinaldi, Bo. *The Complete Idiot's Guide to Green Smoothies*.

Schinner, Miyoko. *Artisan Vegan Cheese*.

———. *The Homemade Vegan Pantry: The Art of Making Your Own Staples*.

Specialty Foods and Products

www.veganessentials.com

The ultimate vegan superstore with everything from cosmetics to clothing, to household products, supplements, and more. When it comes to vegan—you name it, they have it.

www.livesuperfoods.com

The go-to site for all of your raw food needs, from food and supplements to appliances, such as juicers, blenders, dehydrators, and spiralizers.

www.vitamix.com

Find the latest Vitamix blenders here on the official site, including factory-reconditioned models that still come with a seven-year warranty. For free shipping in the continental United States, enter code 06-002510.

www.877myjuicer.com

This website carries way more than juicers, including everything kitchen related, plus air purifiers, books, and articles.

www.tribest.com

Award-winning juicers, Sedona dehydrators, and lots of cool kitchen gear.

For our free vegan starter kit, as well as a comprehensive resource guide to our recommended vegan health and wellness websites, vegan lifestyle websites, raw food websites, organic and gardening websites, and a list of our favorite movies and documentaries, please visit www.doctorchefresources.com.

METRIC CONVERSIONS CHART

The recipes in this book have not been tested with metric measurements, so some variations might occur.

Remember that the weight of dry ingredients varies according to the volume or density factor: 1 cup of flour weighs far less than 1 cup of sugar, and 1 tablespoon doesn't necessarily hold 3 teaspoons.

General Formula for Metric Conversion

Ounces to grams
  multiply ounces by 28.35
Grams to ounces
  multiply ounces by 0.035
Pounds to grams
  multiply pounds by 453.5
Pounds to kilograms
  multiply pounds by 0.45
Cups to liters
  multiply cups by 0.24
Fahrenheit to Celsius
  subtract 32 from Fahrenheit temperature,
  multiply by 5, divide by 9
Celsius to Fahrenheit
  multiply Celsius temperature by 9, divide by 5,
  add 32

Volume (Liquid) Measurements

1 teaspoon = ⅙ fluid ounce = 5 milliliters
1 tablespoon = ½ fluid ounce = 15 milliliters
2 tablespoons = 1 fluid ounce = 30 milliliters
¼ cup = 2 fluid ounces = 60 milliliters
⅓ cup = 2⅔ fluid ounces = 79 milliliters
½ cup = 4 fluid ounces = 118 milliliters
1 cup or ½ pint = 8 fluid ounces = 250 milliliters
2 cups or 1 pint = 16 fluid ounces = 500 milliliters
4 cups or 1 quart = 32 fluid ounces = 1,000
  milliliters = 1 liter
1 gallon = 4 liters

Volume (Dry) Measurements

¼ teaspoon	=	1 milliliter
½ teaspoon	=	2 milliliters
¾ teaspoon	=	4 milliliters
1 teaspoon	=	5 milliliters
1 tablespoon	=	15 milliliters
¼ cup	=	59 milliliters

Volume (Dry) Measurements cont.

⅓ cup	=	79 milliliters
½ cup	=	118 milliliters
⅔ cup	=	158 milliliters
¾ cup	=	177 milliliters
1 cup	=	225 milliliters
4 cups or 1 quart	=	1 liter
½ gallon	=	2 liters
1 gallon	=	4 liters

Weight (Mass) Measurements

1 ounce	=	30 grams		
2 ounces	=	55 grams		
3 ounces	=	85 grams		
4 ounces	=	¼ pound	=	125 grams
8 ounces	=	½ pound	=	240 grams
12 ounces	=	¾ pound	=	375 grams
16 ounces	=	1 pound	=	454 grams

Linear Measurements

½ inch	=	1½ cm
1 inch	=	2½ cm
6 inches	=	15 cm
8 inches	=	20 cm
10 inches	=	25 cm
12 inches	=	30 cm
20 inches	=	50 cm

Oven Temperature Equivalents, Fahrenheit (F) and Celsius (C)

100°F	=	38°C
200°F	=	95°C
250°F	=	120°C
300°F	=	150°C
350°F	=	180°C
400°F	=	205°C
450°F	=	230° C

ABOUT THE CONTRIBUTORS

Elizabeth Arraj, recipe tester and food photographer. Elizabeth Arraj has trained under award-winning Vegan Fusion chef Mark Reinfeld. She has received the T. Colin Campbell Center for Nutrition Studies Certificate in Plant-Based Nutrition. She works as a vegan cook for a small coffee shop and café. She teaches plant-based culinary classes at her local community college, where she loves to inspire people how to cook nutrient beneficial foods. When she is not working in kitchens, she loves to contribute recipes to various publications and provide culinary support to local CSA farm members. etar73@hotmail.com

Lisa Parker, recipe tester. An alchemist at heart, Lisa loves plants, colors, flavors, textures, and smells. She loves measuring and stirring and filling the kitchen with delectable fragrances. These days, she makes macadamia nut butters, raw chocolates, grows vanilla, and works with her husband to create a tropical food forest and sanctuary at their home on Kauai. www.tinyislekauai.com

Roland Barker, recipe tester. Roland is inspired by nature's abundance and ability to nourish and heal, and as a cook, he tries to add to that his intention for healing and joy in the preparation of natural, whole foods. Xnau Web design: www.xnau.com

Suzanne Prendergast, recipe tester. Suzanne is an avid world traveler with a lifelong passion for food. Her palate has been strongly influenced by the cuisines she has eaten while on trips to over fifty countries. Suzanne divides her time with catering and teaching classes for home cooks at the Auguste Escoffier School of Culinary Arts in Boulder, Colorado. www.thelifeofsmiley .com

Lisa Portnoff, recipe tester. Having eaten and cooked vegetarian, vegan, and raw foods for many years, Lisa finally devoted herself to the culinary world after a long, successful career as a ceramic and textile artist. She completed the New School Culinary Program in New York City, studied at the Natural Gourmet Institute, the Institute of Culinary Education, and is a proud certified Vegan Fusion chef. She has worked as a chef, caterer, personal chef, cooking instructor, and recipe tester and developer, and is now studying to become a holistic nutrition therapist. lisaportnoff@hotmail.com

ABOUT THE AUTHORS

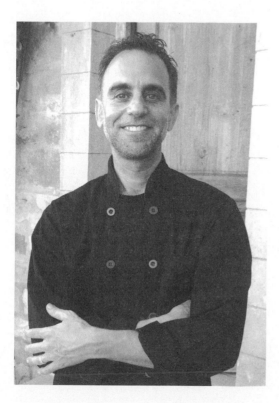

Mark Reinfeld

"The male equivalent to a vegan Rachael Ray—Mark Reinfeld's recipes are flavorful and approachable and certainly have the same potential for mass appeal."
—*Publishers Weekly*

Mark Reinfeld is the 2017 Inductee into the Vegetarian Hall of Fame. He is a multi-award-winning chef and author of eight books, including the best-selling 30-Minute Vegan series and his last book, *Healing the Vegan Way*, selected as the #1 book for Vegans in 2016 by Philly.com. Mark has over twenty-five years of experience preparing creative vegan and raw cuisine. Since 2012, he has served as the executive chef for the North American Vegetarian Society's Summerfest. He has offered consulting services for such clients as Google, Whole Foods, Kroger, the Humane Society, Bon Appétit Management, Aramark, Sodexo, White Wave, and more. Mark was the founding chef of the Blossoming Lotus Restaurant, voted "Best Restaurant on Kaua'i."

His first cookbook, *Vegan Fusion World Cuisine*, coauthored with Bo Rinaldi and with a foreword by Dr. Jane Goodall, has won nine national awards, including Best Vegetarian Cookbook in the USA. Mark is the recipient of Aspen Center for Integral Health's Platinum Carrot Award for living foods—a national award given by the center to America's top "innovative and trailblazing healthy chefs." He is the winner of Vegan.com's Recipe of the Year Award and is described by VegCooking.com as being "poised on the leading edge of contemporary vegan cooking." In addition, Mark coauthored *The Complete Idiot's Guide to Eating Raw*.

Mark received his initial culinary training from his grandfather Ben Bimstein, a renowned chef and ice carver in New York City. Through his Vegan Fusion company, Mark specializes in vegan recipe development and offers culinary workshops, a plant-based chef certification program, chef trainings, and consulting services internationally. His two-part online culinary course, offered in conjunction with *Vegetarian Times*, is available at veganfusion.com.

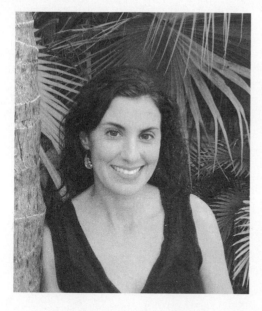

Ashley Boudet, ND

Ashley Boudet is a naturopathic doctor trained in primary care medicine, with a background in social work, behavioral health, and research. While nutrition is a major focus of her naturopathy practice, she acknowledges that self-care is truly the best care, and uses a personalized approach in helping others achieve and maintain their health goals. She is fully committed to promoting a connection to nature as a pathway to healing, both personally and globally. She enjoys learning and research, and views aging as an exciting opportunity for continued growth and expansion both professionally and personally.

She currently teaches both live and web-based classes with her husband, Mark Reinfeld, through The Doctor and the Chef, and also offers private phone and Skype consultations. Visit www.doctorandchef.com to learn more. Ashley also serves as an active board member with the International Congress of Naturopathic Medicine, and as an executive organizing committee member for a yearly gathering to unite natural health-care experts and the global natural medicine community worldwide. http://icnmnaturopathy.eu/en/About

ABOUT MICHAEL A. KLAPER, MD

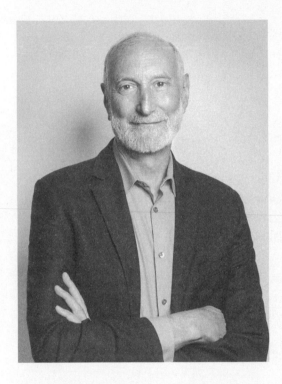

Dr. Klaper is a graduate of the University of Illinois College of Medicine in Chicago and has practiced acute care medicine in Hawaii, California, Florida, Canada, and New Zealand.

Far more fulfilling to him is his current practice, focusing on health-promoting food and lifestyle choices to help people stay out of hospitals and off operating tables. He has authored numerous articles on plant-based nutrition and is authoring a book on using plant-based medicine to arrest and reverse disease.

A longtime radio host and a pilot, Dr. Klaper has served as nutrition adviser to NASA's programs for space colonists on the Moon and Mars and on the Nutrition Task Force of the American Medical Students Association.

To improve the health of his patients as well as his own, and to minimize suffering of sentient beings, Dr. Klaper adopted a plant-based diet in 1981. He makes the latest information on health and nutrition available through his website, DoctorKlaper.com, where visitors can find the numerous videos and DVDs he has produced, as well subscribe to his free newsletter, *Medicine Capsule.*

INDEX

A

acid reflux, 28–30
adrenal glands, 87–88
Age-Defying Advice, xvii
aging process, 6–8
algae foods, 18, 74
allergies, 29
aluminum, 20
Alzheimer's disease, 3, 5, 9,
    11–14
The Alzheimer's Solution, 14–15
anemia, 29
angina, 52
animal-based diets
    cholesterol in, 54
    growth hormones in, 91
    scientific evidence on, xvi, 5, 8
anthocyanins, 19, 25
antioxidants
    for eye health, 24
    for heart health, 60
    in plant foods, 7–9
    reducing inflammation with, 41
    reducing radiation damage with,
      57
    for skin health, 74
anxiety, 16
apples, 34
argan oil, 78, 79
arrhythmias, 51–52
art, engaging in, 22
arthritis, 4, 40–42
atherosclerosis, 51
atrazine, 90–91
avocados and avocado oil, 76, 78

B

B_{12}, 17–18, 25, 29, 46
bare feet, and "Earthing" theory, 59
beans, 48
benign prostatic hyperplasia (BPH),
    65–66
berries
    for brain health, 19
    health benefits, 9
    for heart health, 57
    for kidney health, 67
    for skin health, 76
Bifidobacteria, 32
biological age, xiv, xvi
bisphenol A (BPA), 90
bladder, 64–66
blood glucose, 18, 84
blueberries, 9, 19
Blue Zone diets, 10
bones
    Age-Defying Advice, 48–49
    remodeling process, 39–40
    strengthening, 40
    and tooth loss, 42
    top nutrients for, 45–47
    weak (osteoporosis), 40
brain-derived neurotrophic factor (BDNF), 19
brain health
    Age-Defying Advice, 25
    exercise for, 21–22
    and heavy metals, 19–20
    nutrients for, 12, 15–19
    studies on, 12–15
    superfoods for, 9, 10
breakfast, and weight loss, 34

fiber
  for balancing hormones, 92
  for digestive health, 35
  easing constipation with, 30
  for longer telomeres, 7
  for skin health, 74, 80
  for weight loss, 33–34
fish, mercury in, 20
flaxseeds, 9–10
fluid buildup, 65
Fountain of Youthers, xvii
  Babette Davis, 81
  Cherie Soria, 69
  Ellen Jaffe Jones, 50
  Joel Kahn, 61
  Lani Muelrath, 94
  Miyoko Schinner, 36
  Victoria Moran, 26
frailty syndrome, 43
Framingham Heart Study, 55–56
free radicals, 6
fruits, 41, 48, 76

G

garlic, 57, 76
gastrointestinal reflux disease
      (GERD), 28
ginger, 57
ginkgo biloba, 24
ginkgo tea, 25
glucose, 18, 84
glycemic index, 18
goji berries, 24
grains, whole, 10, 18, 35, 48
grapes, 57, 86
greens, 10, 19, 48
green tea, 58, 76, 80
gum inflammation, 42

H

hair, 78–79
hawthorn berry, 57
Healthy Brain, Happy Life (Suzuki), 21

hearing loss, 24
heart attack, 52
heart disease
  assessing overall risk of, 56
  cholesterol and, 53–56
  impact on longevity, 3, 51
  risk factors, 52–53
  types of, 51–52
heart failure, 5, 52
heart health, 55–58, 60
HeartMath Solution, 59
heavy metals, 19–20
herbal infusions, 48
herbal medicines, 67
herbal teas, 48, 67–68, 93
herbs, beneficial, 35, 93
hibiscus tea, 58
high blood pressure. *See* hypertension
high-density lipoproteins (HDL), 53
Himalayan salt, 48, 58
homocysteine, 56
hormone replacement therapy (HRT), 87
hormones
  balancing, foods for, 91–92
  endocrine disruptors and, 90–91
  functions of, 83–85
  produced by adrenal glands, 87–88
  reproductive, 85–86
  for sleep, 88–89
hydrating elixir, 80
hydration, xviii–xix, 73. *See also* water
hydrotherapy, xix, 68, 74, 78
hypertension, 4, 51, 58
hypoglycemia, 84

I

immune system, 27, 44
indigestion, 28–30
inflammation
  anti-inflammatory foods and herbs,
      80
  anti-inflammatory supplements, 68
  in joints, 4, 40–42

inflammation (*continued*)
from meat and dairy, 15
role in degenerative diseases, 16
inflammatory bowel disease, 31
infusions, herbal, 48
insulin resistance, 84
intention, xviii
intestinal bacteria, 29
iron, 19, 29
irritable bowel syndrome
(IBS), 29
ischemia, 52

J
joints
Age-Defying Advice, 48–49
inflammation in, 4, 40–42
top nutrients for, 45–47

K
Kahn, Joel, 56, 61
Kegel exercises, 64–65
kidney disease, 5
kidneys
best foods for, 67–68
function of, 63
stressed, 63–64
kidney stones, 66

L
Lactobacillus, 32
legumes, 34, 48
liver-supporting foods, 93
longevity factors, 3
low-density lipoproteins (LDL), 53, 55
low-GI foods, 18
lung disease, 5
lycopene, 76
lysine, 71–72

M
magnesium, 15–16, 25, 47, 57
massage, abdominal, 31

massage, oil, 78
meat, 15, 54, 91
meditation, 59
melatonin, 88–89
MEND study, 12–14
menopause, 84, 85
mental exercises, xviii, 12, 22
mercury, 20
metabolism, 43
microbiome, 31–33
mineral deficiency, 29
minerals
for balancing hormones, 92
for endocrine health, 93
for skin health, 74
trace, 47, 48
mitochondria, 6, 19, 44
mortality rates, 3
movement, 21, 41–42, 44, 89. *See also*
exercise
muscles
Age-Defying Advice, 48–49
degenerative (sarcopenia),
42–43
skeletal, 43–44
strengthening, 42–44
top nutrients for, 45–47
music, 22, 24

N
nails, 79
neuroplasticity, 12
neurotoxins, xvii
nitric oxide, 56
noise pollution, 23
NOURISH philosophy, xvii–xix
nutrient-dense foods. *See* superfoods
nutrition, xvii
nuts, 48

O
obesity, 53, 65
oils, 54

omega-3 fatty acids
    for bone and joint health, 47
    for brain health, 16–17, 25
    in chia seeds, 76
    for eye health, 24
    for healthy joints, 41
    for kidney health, 67
    low levels, and heart disease, 56
    and telomere length, 9–10
omega-6 fatty acids, 67
oral hygiene, 14
organic food, xvi–xvii
organophosphate pesticides, 91
Ornish, Dean, 7–8, 58–59, 60
osteoarthritis, 40
osteoporosis, 40, 43
overactive bladder (OAB), 64–66
oxidative stress, 6, 40–41
oxygen, 89
oxytocin, xvii–xviii

P

parabens, 90
Parkinson's disease, 16
parsley, 75
pelvic muscles, 64–65
perchlorate, 91
perfluorinated chemicals (PFCs), 91
periodontal disease, 14
pesticides, xvii, 20
phosphorus, 46–47
physiological age, xiv, xvi
phytochemicals, 7
phytoestrogenic foods, 67
phytoestrogens, 65, 85
ping-pong, 21
plant-based diets, xiii–xiv, 8–10, 55
polychlorinated biphenyls (PCBs), 90
polyps in the colon, 31
posture, 45

potassium, 47, 58
prebiotic foods, 32–33, 35
probiotic foods, 77, 92
probiotic microorganisms, 32
processed foods, xvii
    brain toxins in, 20
    phosphorus in, 46
    scientific evidence on, xvi, 8
    sodium in, 58
    weight gain from, 34
progesterone, 85
prostate gland, 65–66
prostate specific antigen (PSA) test, 66
protein, 10, 45–46
pulse, checking, 59
pumpkin, 75
pumpkin seeds, 76

R

relationships, xviii
reproductive hormone health, 85
resistance training, 21, 42, 44
resveratrol, 9, 86
rheumatoid arthritis, 40
rosemary, 25

S

salts, 48, 58
sarcopenia, 42–43
saturated fats, 54
seed cycling, 91, 93
seeds, 48
selenium, 67
senescence, 6
serotonin, 15
silence, 23
silica-rich foods, 74–75
skin
    Age-Defying Advice, 77–78, 80
    best foods for, 74–76
    brushing, 77
    damage, slowing down, 73–74
    effect of aging on, 71, 72

Recipes

M

Maca Pepita Elixir, 118
Mango
  Creamy Tropical Bliss, 118
  Rice Pudding with Salted Caramel, 293
Maple Marinade, Smoky, 256
Marinades
  Cilantro Lime, 256
  Smoky Maple, 256
  ways to use, 255
Mayonnaise
  Aqua, 272
  Chipotle, 273
  Sriracha Aioli, 275
  Vegan, 273
  Wasabi, 222–223
Meal prep tips and tricks, 97–99
Mexican Spice Mix, 252
Milk
  Oat, 116
  Pumpkin Seed, 116
Millet
  Ancient Sunrise, 135
  Kale Tabbouleh, 164
Miso
  Ginger Glazed Eggplant, 202
  Roots Soup, 142
Moroccan Spice Mix, 252
Mousse, Berry, 290
Mushroom(s)
  Asian Couscous, 208
  Braised, Stroganoff, 240–241
  El Tortilla Pizza, 224
  Grilled Vegetables Extraordinaire,
    178
  Leek Gravy, 276
  Medley, Magical, 184
  Portobello Cheez Steak Stuffed
    Peppers, 232
  Risotto, 233–234
  Shiitake Hot Pot Noodle Soup,
    149
  Smoky, 254–255

N

Nachos, Loaded, 206
Noodle(s)
  Brats and Kraut, 243
  Shiitake Hot Pot Soup, 149
Nourishing Tonic Tea, 122
Nuts. *See also specific nuts*
  soaking, 106–107
  toasting, 106

O

Oat(s)
  Milk, 116
  Raw Fig Thumbprint Cookies, 282
  Superfood Granola, 128
  Walnut Flapjacks, 286
Okra Tomato, Santorini, 177
Onion, Pickled Red, 262
Oranges
  Citrus Cleanse, 117
  Rosemary Star Anise Tea, 113

P

Pancakes, Superfood Buckwheat, 132
Panini, Hummus, with Balsamic Massaged
    Kale, 239
Papaya
  Creamy Tropical Bliss, 118
Parsnip(s)
  Garlicky Whipped, 192
  Leek Soup, 151
Pasta
  Mac n Cheez, 230
  Roasted Butternut Squash Penne with
    Sage, 242
  Salad, Club Med, 168
Peach(es)
  Berry Smoothie, 121
  Chia Pepper Jam, 258–259
  Fruit Compote, 287
Pecan(s)
  Raw Choco-Cherry Bombs, 281
  Sage Holiday Loaf, 244–245

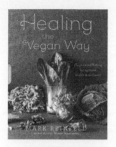

If you have enjoyed *The Ultimate Age-Defying Plan*, please check out the companion book, *Healing the Vegan Way,* and the books in the 30-Minute Vegan series.

Healing the Vegan Way by Mark Reinfeld

> Paperback: 978-0-7382-1777-2
> Ebook: 978-0-7382-1778-9

The 30-Minute Vegan Series

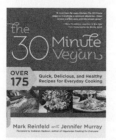

The 30-Minute Vegan by Mark Reinfeld
and Jennifer Murray

> Paperback: 978-0-7382-1327-9
> Ebook: 978-0-7867-4814-3

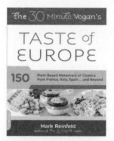

The 30-Minute Vegan's Taste of Europe by Mark Reinfeld

> Paperback: 978-0-7382-1433-7
> Ebook: 978-0-7382-1616-4

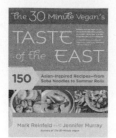

The 30-Minute Vegan's Taste of the East by Mark Reinfeld
and Jennifer Murray

> Paperback: 978-0-7382-1382-8
> Ebook: 978-0-7382-1416-0

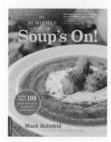

The 30-Minute Vegan: Soup's On! by Mark Reinfeld

> Paperback: 978-0-7382-1673-7
> Ebook: 978-0-7382-1674-4